D1283825

International African Library 23
General Editors: J. D. Y. Peel, David Parkin and Colin Murray

DEATH IN ABEYANCE

The *International African Library* is a major monograph series from the International African Institute and complements its quarterly periodical *Africa*, the premier journal in the field of African studies. Theoretically informed ethnographies, studies of social relations 'on the ground' which are sensitive to local cultural forms, have long been central to the Institute's publications programme. The *IAL* maintains this strength but extends it into new areas of contemporary concern, both practical and intellectual. It includes works focused on problems of development, especially on the linkages between the local and national levels of society; studies along the interface between the social and environmental sciences; and historical studies, especially those of a social, cultural or interdisciplinary character.

International African Library

General Editors

J. D. Y. Peel, David Parkin *and* Colin Murray

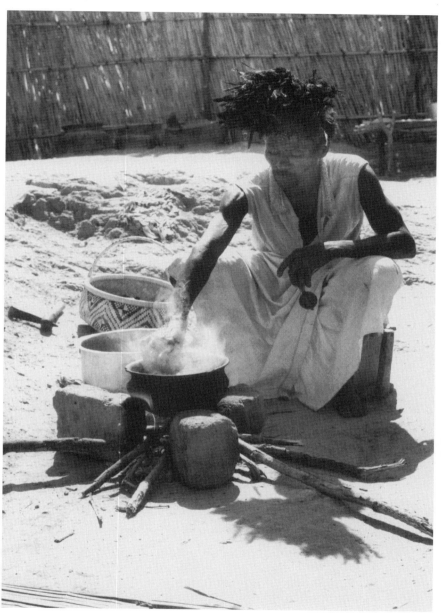

Kawele divining with boiling water

In memory of my parents

God keep me from ever completing anything.
This whole book is but a draught – nay, but a
draught of a draught. Oh, Time, Strength,
Cash, and Patience!

Herman Melville

DEATH IN ABEYANCE

ILLNESS AND THERAPY AMONG THE TABWA OF CENTRAL AFRICA

CHRISTOPHER O. DAVIS

EDINBURGH UNIVERSITY PRESS
for the International African Institute, London

© Christopher O. Davis, 2000

Edinburgh University Press Ltd
22 George Square, Edinburgh

Typeset in Plantin
by Koinonia, Bury, and
printed and bound in Great Britain by
The Cromwell Press, Trowbridge

Publication was made possible in part by
a grant from the Netherlands Organisation
for Scientific Research (NWO)

A CIP record for this book is available
from the British Library

ISBN 0 7486 1305 6 (paperback)

CONTENTS

LIST OF MAPS, TABLES AND FIGURES

ACKNOWLEDGEMENTS

When a book has been this long in the making, one must begin with an apology. The list of acknowledgements may seem long, but surely longer is the list comprising those robbed of recognition by a trick of recollection or of space.

Funding for this study was generously provided by a US Public Health Service Training Grant, a Social Science Research Council Foreign Area Fellowship and a Wenner-Gren Foundation Grant-in-Aid. A fellowship from the National Endowment for the Humanities first allowed me to develop the perspectives emergent from fieldwork.

Murray Last was guardian of the memory and hope that kept alive the possibility of the draft before you now. My colleagues here at SOAS restored to the practice of anthropology its status as a gift; none more so in this regard than John Peel and David Parkin. In so doing, they completed an arc begun by Irving Goldman and then continued by Victor Turner, Bernard Cohn and Raymond Smith. The manuscript benefited enormously from the close reading and kind criticisms of John Janzen.

Although the writing follows the ethnographic convention of the first person singular, the project itself would not have had the qualities it did were it not for the generosity of many. Allen Roberts was an amiable companion. His research interests parallelled my own; and as a partner in life's adventures he could not have been bettered.

In Kalemie, Kalunga Twite took us into his family for three months while we found our feet. Geneviève Nagant, long resident there, shared with us much that she had learned during the course of her own research. Through her we made the initial contacts that eventually took us to Mpala; the place where we lived for roughly four years. Later, our intermittent visits to Kalemie were enlivened by the company of Guillame Kinyongo, among others.

Halfway through our stay, it was our good luck to meet by chance three colleagues from Japan. With Swahili as our common language, Makoto Kakeya, his wife Hedeko and Hideaki Terashima renewed my attention to the world around us and restored my enthusiasm for its detail. One part of this was interest in medicinal plants themselves. Makoto showed me a better way to preserve them than the one I had been using and encouraged me to be more focused in my approach. The result was a collection of around 225 specimens which were submitted to and identified by colleagues at the East

African Herbarium in Nairobi, whose interest in the project was and is much appreciated.

The foundation for the text itself was laid by collective effort and conversation with many people in Mpala and elsewhere. I hope their teaching shows in this book; and I hope to make it even more directly a part of the one to come.

Starting at the University of Michigan and continuing since that time, I have been graced by the lively intellects and good company of my postgraduate supervisees. In addition, there are a number of people whose work and whose casts of thought and character have been continuing influences on my own. Included among them are Walter Allen, Ann Anagnost, the late Richard Burghardt, Augustus Casely-Hayford, Ross Chambers, Jane Guyer, Thomas Holt, Alcinda Honwana, Philip Jones, Ali Mazrui, Don Merton, Valentin Mudimbe, Akira Okazaki, Stefan Palmie, Pamela Reynolds, Rosemary Singleton, Edith Turner, Roy Willis and Joy Wolf.

Elizabeth M. Taylor has been a moral/political compass for me for decades; and she continues to be. Audrey Cantlie and Veena Das have been unfailing in their support (and gentle pressure). They are my most immediate companions in thinking. Peter Bate's devotion has seen us through more than one hard time. Avery Davis-Roberts has been a beacon of sanity and a source of delight across the years and miles connecting one home to another.

BY WAY OF AN INTRODUCTION

the *page* [surrounding a poem] is a visual unity. ... [it is] addressed to the glance that precedes and surrounds the act of reading – and 'notifies' the movement of the composition. By providing a sort of material intuition and by establishing a harmony among our various modes of perception, or among the *rates of perception* of our different senses, it should make us anticipate what is about to be presented to the intelligence.

Paul Valéry on Mallarmé's 'A Throw of the Dice'

Telling stories is a way of disarticulating an author's pretensions, as well as of reformulating the supposed logical derivations of even a mathematical demonstration. In effect, the story organizes its own basis, operations, objectives and anticipations. The master of the storytelling performance is the listener who, when bored, can stop at any time or simply cease to listen.

V. Y. Mudimbe

By convention, the introduction is the place where the writer of a text becomes the one who ushers it into a world of imagined or anticipated readers. By convention, their variety is reducible to two kinds of cast of mind: the gladiatorial and the sociable. For the former, the writer tries to make the introduction something that will forestall misreading and perhaps pre-empt foreseeable criticisms. In this capacity, the introduction will come to function as do those margins of silence by which the page surrounds a poem and so allows it to make visible to us the singularities of its speakings. With reference to the latter cast of mind, the writer evokes through her introduction the circle whose terms of reference may be expanded by her *prise de parole*.

In each case, then, the introduction is the place where the writer turns up to explain herself and give some indication of what she thinks she's doing. Her representation of this can resemble a window opening onto the world of the work, or it can suggest the opening of a door into a room, with a desk in it, and papers on that and a writer who turns (Certeau 1980, 1983; Demos 1994) to look at you, the reader – and who says:

'BEAR WITH ME A MOMENT WHILE I READ YOU THESE'

9 May 1977
(7 May)

Just a few notes on a couple of interesting conversations overheard the other day:

In the morning, when everyone was outside shelling peanuts and making soap, I could overhear animated discussion – with Muzame, as usual, taking the principal part. I didn't pay too much attention to what was said, but just noted that everyone seemed to be having a good time – were laughing, etc., and that it was about Bulumbu. I commented to Al that having Muzame around seemed to add a good deal of spirit to the work. And, a few minutes later, Al pointed out that that had two sides, because shortly after laughing together like that, everyone had seriously quarrelled – stopped talking, and stomped off in different directions.

In the afternoon, Luvunzo came back with the news that the two Bulumbu diviners with whom I wanted to talk had agreed to come to the house the following Monday afternoon. One, he said, had thought I wanted her to come, and have her pepo *mount her so I could talk with it. I said that this was not the idea, but that sometimes* pepo *knew more about Kibawa, etc., than the people did themselves. Muzame, hearing this, took up the argument again.*

In the morning, he told me, they had had an ubishi. *Some people (notably Luvunzo) had said that the strength of a person when his* pepo *mounts him is the strength of the man himself. Others (i.e., Muzame) said that it was the strength of the* pepo. *Muzame was taking the occasion to argue his case again, to me – in a situation where the others were absent, and so couldn't speak.*

In addition to Luvunzo, Kalolo's wife was also there, however, and I immediately set about asking everyone present (including Manda and Kabepa) which side they were on. Muzame cited as proof of his argument the fact that a dying Bulumbu practitioner can rise up from his death-bed and dance and sing his songs, only to lie down again, and die on the spot. Luvunzo pooh-poohed this, saying that one has seen that even normal people, especially just before they die, can arise from their beds and sometimes have to be forced to lie down again by several people – and they too then die.

At this, the discussion got rather good, but was rather typical in that everyone was talking and shouting at once, and no one was listening to anyone else – and so no conclusions were drawn. Muzame was especially disagreeable and disorderly – he talked continually. Whenever a question was put to him he responded by (a) continuing his story in a louder voice or (b) going into the kitchen and not listening or (c) starting a new story or (d) some combination of all of the above.

Well, Muzame went on, what about the way in which people, when possessed by their spirits, were able to walk on fire? They were never burnt – and this was from the strength of the pepo. *Luvunzo snorted. With the agreement of Kalolo's wife, he said this was just* viezia *(i.e.,* dawa*). While Muzame went off into a loud, irrelevant description of the* viezia *in which people appeared to cut their tongues, Manda came around the corner and said that it was* dawa *that enabled the people to do this. But, and here's where his argument was interesting, he meant to say that the derivation of this power from* dawa *was the same 'otherness' (my word) as that of* pepo *derivation. Luvunzo, on the other hand, was arguing that the use of* dawa *was the opposite of mystical derivation – it was the strength of men.*

Kalolo's wife wanted to give Muzame an example (kumupa mfano). She called him several times, but had difficulty getting his attention – every time she would start talking, he would go into the kitchen. The rest of us were listening, though.

When you send an arrow to an mfumu, *she said, and the* mfumu *tells you to come the next day, you go the next day. When you get there, he starts loudly belching (which she did several times in an exquisite combination of comic relief, mild mockery, and demonstration). Then, he goes and dresses himself, and puts* pemba *(which – in the same combination of the first three attitudes – she called 'flour' (*bunga*)) on his face. He comes back out. Do you think, she asked Muzame, his* pepo *has come to him then? Do you think he is a* pepo? *No, he just does that because he sees you coming.*

*Muzame never replied – he'd scuttled off into the kitchen so as to avoid having to answer. Luvunzo replied that the person was 'not a bit' possessed (*hata*). He was, the two of them agreed, only acting. Luvunzo went on to say that the real divination had taken place the night before, in his dreams – he had obtained* malosi *through the use of medicines with which he was* chanja'ed. *There, Luvunzo continued, he had seen and spoken with all your dead kinsmen – all the people involved in the case. Through the use of these medicines, in dreams they had come to him and told him what the situation was – and then the next day at the moment when you saw him, he was just saying in the guise of a* pepo *the things he had already dreamed. He said these thing in this guise 'that you believe him' (*upate kusadiki*) – but it was not the* pepo *which did it.*

*Muzame never put himself out there enough to answer the question directly. After their discussion was finished (and Manda had again put in his idea that powers derived from medicine are not the 'strength of men' (*nguvu ya watu*)), Muzame came out of the kitchen again to point out that if dreaming were the place of the real divination, how could they and Luvunzo account for the fact that one could send an arrow and have the divination done on the spot, without dreaming?*

Kalolo's wife started to respond that if one really noted, whenever one sent an arrow for on-the-spot divination, one was frequently told that the divination could not be completed at that time, and one must return the next day. But again Muzame whipped off, so as not to have to listen. I was dipping in, too, to try to get him to listen, but he evaded me.

He hid around the corner again, and then came back with the point that they said all these things, but when the time came to fall ill, they'd be right there getting a divination made all the same. Luvunzo laughed wryly at the truth of this – but Kalolo's wife insisted that she was not fond of divining because one was told so many lies.

Muzame asked her, if your husband were ensorcelled would you not go to divine? No, she replied, she would not. In that case, he said, in what I thought was a nasty remark, indicative of his sense that he was losing, you're a mukalamusi *– a clever person – but also a troublemaker or somewhat tricky – this was rather an insult. But she let it pass and replied only that if you went to divine in that sort of case you might be told that it was your* mkubwa *who was ensorcelling you, and then you'd fall out with that person for no reason – only because you'd been told. Or, you would be told that it was a* mukalye *that had made you ill. How, she wanted to know, could a bit of cloth and some beads make anyone sick?*

Muzame cited as ultimate proof that a pepo *was different from the person the fact*

that if one commits adultery and has a pepo, *frequently it is the case that that very
night the spirit will mount you and announce to your wife what you have done.
Would a person do that himself? Impossible. Therefore, argued Muzame, it must be a
different thing from the person himself.*

*Luvunzo said that the whole discussion of the morning had started with
Muzame's saying that he had seen a Bulumbu go to urinate. Luvunzo had replied
that this (a) could not have been a Bulumbu spirit – or, if it was, it just proved that
(b) the thing was just the strength of men, anyway. Muzame quickly conceded that
perhaps that one had been phony – but went on to say that a real Bulumbu could go
on all night, etc., without urinating – and could even go for a month without eating –
etc. At this, the discussion petered out, and I started over to Polombwe's and
Lukena's.*

When I got over there, I told them that the reason I was late was because of this
ubishi. *This started them off, as well. At first Lukena and Polombwe were saying
that the divination was by the strength of the* pepo *itself. But then, they went on to
say that* pepo *didn't last a long time, in any case. Usually, they were really good
only for a year or two and then fled the person. They hardly ever lasted more than
five years – after this, they would flee their* kapondo. *But the* kapondo, *being used
to their methods (and the money), would continue to divine. This led to more general
discussion of the shortcomings of various diviners – or types of divination....*

*Back at the house, I met Kapelumo, who was talking to Al. He said that these
days there are no real Bulumbu left. And by real, he meant those who are able to
perform* mwigiza. *A real Bulumbu, he said, could be closed in the house, with people
all around the outside – at every window and door. He would sing one song within
the house, after which there would be silence – and then singing far off in the distance.
How the diviner would have got out of the house would be a mystery to everyone.*

*Or, again, he could be sitting there in the room – and then suddenly, with his
fingernails, begin to dig a hole in the ground. It would rapidly become so large that
soon the whole person would be lost to sight – and would come out beyond the house
somewhere. One does not see this any more, and those people who think they have*
pepo *these days are only deceiving themselves (*wanajidanganya tu*).*

*There is no one today who can go from Katenge to Kamucheli or beyond entirely
underground – as Kapelumo said he earlier did, going from Tembwe to Kabwema.
All of these are things that were done by* pepo *of* zamani, *but not now. Also a* pepo
never, he said, lasts longer then five years at most. For the pepo *of today, and those
of greater age than five or six years, it is really just 'theatre' and not possession at
all.*

28 July 1977
(page 2)

*A couple of weeks ago, as I was finishing off the outline of my dissertation, I had put
in this idea that the medicines in a* mwanzambale *or similar medicine (including
sorcery) constitute a kind of microcosm of the world as a whole. One tries to include
such things as all snakes, all predators, all winds, etc. I had commented in my
analysis that the medicine works because it is a kind of metaphor – but that the
relation of the person to his medicine is as God's to the larger world. After thinking
about it a bit, I decided to ask people about this, to see if they would agree.*

I went outside and found Mwalimu Fredi, the landlord; Muzame; Manda; and Luvunzo. I put the analysis to them by saying that everyone said that a mulozi was God. At first everyone resisted this idea. Mwalimu Fredi said that God was bigger than a mulozi, because perhaps the sorcerer would have the intention of killing one, but this could not happen without God's agreement. And if God refused, one could not die.

Well, I replied, even if his strength was not the same as God's one could still say that it worked like God's, could one not? I pointed out that people had said that both God and a sorcerer could put illness into one's body in mysterious ways. One would feel nothing enter, would see no lesion or other sign. All one would know is that one would suddenly become ill.

This analogy was conceded, but Muzame, Luvunzo and Mwalimu Fredi still refused to agree that a sorcerer was God. Mwalimu Fredi said that when a sorcerer throws medicines upon one, he had to call upon his God to help him. Thus, it was really by this power, and not by any power of his own, that he worked. Perhaps he would throw medicines upon you, and your God would protect you. You get sick, but do not die. He then calls upon a greater sorcerer, whose strength is superior to his. This man throws medicines on you, and you become worse. But you still have not died. Finally, they go to an even stronger doctor, and he throws medicines on you, and then you die.

I said that, in this case, it would seem that the real God was the last sorcerer. And after a moment's pause, everyone burst into laughter. They said that the differential abilities of sorcery to work did, ultimately, have to do with the differential strengths of the mipasi *of the practitioners.*

It was finally concluded that the medicine could be seen as a small world. Mwalimu Fredi went on to add that, just as the medicine contained such things as snakes, etc., so could one's mipasi *work through such things as snakes, etc., which might be sent to bite one as punishment for some wrongdoing. So, in so far as one could will events through the medicine, it was a little world and one was God. After hearing my explanation, Luvunzo readily agreed with this.*

But people were very emphatic on the point that one's will alone is insufficient to assure success – though it is necessary. If one's medicines ultimately succeed, it is because of the larger will of God. Muzame concluded by saying that a sorcerer and God were indeed alike. But God is the greater. The sorcerer is only the younger brother.

In this same conversation, we talked about the kinds of people who used to be sorcerers, and those who are likely to be them now. Mwalimu, with the concurrence of Luvunzo, said that even when they were growing up, it was not common, as it is now, for sorcerers to be around. They were few, and they ensorcelled within their own families, and according to certain rules.

At this time, most sorcerers were old people, and having grey hair was indicative of sorcery – though it was not a definite proof, and one's character was the more decisive marker. Also a person who was dirty – who did not wash himself or his clothes, who allowed his hair to grow long, to be dirty, and uncombed – would be thought to be a sorcerer on this basis.

Mwalimu Fredi said that even after independence there were not so many youths with sorcery as there are now. He remembered distinctly the time when all of this began *to increase. Year before the year before last, it was (*juzi kutwa*). He was living at Kapakwe at the time. A lot of young men from there went down to Molilo during the dry season to fish* dagaa. *They had a good season, and made a lot of money. A good number of them took this money, and crossed over to Tanzania, where they used it to buy* djin *medicines. When they came back to Kapakwe, they made much noise about their medicines, and a lot of people, especially old people, died at this time. For this reason there are not many old people left in Kapakwe now. And this was the beginning. Now, a person with sorcery can be young as well as old – and they ensorcell 'anyhow'.*

Manda made the same remark, saying that young people had so much money these days from fishing. And yet, where did it all go? You look at them, they don't wear nice clothes – what have they spent their money on? They've gone to get medicines, 'wabakie kwa milele' *(that they live forever).*

Luvunzo said something similar, adding that people could see in their behaviour signs that would indicate their sorcery. Principal among these was arrogance. They could be rude or insolent to others, particularly their seniors. They could quarrel with or insult people openly, etc. Seeing this, people begin to ask themselves – a person who behaves in this way must have something, that he think of himself as so free of the necessity to remain in the good graces of others. He must have medicine – otherwise he would be thinking about what he'd do if his children fall sick or he gets in trouble, etc.

As part of a talk with Lubeni, the question of mulozi *as Mungu (sorcerer as God) and God as a sorcerer came up as well. Lubeni had just been having a similar discussion earlier that afternoon, with a group of young guys. Al has written in his notebook Lubeni's comments on God as sorcerer. I note here only that when I presented my microcosm idea (*kadunia*), Lubeni was so far ahead of me that he did not even pause to state his agreement. Nodding, he laughed, and wryly said 'yes, but it isn't a microcosm of great continuity, because if they want to kill you, they'll get you all the same' (*Si kadunia cha kuendelea; wakikutaka watakupata vile-vile*)....*

Lubeni also spoke of a couple of cures he was working on, adding that this was why people called him a sorcerer – because he cured people whose illnesses were very great. He also commented that his ability to throw people in the bush successfully derived from his mipasi, *who fixed it so that then he threw a person in the bush, the* kibanda *remained* lalisha'ed ....

OPINIONATION

Of all kinds of exchange, the exchange of economic values is the least free of some tinge of sacrifice. When we exchange love for love, we release an inner energy we would otherwise not know what to do with. Insofar as we surrender it, we sacrifice no real utility ... When we communicate intellectual matters in conversation, these are not thereby diminished. When we reveal a picture of our personality in the course of taking in that of others, this exchange in no way decreases our possession of ourselves. In all these exchanges the increase of value does not occur through the calculation of profit and loss. Either the contribution of each party stands beyond such a consideration, or else simply to be allowed to contribute is itself a gain – in which case we perceive the response of the other, despite our own offering, as an unearned gift. In contrast, economic exchange ... always entails the sacrifice of some good that has other potential uses, even though utilitarian gain may prevail in the final analysis.

Georg Simmel

There are a number of reasons why passages from fieldnotes, and these passages in particular, should introduce the introduction. Taking each reason in turn will structure our discussion here, much as the larger body from which the notes have come has structured the text as a whole.

I wanted to begin with these because they represent what was one of my deepest pleasures in Zaire – as it has always been one of my deepest delights in life – a shared play with words and ideas, in a situation where everybody talks at once and no one gives the appearance of listening to anyone else; and of course no conclusions are drawn, because everybody already knew everything in the first place and had no intention of changing their minds. Here, the amusement lies especially in the fact that *nothing is at stake* other than people's tempers and the opinions they have of each other's opinions, matters important and insignificant at the same time.

Taken in its aspect as the starting point for a game, the question around which this *ubishi* was formed is one of a number of similar types of problem or puzzle. We can say these form a continuum at one end of which are the satisfying, if transient, complexities of daily news and gossip. At the other end would be generic puzzles (are bats birds or mice?), problem scenarios (if you're treated simultaneously by several doctors, how will you know which one you should pay?) and dilemma tales. For none of these is there a right answer; rather they are engines well built for proliferating points of view (Bascom 1975; Fernandez 1986). As such, they provide resources for discussion as an amusement, making conversations into arenas where judgement is trained and kept in condition. In turn, the discussions are one source for the cumulative backlog of judgements and judging – of issues, of others and of others' manners of judging – against which arguments about life's *truly* important events are made and decisions taken.

An attentive reader will note that every single individual who spoke to the issue of spirits (*pepo*) had a slightly different point of view, so in that sense I now see that I was wrong when I set out to see 'which side' everyone was on, as though there might be just two. Since no two people were exactly in accord, there were as many 'sides' as there were people, and the evocative figure would have had to have been some complex geometric form. Each person's individual opinion had been composed by thought about as well as with the heterogeneous array of culturally provided possibilities.

That culture underwrites contestation has long been recognised in our understanding of local politics (Gluckman 1955; Epstein 1958; Turner 1957), where we would expect competition to enhance differences of opinion. Here, however, my concern has been to place opinionation in a different empirical and in a broader theoretical situation; viz., *that of knowledge production and self-realisation in the contexts of mortality and of being.* For me, the terms of reference by which we are to locate the study of illness and therapy amount to nothing other than these, and understanding them in some depth has informed the shape and scope of this book.

What the passages bring us, then, is a close view of ordinary singularisation (Guyer 1993, 1995; Guyer and Eno Belinga 1995; Kopytoff 1986; Simmel 1971), the name we may give to that process by which incommensurabilities of outlook are taken for what they are: viz., originalities of human being. This is to say that it is not only that everyone has formed their own opinion, created a particular compositional medley of argument. More important, it is that such composition (Fernandez 1982; MacGaffey 1986, 1988, 1993) and singularisation are expected, taken for granted. They are fundamental to the way knowledge works and, indeed, to how knowledge is – that is to how it is systematised, transmitted, and expanded or amplified.

That people are learning all the time is presumed in the discussion of sorcery in the second passage from notes. In that conversation, which centres upon relations between sorcery and divinity (i.e., between proximate and ultimate causes), what goes without saying is the parcellation of knowledge and power among members of a social network, such that even a sorcerer would normally seek help and information from a colleague. Hence, also presumed is a fundamental limitation of individual capacities. However, these and their limit are measured not so much by reference to some absolute standard as by comparison to shifting combinations of the capabilities of others and their ancestors' relative power. What is not strong enough today, though itself unchanged, may yet be strong enough tomorrow. The manifest uncertainties and astonishments of life's events are the result of this ever-shifting terrain.

Thus, heterogeneity and heteronomy condition human being, knowing and doing. Therapeutic knowledge in its systematic and technical senses is grounded in and informed by this. A science of (un)anticipated outcomes, therapeutic attention focuses on the unique rather than upon the typical occurrence; it is not directed so much towards the understanding of what things are in general as to how things will have turned out in particular (Evans-Pritchard 1937; Tambiah 1973, 1990). In this regard, the relationship between knowledge and singularisation goes, so to speak, all the way down, as we will see.

FIELD SCIENCES AND DOCUMENTARY ARTS

anthropology reconciles a number of divergent personal claims. It is one of the rare intellectual vocations which do not demand a sacrifice of one's manhood. Courage, love of adventure, and physical hardiness – as well as brains – are called upon. It also offers a solution to that distressing by-product of intelligence, alienation. Anthropology conquers the estranging function of the intellect by institutionalizing it.

Susan Sontag

Inserting the passages from fieldnotes also at least evokes the possibility of dislocating the generic relationship between the writer and the reader of ethnography. In the notes, the elements of the conversation that are of most interest to the participants are precisely the bits that have been, until recently, of least use to the ethnographic monograph as such (Asad 1986; Rabinow 1986). While our expectations of non-fiction allow us readily to recognise as knowledge the representation, as generalities, of rules and their objects, these same expectations effectively prevent our recognising as knowledge the interplay of provocations with the understanding of what happens next. While we are willing to be plunged into confusion as field-workers and readers of novels, as readers of non-fiction we usually feel entitled to know immediately what's going on and why that's important. We are averse to waiting for the point to make itself plain.

In this, our attention as readers is consistent with the genre, with the metaphysics of science (Dupré 1993) implicit in it, and with the eliciting as verbalised rules of knowledge usually realised in/as practice (Bourdieu 1977). The reflective awareness that knowledge is a kind of writing (Rorty 1982), that strategies of exclusion pre-exist criteria of truth (Foucault 1970, 1972; Hacking 1982, 1985), and that genres are social constructions (Ricoeur 1981) does not seem to have a bearing on our responses. Yet in part it is precisely this resistant inclination (perceptible as boredom or impatience with the representation of stories) that marks as ideological a type of epistemological closure in us as readers. Even when we assert that it is a process, the necessities of our representational genre reduce a 'tradition' to an enclosed/enclosing set of rules; the limits of rather than the starting point for the formulatable.

In contrast, the discussions of spirits and of sorcery place us at that growing edge where the thought and the formulatable coincide. By 'the thought' I mean to refer to what is held in consciousness either as the particular compositions of individuals (e.g., medicine is not the strength of men) or as the potential components of compositions – items which we might here refer to as matters of public opinion, clichés or commonplaces (e.g., that diviners are charlatans). By 'the formulatable' I mean those new compositions which can come or be brought into being in response to the radical novelty of events.

This dimension of invention is a privileged location in any science, inasmuch as it is the place at which events are not mere instantiations of known qualities and properties (Bennett 1988), and where, instead, events come to modulate the terms through which they were initially understood, if only as a by-blow of the effort required to domesticate them. Muzame's having seen a Bulumbu spirit go to urinate was one such event, the anthropologist's pursuit of analogies for amulets was another. Here, the image evoked by chess pieces is useful. The pieces contain rules as much as the rules contain pieces. Each is a little bundle of limitations and possibilities. With reference to the others, each forms part of the living landscape (Wallman 1997). Inversely, it is in part with reference to that landscape that the capability of each piece is defined.

Thus, what is at stake, what is going on in the sort of talk represented here, is not just the relating that is the point of the relating, i.e., the relationship that is created or modulated by the narrative (Chambers 1984, 1991; Das 1992; Jackson 1982, 1989), although that is important in itself. There is also an agreement that the effort will be to retain the instability of the new; that is, rather than allowing it to be dissolved in pre-existing categories of comprehension, we will make of it the foundation for further thought. We agree to see what happens if we fabricate compositions around it.

'Collage' rather than 'bricolage' is what I mean (Coombes 1994), and the image may be particularly suited to modelling the innovative aspects of those forms of knowledge that are specifically about – and indeed can be defined as systematics or sciences of – (un)anticipated outcomes. In these sciences, exemplified by therapeutics (Canguilhem 1991; Reznek 1987), war (Clausewitz 1984; Gibson 1986; Gray 1997) and farming, each application of a principle is also an experiment with it. Practitioners engage with the situation, then see what happens. Part of what does is conditioned by an 'other'; an event-generating agent whose reactions include summative responses to or awareness of shared conditions and which can never fully be predicted – in part if only because they are informed by what the other thinks the practitioner is thinking (Lacan 1972b).

Like *ubishi*, ethnographic field research also privileges unique events and singularisations, also knits together the thought and the formulatable. Indeed, this, our formative practice, is designed to do little other than provoke and interweave them. Placed in this context, ethnography becomes recognisable as a mediate science of meaning (Ricoeur 1970), whose claims to authenticity rest upon the attempted application of a conscious method of ciphering or formulation to the immigrant's personal experience of consciously deciphering life – encounter by encounter.

Indeed this, our intellectual manual labour, seems to be emerging as that which remains distinctive in our formation. Although the notion of 'the field' has been linked to the idea of travel over distances short as well as long

(Gupta and Ferguson 1997; Clifford 1997), I would argue that it is not the travel but the 'work' and the conditions under which it is conducted which make the field.

By this I mean to include not just the practice of daily writing, not just the discipline of systematic questioning, but primarily the consequence of their action on the intention-to-dwell that conditions an immigrant's sensibility. Over time, by means of the method, the fieldworker's subjectivity becomes the medium in which ethnographic understanding develops (Ellen 1984), in the photographic sense of the term (Pinney, Wright and Poignant 1995; Davis 1995).

Unlike immigrants, who are inclined to make themselves comfortable by reproducing the familiar in their immediate surroundings, we make ourselves uncomfortable, hoping that with luck, we'll come to feel at home. We gather data which take the forms of maps, genealogies, kinship terms, case histories, life histories, animal categories, descriptions of religious practices, court cases, gossip, etc. In the process, we make friends. Regularities emerge from the repetition of particulars; and we attain some sort of fluency, not just with the language, but also with the culture. We remember what we had to learn in order to get that far; and this is our ethnographic knowledge. On the basis of our fluency's imperfections, sometimes including an awareness of what we do not know, we begin to ask the kind of question, to raise the kind of objection, that makes conversations really good.

Our best questions are the ones which place the unthought in the position of the formulatable. They are the kinds of question natives wouldn't ordinarily think to ask, but ones for which the process of generating an answer is itself intriguing. They are questions about conjunctions or disjunctions of which natives ordinarily take no notice.[1] Like long-term denizens, fieldworkers are often the ones who, having learned the culture in adulthood, come to notice the regularities in discrepancies, to wonder and so raise questions about them. This is the generative capacity of ethnographic ignorance, and there is a new anti-heroic representation of discursive authority (Clifford 1983; Rabinow 1977; Sontag 1966) which attends it.

It is fieldwork's methodological intervention in ourselves, in our memories, as much as in the lives of others that authenticates the discipline's claim to realism in/as science (Hacking 1983). In turn, the intervention underwrites an appropriate redefinition of realism in ethnographic representation – that is, the consideration of ethnography as a documentary art.

In ethnography as in art (or in documentary art), realism takes as its object the image of the thing, not the thing the image is of (Hobson 1982; Klein 1970). In presenting the image, realism simultaneously shows itself as a technique or style of disclosure. It makes itself plain as a device by which is represented, in miniature so to speak, a summation of a past activity, itself rendered in terms of an attributed significance (the 'point'). In art or aesthetic theory, this would be the 'truth' of the work (Heidegger 1971). In Lévi-Strauss's terms, it would be a knowledge of the thing (1966). In a documentary art, created out of ignorance, framed by doubt (Sontag 1966; Lévi-Strauss 1978), our claims are, of course, more limited; it is what we have come to understand.

The approach of the Manchester School exemplifies one style of realism in ethnography or documentary art. Their heterogeneous output was unified by a commitment to the comprehension and representation of what was there to be seen on the surface, so to speak, in individual cases (Werbner 1990; Gluckman 1958). As a consequence of this commitment, the focal object of study changed (as did the relationship of the general rule to the unique event), the analytic language changed (as did the relationship of ethnographic to local understanding), and the ethnographic present changed (as did the relationship between anthropology and history).

Turner's *Schism and Continuity* (1957), *Forest of Symbols* (1967a) and *Drums of Affliction* (1968) can be taken as demonstrative of a style in which the representation of the field science formed an integral aspect of the documentary art. Of this body of work, 'A Ndembu doctor in practice' (1967c) is a particularly remarkable piece. Although the information it contains centres upon the articulations among the political, the moral and the therapeutic, the work is actively constructed as an appreciation of Ihembi's genius. What we learn about the dynamics of social (dis)order is presented as what we need to know in order to understand what Ihembi was doing. The piece finds its climax in a passage from fieldnotes, inserted in the text to preserve and convey the drama of the moment:

> Kachilewa now held his hand poised over the leaf-concealed calabash while all of us waited intently. He removed the leaves and dredged with his hand in the bloody mixture. After a while he shook his head and said 'Mwosi' ('Nothing in here'). *We were all disappointed.* But Ihembi with a gentle smile took over. He plunged his fingers into the gruesome liquid and when he brought them up I saw a flash of white … It was indeed a human tooth, we had to say. It was no bush pig's tooth, nor a monkey's. Jubilantly we told the women, who all trilled with joy. Men and women who had been on cool terms with one another until recently, shook hands warmly and beamed with happiness. (Turner 1967c: 391; emphasis added)

That emphasised line, with its willing sociability, set out what I wanted to achieve during the years of living in Zaire. I added to this a determination to understand how Bemba women could say of Chisungu that the ceremony literally 'grows the girls' (Richards 1956; Turner 1967b). Thus, with regard to documentary arts, this study is an extension and completion, in the domain of medical practice, of studies which have understood therapeutic events primarily or almost exclusively in so far as they support events social, political and moral.

REFLECTING SURFACES AND HABITABLE SPACES

Between the *language* (*langue*) that defines the system of constructing possible sentences, and the *corpus* that passively collects the words that are spoken, the *archive* defines a particular level: that of a practice that causes a multiplicity of statements to emerge as so many regular events, as so many things to be dealt with and manipulated. It does not have the weight of tradition; and it does not constitute the library of all libraries, outside time and place; nor is it the welcoming oblivion that opens up to all new speech the operational field of its freedom; between tradition and oblivion, it reveals the rules of a practice that enables statements both to survive and to undergo regular modification. It is *the general system of the formation and transformation of statements*.

Michel Foucault

The notes are dated. They are labelled with reference to the point in some external chronology at which they were written. More significantly, the notes are locatable from 'within'. That is, they are placed at a certain fixed distance from the occurrences which they describe. 'The other day', 'a couple of weeks ago', mark the spot – the point of exodus or entry – the rhizome or umbilicus (Freud 1958) – linking the act of writing to the occurrences informing although not occasioning it. Itself dispersed, the occurrence is recollected on the page, the place of production not just of notes but of the ethnographer-as-subject, and of her artefactual memory. Fieldnotes are thus our primary ethnographic text, and the moment at which they are written is our actual ethnographic present.

What I am trying to get at here is the interplay of experience and rumination linking writing as a daily practice (as a series of articulated operations both gestural and mental; an itinerant, progressive, regulated, repetitive process (Certeau 1984)) to the development of a memory that is a created object – a mental archive of which the notes themselves are both the residuum and the armature. The notes are an artefact of the memory, the trace of daily recollections, yet the memory that is an artifact of the notes – of the systematisation that is the consequence of the writer's reflections (cf. Ellen 1984) – is the more important of the two.

In the 'lore' of the profession there is the story of Edmund Leach (1954), which lets us know that it is possible to write a monograph with memory but without the fieldnotes which formed it. With the foreclosure of armchair anthropology, we have founded ourselves as a community on the premise that it is not possible to write a monograph with notes but no living memory of their construction. What we come to know as the culture we are transcribing is a knowledge brought into being in the displacements of thought that are mediated by writing as a practice. Ethnography's arts and landscapes of memory (Yates 1966; Connerton 1989; Halbwachs 1992; Certeau 1984; Mudimbe 1988; Kirmayer 1996; Fischer 1986) are caught up and kept alive on the reflecting surfaces and in the habitable spaces of the notebooks.

If we press the point that there is no speech without a listener (Bakhtin 1984; Lacan 1972a, 1977a), we may come to claim that there is no genre of 'speaking' (Bakhtin 1986) without its culturally constructed 'ear'. Neither letter nor diary – less public than one, more public than the other – the fieldnotes inscribe a language practice somewhat like soliloquy. Suspended between 'scenes', separated by margins of silence from the world of voices that otherwise possesses us, fieldnotes, like soliloquy, are duplicitous, directed to 'no one' but nevertheless meant to be (over)heard by eaves-droppers imagined and unexpected – ourselves in multiple guises.

There is the 'other' whose 'being there' guides our scrutiny of the day's residues as we recall, select among and inscribe them (a device or quality of attention we might regard as the positive unconscious of the discipline as a community). There is that 'other' which is the source of a 'deferred action' (cf. Laplanche and Pontalis 1973, from Freud 1958 and Lacan 1977a), by virtue of whose revisions and reconstructions we come to make first note of the *repetitions* of incongruities that, in their turn, become gateways to insight – the primary process that *is* the education in the educated guesses of Geertz's 'thick' description (1973a). Finally there is that 'other' – unknown in herself – for whom the fieldnotes will serve as an archive, viz., the future ethnographer as she is imagined by herself in the present.

We can say that this accumulation of recollections towards the virtual space of a future anterior being is what the discipline adds to us outright. In the manner of an adulthood added by initiation, it is a change of state putatively unmediated and absolute, but whose effects are demonstrable in their later unfolding. In this sense, fieldwork is an event whose significance lies in the options for being to which it gives place (Certeau 1997); our memories of it are the localised authorisations underwriting their reality, and our notes are both their objective correlatives and the dwellings or habitable spaces (Certeau 1984) in which the memories live.

Once 'home' we are moved away from the constitutive event by passages through three different registers of time: (1) the passage of days, (2) the passage of thought through the significations (meanings) of the options for being – the acculturations – to which we have been exposed, and (3) the passage of ephemeral, fragmented recollections through the hypostasisation that makes them into culture, written. The singularity of each field experience leaves its imprint here: in the ways the registers articulate, in the changing blends of agency and patiency in each, and in the shifting effects of each element upon the others. 'Ending' is the situation emergent from this mix and the text is its public manifestation.

In this sense we may place the progress towards the monograph in a larger family of transfigurative memory practices or disciplines and the subsequent memory work to which they give rise: psychoanalysis (Freud 1958; Lacan 1972a), missionary conversions (Mudimbe 1991, 1994a, 1994b, 1997), training for and experience of war (Gibson 1986; Feldman 1991; Young 1995), and surviving individual and collective trauma (Frankl 1985; Kirmayer 1996; Antze and Lambek 1996; Young 1993, 1995), among others (Althusser 1971; Connerton 1989; Butler 1997). In this context the progress towards hypostasisation is a progress towards 'having done' with a memory, as measured by a capacity to make it real, to have it taken by others as veridical. Seen from this perspective, the ethnographic library's processual interior becomes a socially shared, culturally conditioned landscape of memory (Kirmayer 1996; Halbwachs 1992; Connerton 1989), which acknowledges some types or forms of recollection but not others (cf. Stoller and Olkes 1987).

With boundaries enforced by relegation to silence, the landscape is a matter of genre as well as of style of reasoning (Ricoeur 1981; Hacking 1982, 1985; Foucault 1970, 1972; Canguilhem 1988). The admissibility of the recollection depends in part upon the balance the narrator can strike between the idiosyncrasies of the experience and the broader regulative understandings uniting the community as a whole. These are perhaps discernible as the underlying question, itself suppressed from the text, whose terms shape the answer that is the text. The changing qualities of our landscape – one consequence of the community's lineage or descent systems (cf. Haraway 1991, 1992) – are measurable by the ways in which this question has changed:

1. How can this be? (functionalism)
2. What does this mean? (structuralism/interpretative anthropology)
3. What does the world have to be in order for this to be so? (locationism)

As evidenced by the long list of 'new'-style ethnographies, the last question increases the singularities of ethnographic writings, their incommensurabilities, and their loyal adherences to the local authority of the communities created by or existing among ethnographers and the people who tried to teach them something. With the decline of the generalising theory, the value, if not the power, of a discursive regularity running across and uniting diverse representations is diminished; and there is a concomitant increase in a particular type or tone of contestation. The veridicality of the work is measured as much by the limits of what it can represent as by what it succeeds in representing. This reference to our professional disputations about relations between illusion and truth (cf. Kleinman 1995) – about the morality of representation and about the training of judgement and of discernment – brings us back to the discussion with which this gesture at introduction began: an *ubishi* in which the same set of issues is in play, and in not dissimilar terms.

As importantly, admission to the landscape of monuments means a writer's dispossession; it is a passage from recursive movement in the habitable space of memory to exclusion from the closed counter-memory captured by and in the monument (cf. Lacan 1977a). Although prompted, if not informed, by contingency and experience, the monument is made none the less to endure as a caption point for collective recollection and inexperience; it is not a dwelling for the domesticity of remembering, but a public site for not forgetting – a book in a library.

The price of this little piece of endurance is identification with the experience on which it has been based. The writer has no greater claim to what the book remembers than do any of its other readers – perhaps, actually, less. We all remember the same 'Azande'; we are yet to have done with that granary.

TEACHING A STONE TO TALK

Psychoanalysis and ethnology occupy a privileged position in our knowledge – not because they have established the foundations of their positivity better than any other human science, and at last accomplished the old attempt to be truly scientific; but rather because, on the confines of all the branches of knowledge investigating man, they form an undoubted and inexhaustible treasure-hoard of experiences and concepts, and above all a perpetual principle of dissatisfaction, of calling into question, of criticism and contestation of what may seem, in other respects, to be established.

Michel Foucault

Summations of our moment show that it is characterised by the transposition of the values adhering to fundamental opposites (work/play, depth/surface, identity/difference) (cf. Harvey 1990). In writing, ours is the era of the gerund, or, more broadly, of the verbal noun; a device intended to stress our recognition of the contingency and situatedness of all identities, with much invented, located, dislocated. With time defined by allusions to place, there are multiple opinions on when or where 'now' began: Woolf's December 1910 (Bradbury 1976), Jameson's late 1950s/early 1960s with the appropriation of modernism by institutions (1991), Robert Young's Algerian war (1990), Harvey's (following Jenck's) demolition of low-income housing in 1972 (Harvey 1990) – all are seizing a moment when the accumulated weight of smaller changes opened onto an irreversible break.

For contemporary anthropology, such a point must be the first six months of 1968. Early February saw the Tet offensive in Vietnam; in spring there were the assassinations of M. L. King and R. F. Kennedy, the creation in Washington of 'Resurrection City' (the expansion of the civil rights movement into the pressure for economic justice), and in Paris the events of May. These were a series of 'critical events' (Das 1995b) by virtue of which new modes of action came into being, redefining traditional categories and opening new forms to political actors (Das 1995b; Certeau 1997). In a rough-and-ready sort of way, we can say that this is the year marking the switch in ethnography's disciplinary 'mentality' (Horton 1967, 1982; Lloyd 1978, 1990; Vickers 1984) from an anxiety about difference, with its fundamental project as the search for universals, to a fear of the same, with its corresponding project – the valuation or appreciation of singularities.

Paul Rabinow's fieldwork in Morocco began in 1968, and his re-presentation of it in his later study (1977) crystallised this concern, while simultaneously introducing the experience of antagonism (Laclau 1990) into the discipline's constituting myth (cf. Clifford 1983, 1988). This is to say that although the fact of conflict had not been excluded from earlier characterisations of the experience of fieldwork, it had been relegated to the margins of the work: the validating introduction (Evans-Pritchard 1940; Geertz 1972), the private diary (Malinowski 1967), the novel (Bowen 1954), the preparation for 'culture shock' (Ellen 1984). Rabinow's *Reflections on Fieldwork in Morocco*, however, took the problem of antagonism and of misunderstanding – the limits of objectivity – as the central problematic of ethnographic knowledge. As such, it reflected not only the uncertainties but also the maturation of a cohort for whom ethnography is not to be separated from a social setting or broader social purpose.

All of 1968's critical events were challenges to the authenticity and legitimacy of representation and/or representative government as it had been practically constituted prior to that time. With the two post-revolutionary societies on/in which the events had bearing (the United States and France, their conservatist pulls notwithstanding), the matter or gesture of authentication is construed as prior to and/or more fundamental than any particular representation – it *is* the just consent of the governed. Hence, in terms of politics, the point giving foundation to representative democracy was not whether you can see the 'other', but whether you can see 'yourself' in it (a construal whose operation can be said to have become critical to most forms of civic contestation in the United States since that time). This is a problematic of continuously compelling interest in post-revolutionary social orders, which always need to know the foundation of compliance or the terms of the social contract on the basis of which they are operating, and which press the human sciences into the service of disciplined self-reflection with regard to it.

In terms of writing, the experience of being misrepresented translates into a concern about the criteria by which authentication can be achieved – the terms under which the citizens of the republic of the written can be made equals and the constraints/conditions under which claims for or aspirations towards freedom operate. Since unity is precisely what is not foregone but must be forged, the discovery of common cause as the basis for federation (US) or of a 'natural reason' commonly shared as the basis for equality and fraternity is the gesture or proof with which any work must begin. The two books Rabinow recalls, in 1977, as having most influenced him in 1968 were Kuhn's *Structure of Scientific Revolutions* (1962) and Lévi-Strauss's *Tristes Tropiques* – texts with dislocation, contestation and the problematic nature of understanding as their central themes.

Britain has eschewed the political model of revolution as rupture or fragmentation, and instead deploys metaphors of tradition or continuity and the device of radical recursion as a means of encoding and containing change in the idiom of endurance. Hence, the allure of self-scrutiny, of doubts about belonging, epistemological or otherwise, found little resonance in British social anthropology. In Britain, faith in empiricism remains basically unshaken, and provides its own style of critical awareness (cf. Asad 1973, 1986, 1991; Fardon 1990, 1995). Disciplinary reflection on the domestic social order has not been excluded from ethnographic practice (cf. Douglas and Wildavsky 1982; Frankenberg 1982; Werbner 1990), but criticism derives more strongly from work in British cultural studies (cf. Turner 1996; Hall and Jefferson 1993; Hebdige 1994; Gilroy 1992). This draws upon an historicist, socialist, oppositional tradition of its own and its critical observations on the representations of class interests have been put to use in the United States.

Solutions to the problem of hierarchy and authentication in knowledge have taken several forms, all of which have to do with visibly delimiting the claims of the knower in the text – making evident the elements of which the knowledge was constructed, keeping everything in something like the 'same' register or order of value. The metaphor of archaeology (Freud 1958; Foucault 1972) or the archaeological site is, in this sense, the mark of the new self-consciousness. Linking the thought to the unthought through an idiom of visibility, the idea of archaeology attempts to display the process by which one pattern of thinking is imposed upon another that is already there (Canguilhem 1988; Geertz 1973b). Democratising a hierarchy that it is impossible not somehow to maintain, archaeology's claim is renunciation of the power of the hidden; it therefore puts the role of the interpreter into circulation – the unthought becomes less a manifestation of the 'primitive' or the resistant and more a type of residuum brought to the surface at the moment in which there is expression of originality (Ricoeur 1970, 1974, 1981; Foucault 1970). Although the forms of texts may not vary radically from what we presented before, the tacit understanding with which readers come to texts, and the manner in which we present them, have changed in a fashion informed by the metaphor.

In this respect what become worthy for thought are not merely the patterns by which we place ethnographic 'things' together, to make sense of them (e.g., one can't have sex before making peanut oil, therefore some relationship between the two processes exists, although the specifics of its content remain to be determined by comparison with other 'things' including principles of construction deriving as much from the discipline as from the social order represented). We also become conscious of the 'economy' tacit in our combinations and compositions: that is, we become aware that the domain or order which will be the foundation of our study ('knowledge', 'the social', 'the political', 'the religious') is our choice; we are conscious of whether we are emphasising the determinacy or indeterminacy of the knowledge; whether we view its end as the (re)production of itself, or of innovation and the production of a new social moment, and of the amenability of each approach to the process not of non-fiction writing but rather of non-fiction reading. It is, after all, in the reading that the writer finds her voice; and in this regard, the present volume is intended as one of two, the second of which will cover much the same ground as this, but in an entirely different way.

For this study, I have been concerned both with the individual minds whose practical reasoning has held death in abeyance some of the time, and with the 'mind' inhering in the knowledge of illness and therapy used by those individual reasoners – the *'langue'* from which their *'parole'* emerges, and, to which, in their 'speaking', they add. This second 'mind' I have composed on the basis of our contemporary ethnographic habitus (cf. Bourdieu 1977; Lévi-Strauss 1966), but with the exception that I have tried to describe things in their positivity – in terms of what they produce, do, create, make possible; not in terms of what they do not do or are not. I have attempted to represent therapeutic knowledge not as a closed totality, but as a living resource which adults learn from and teach each other, and with which people can try to live up to the undecidability of the vital moment.

The elimination of negative or framing words ('beliefs', 'notions') or of representations couched in terms of how 'they' vary from 'our' expectations makes ethnography harder to write. If 'they' are not a non-version of 'us' we are also forced out of the comforts of home – we must exchange the familiarity of known categories (Evans-Pritchard 1937, 1940; Geertz 1988) and relocate to a linguistic 'elsewhere'. I found the language and the interpretative economy best suited to my ends outside of anthropology's ongoing debates (cf. Valéry 1972; Gilman 1978; Klein 1970; Hobson 1982; Manuel 1959; Stewart 1993; Rajchman and West 1985). The processual structures I found most directly compatible were those emphasising the

indeterminate, constructed qualities of knowledge as the realisation of mind
or thought (the usual suspects). I have not been particularly concerned to
globalise this locality so much as to have racinated the body, illness and
therapy radically in a representation of material being proper to them. In
these respects, I have attempted to make clearer the bonds uniting the
'symbolic' and the 'instrumental' by writing around them and writing them
into a substantial world that would have to exist in order for their union to
be so.

STORIES ABOUT PLACES ARE MAKESHIFT THINGS

> Arguments, theories, terms, points of view and debates can therefore
> be clarified in at least two different ways: (a) in the manner ... which
> leads back to the familiar ideas and treats the new as a special case of
> things already understood, and (b) by incorporation into a language of
> the future, which means that one must learn to argue with
> unexplained terms and sentences for which no clear rules of usage are
> as yet available.
>
> Paul Feyerabend

A text's evocations of predecession (one form of which is referencing) give
indication of the intertextual community (or collection) in which its contribution is meant to be located. Here, I am working through a conception of
text that accords to it the 'elemental' qualities of 'flesh' as phenomeno-
logically rendered:

> a *general* thing, midway between the spatio-temporal individual and
> the idea of a sort of incarnate principle that brings a style of being
> wherever there is a fragment of being ... Not a fact or a sum of facts
> and yet adherent to *location* and to the *now*. Much more: the
> inauguration of the *where* and the *when*; the possibility and exigency
> for the fact; in a word: facticity, in what makes the fact be a fact. And
> at the same time, what makes the fact have meaning, makes the
> fragmentary facts dispose themselves about 'something'. (Merleau-
> Ponty 1968: 139–40)

So, the here and now of the hermeneut's transfigurative change in horizon
(Ricoeur 1981) can rest on your lap, be held in your hand, or stuffed back
into a bag when your flight is announced.

I am reading of domestication and the conflict of memories (Mudimbe
1994b) when I run across his name: Morlion. Not indexed. It is the only
mention. The text tells me that in 1940 he succeeded Victor Roelens as the
head of the vicarate, a powerful, populous enterprise of conversion; paradigmatic of a presumptive right to colonise.

As I remember him, Morlion was eighty-six or more – a background figure
in the life of the small, ageing community of White Fathers up the mountain,

at the mission in Moba (called so again, after having been, for a time, Baudoinville). The men accumulated a month's vacation every year, but took these every six years in six-month periods that they would spend in Europe.

I remember Morlion's letter, written just after his return from his stay in Belgium. He said he was relieved to be back again. The whole time he'd been away he'd been anxious that he would die there; far from home, among strangers. Now, given his age, it seemed likely he would never have to go again – or at least he was safe for another six years – and the thought was a comfort to him.

Further up the lake, in the village that bore his name, was Kizumina. Older than Morlion, in his nineties, blind and frail in body, Kizumina Mkubwa was 'mother's brother' (*mjomba*) to Mpala and a renowned historian. He could remember as a boy having seen not the first but the second missionaries to the area. By rights he should have been a chief, and people acknowledged him as such, but correct succession had been overturned by the colonial authority and never restored after Independence.

One evening after dark, coming back from somewhere further down the lake, we pulled into his place, to pay him a visit. The village was black; deserted and nothing stirring. When we shouted, people came down from the mountainside. Everyone had run to hide, thinking we might be the government or the rebels, but, either way, bad news. Kizumina himself they had tucked up into a corner of a darkened house, hidden. At the time, sitting around together afterward, we all thought it was pretty funny – not because the fear had been unreasonable, but because, this time, it turned out to have been so unfounded.

Fragments of recollections are here represented as the indices of our dilemma. At the interface of two opposed domesticating orders, each of two memories contains the entirety of the colonial period, and then close to two decades beyond. Colonialism is a 'normal' displacement – contained, endured, outlived, survived, 'bested' – across the span of a single life. Yet the trajectory of each life has also been radically deflected; each man is dwelling in a here and now that would not have happened without the specificity of the colonial intervention there and then.

I have yet to formulate a name for this local habitation, this 'dwelling' in the here and now that is one's own body in maturity and age, in the space conditioned by so many intercalations of outcomes with origins. This is the third pass the introduction has made by the issue of labile being and its entrainments: (1) deferred action in which the future plays a vital role in the reconstitution of what we think of as having been our past, (2) composition of knowledge through devices highlighting its limits, and (3) intercalations of origins and outcomes such that nothing is what it would have been. The perspective we are developing resembles the type of dynamic (in)stability taken for granted in the *ubishi* and in other conversations in Mpala: the

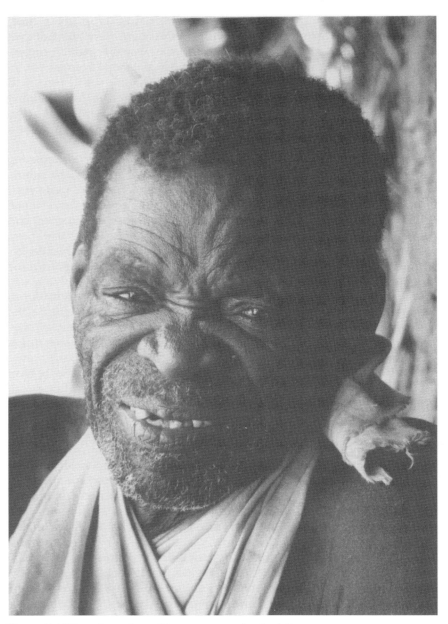

Figure I.1 Kizumina, whose life encompassed colonialism

shifting location of any situated knowledge, the absolute (im)permanence even of the transcendent, intercalations of truth and falsehood, falsehoods that lead to belief in truth, absolute but temporary power, alternate, mutually subverting centres.

The parallel permits us to see more clearly the larger family group into which contemporary theory can be placed. If we designate it less by time than by the relative position of the subject from which it is drawn, the (post)modern is a localised construction of the recognition of certain mortal limits, a position also recognised and made the foundation for knowledge at other times (Nussbaum 1986; Greenblatt 1980; Castiglione 1967; Sorabji 1980) as well as other places (Daniel 1996; Reynolds 1996; Tsing 1993; Scheper-Hughes 1992; Taussig 1987; Lavie 1990; Desjarlais 1992). What we see in the *ubishi* is a comprehension of heteronomy and subjection through an awareness of human frailty and folly – all taken as the accepted *starting points* for dignity and cunning, sociability and selfishness – these among other qualities emergent and changing from person to person and from time to time.

In some respects the theory of our time is also perceptible as the passage into a neutralised or non-specific language of positions that had earlier been articulated with reference to other, more specific situations and subjugated knowledges (cf. Canguilhem 1991; Sartre 1965; Beauvoir 1993; Fanon 1967; Du Bois 1997). One wonders about the link between a generalisable language and the recognition of suffering (cf. Asad 1997; Frankl 1985; Kirmayer 1996); a paradox by which the greater the immediacy of the suffering represented, the less transactible the value of its representation – the less the narrative counts as knowledge about something other than itself (cf. Scarry 1985; Das 1992, 1995a). Thought turns to the necessary relationship between the identification with a historical and social unity and a power which enables speech to resist relegation (cf. Certeau 1997; Arnold 1981; Kesteloot 1991; Cuddihy 1987; Markovitz 1969; Gilman 1993). But with that, the rumination is complete, and I go back to my reading.

There, as in other areas of this project (Mudimbe 1991, 1997), the text (Mudimbe 1994b) establishes for itself a position from which a heterogeneous array of 'things' are accorded equal validity as objects for thought. Under the aegis of the 'sign' and the 'classifying order', we are given as things to think objects which maintain their specific qualities and original locations (what it is/was) while, in their re-presentation, they are also able to carry the weight of abstraction. Thus does Victor Roelens come to be both a life and a paradigm, a specific existence and an object for critical consciousness; missionary conversion both a calling and an enterprise; Africa a location, a signifying function a signified.

I am struck by the respect in which events of record, biographical facts, memoirs, practices and imaginary spaces are put together in a sort of

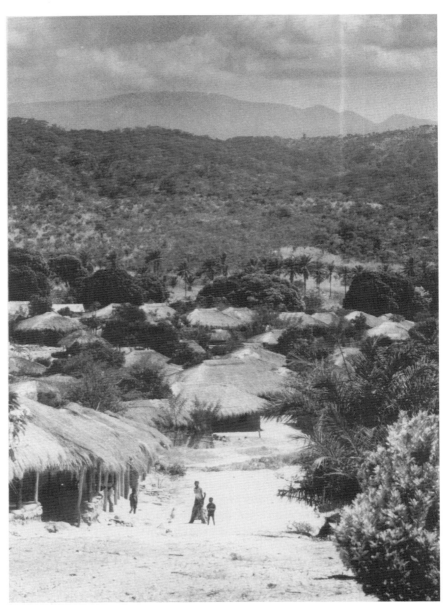

Figure I.2 Mpala, *espace metissée*

heteroglossia of the documentarist's art – an art of relocation. The position, an *espace métissée*, holds them all in a kind of capacious balance between abstract and concrete and in conjunctions that evoke as well as inform. By drawing attention to the 'things' which are now what thought must take into account before beginning, the relocation provides a new foundation. By providing words and figures, the space provides us with intellectual tools for use elsewhere – in places like this one. With the assembly of other voices, the clustered references to other texts, we are given resources with which to sustain ourselves.

This balance between the specific and the ideational is a manner of negotiating the radical irony of being oneself held to account for the injury one has sustained – the price of being heard to speak. The device of storytelling in the midst of argument – the telling here and now of what happened there and then – is a manner of defining the *fracture* as a foundation of the *espace métissée*. To claim identity from it and to insist that it be known is a manner of containing without resolving the dislocation that has brought us here, holding it together with its suffering, then suggesting we build from there.

In his work, V. Y. Mudimbe is walking (1994a, 1994b), with Certeau (1984) on his mind. Spatial practices and scriptural economies blend as he walks from the synecdoche of the mission (by which a right to colonise was extended) to the asyndeton of other('s) order (through which the colonising links were resisted, ruptured), moving (in) the text through two locations – one of which, Kapolowe, is a place where he has been. The other is Mpala, which he, with us, imagines, and whose image he, for us, reproduces.

The *ubishi* with which we began took place on the porch behind the house which still stands on page 138 of *The Idea of Africa*. It is not hard to imagine the philosopher completing his walk in time to participate in the *ubishi*. In the process, his figure establishes for us the intertextual connectedness of the collection (Stewart 1993), a *savoir* with its personal order, knowledge and time standing out from and resisting the library's *connaissance*.

In a compositional gesture meant to be inscribed as much under asyndeton – or resistant disjuncture – as through a synecdoche written from an alternate centre of community, I am here trying to expand an intertext of choice, adding to the comforts of Central Africanist ethnography a companionship of a broader critical community. In it, an ethnography, like the square houses of an *espace métissée* (as in Mpala, not 'traditionally' round, yet in the idiom of the land 'these days'), can become a 'proper' (an 'own') place to dwell even in one's intercalated maturity; can become a position from which to add to a tradition of invention; can operate as a point of 'origin' for a set of questions different from the ones we have asked before.

In its voluntarism, this claim of an intertext 'proper' to itself takes place in

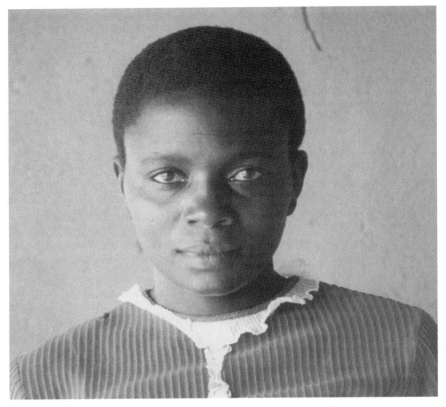

Figure I.3 Kalolo's wife, Kasawa, who didn't believe in divination

the noiseless companionability of an imagined intimacy; one whose identity makes the collection – a spacing in which similitude is the atmosphere emergent from difference. I am making it as I write.

Not only do I not know whether or not this text will be let into any real intertextual community – with its simultaneous speakings, there are other noises also shut out from it: externalities – features of being, of the living reality, that were cut out or written elsewhere, known, remembered, forgotten, but not inscribed. For example, within the world of the *ubishi*:

> Kalolo's wife had a name of her own (Kasawa) although people rarely use own names. She had relatives and children and fields. She also had *kiuu* (an illness characterised by extraordinary thirst – for which it is named – and almost continuous urination – there was sugar in her urine). She had just recovered from a serious illness that had begun as a boil-like lesion, then had seemed for a time to be incurable, before

finally responding to treatment from a brother of her husband's. Her sceptical iconoclasm had been authenticated by her behaviour: no one knew her to have been for divination.

Mwalimu Fredi was a teacher who had not been paid in months. Luvunzo had TB although this was not evident at the time. Muzame had three beautiful daughters, was renowned for his drumming and was in great demand at weddings. During the colonial period he had tended cattle for the priests, and now and then still had a recurring nightmare in which he awoke to discover that, while he had been sleeping, the cattle had got loose and ruined people's fields. Lubeni was in the midst of moving to another village, because his neighbours were giving indication that they considered him a sorcerer, and didn't want him so close.

In the world around the *ubishi*, there is no AIDS as yet, and Luvunzo's death is three years in the future. Although there's a war going on, Kabila's army hovers as it always has done, on the periphery of life in Mpala and somewhat more closely in Kalemie, and, because of the war, on the BBC. From time to time, the rebels come into villages north of Kalemie and take people. Sometimes people you've known or relatives of people that you know are swept into the margins of a hearsay world from which they don't usually return.

You never see them again, but sometimes hear of their life events; they marry, they have babies and the news comes to you by word of mouth. They are not dead, but not alive, actually, either. Their life flares up from time to time until the moment you hear that they have died. When you've been 'home' for a year or two, and people stop having news for you, they tell the teacher doing the writing that it's like that, it's just the same with you: it's as though you've been taken by the rebels. Not dead, but not alive, really, either.

I have tried to make this text an 'element', a 'something', a 'general thing' in the style of therapeutic understanding. On the basis of it we might want to think about where we'd like to begin – and who, for that matter, 'we' is.

AN INTRODUCTION IN THE STRICTER SENSE OF THE WORD

The Tabwa of Zaire occupy part of a large and fairly unified cultural area extending from the lands of the Bemba in Zambia on the south to those of the Bembe (at Kasanga Mtoa, near the border of Kivu region, Zaire) on the north. To the west, this area is bounded by the lands of the Luba-Hemba, and, on the east, by Lake Tanganyika. The whole area displays considerable cultural and historical unity. People say that all groups in the territory participated in different waves of but one migration. The Bwile, Tumbwe, Runda and so forth now appear to be fractions, as it were, of this larger whole. They are groups which have emphasised one or another aspect of their political identity (clan name, chiefly affiliation, etc.), which claim a different 'sub-plot' in the area's history, and which have begun a separate political history. These groups also demonstrate cultural variations which make manifest their combination of unity and diversity.

The people that are known as Tabwa live along the shores of Lake Tanganyika from Cape Tembwe south into Zambia, and inland in the high mountains of the Marungu Massif. Near northern neighbours are the Holoholo and Tumbwe, whose language is quite similar and to whom Tabwa chiefs are related by ties of history and kinship.

Southern neighbours are the Bemba, among whom Zambian Tabwa live and with whom they share many cultural features. Werner (1971: 10) indicates that KiTabwa and CiBemba are mutually intelligible languages, having a 90 per cent 'basic language correspondence'. Like the Bemba, BaTabwa are matrilineal and formerly required uxorilocality and service to in-laws in the early years of marriage.

Also, those of the Bemba were Tabwa *ngulu* land spirits, which took the forms of large snakes and lived in striking outcroppings of rock or other natural formations. Chiefly powers of mediation with ancestors and *ngulu*, and chiefly control over the fertility of the land through the control of ritual coitus and fire, were also common cultural characteristics. In the south people came to identify themselves more and more with the dominant Bemba, so much so that there was an unwillingness on the part of some to speak their own language, with CiBemba becoming increasingly popular.

At other borders, the Tabwa were connected to and influenced by their northern and western Luba and Lubaised neighbours. As one moved north from the Zaire/Zambia border, changes in house and lifestyles were evident. Millet became less significant, and the granaries it required less frequent. At Zongwe, people said they continued to live in communities formed according to the traditional pattern: a man, his children and sister's children living in a small cluster of houses. There, people could also remember and talk about the relationship between the current religious form (of *bulumbu* spirits; possessing and non-possessing) and the former religious entity, the *ngulu*, saying that *ngulu* left their mountainous abodes and came to live among human beings.

By the time one arrived at Moba, much of this had changed. Millet was grown solely for the purpose of brewing beer, and granaries were rarely seen. People had come to live in larger groups than was formerly the case, and few remembered that the *bilumbu* which came from the BaLuba in the thirties met another form of spirit which had been present when they arrived.

At Cape Tembwe, some six hours' walk north of Mpala, self-identification as BaTabwa ceased and that as BaHoloholo began. Though the language remained strikingly similar to that of KiTabwa (and the chief at Cape

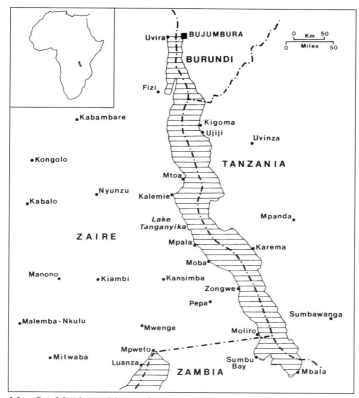

Map I.1 Mpala and its environs

Tembwe recognised his dependence upon Chief Mpala), the influences of KiBembe and other languages were apparent. There were cultural differences as well. Marriage customs, funerary indemnities, secret societies and chiefly office reflected the Luba influence among BaHoloholo and BaTumbwe, an influence which increased steadily as one travelled north of the Cape.

Lying on the cusp, so to speak, between these two great cultural and political traditions (the Bemba and the Luba) is Lubanda and its environs, the area of Chief Mpala and the community in which the bulk of this research was undertaken. Lubanda is the name by which the valley of the Lufuko River delta is called, and Mpala is the *chef-lieu* lying within it.

In 1973–7, the village consisted of some 550–600 houses built on the bluffs overlooking Lake Tanganyika. Immediately north lay the Lufuko River, along whose banks residents of Mpala planted their dry-season gardens, and grew their wet-season rice. With a population of some 2,000 souls, Mpala was the largest community on the shores of the lake, with the exceptions of the railhead and subregional seat at Kalemie, and the Zone location at Moba.

Mpala's increased size seems to have been gained at the expense of villages in the interior, which steadily declined in population after Independence. The constant flow of petty commerce along Tanganyika's shores permitted an involvement in the money economy that had become impossible in regions where roads were no longer maintained. Indeed, this migration was not to Mpala alone, but included movement to and establishment of villages upon every small cove or inlet whose beach would permit building.

The increasingly dense population of Mpala was supported by the farming of manioc, which, as a staple crop, had the benefit of growing well in the poor soil of the hills which rise behind the village as well as in the sandy soil of Tanganyika's shores. In addition, the rich alluvial earth of the Lufuko delta had long permitted the cultivation of crops such as maize, millet, sweet potatoes, yams, beans, peanuts and squash. Small annual crops of rice, potatoes, onions, tomatoes and tobacco were also grown both for subsistence and for sale, mostly locally but also occasionally at Kalemie.

Mpala was the site of one of the first European outposts in this part of Central Africa, that established by Emile Storms in 1883 and turned over to the White Fathers in 1885. Though the mission itself was no longer occupied by priests, the trees and grove behind it continued to bear such fruits as oranges, lemons, avocados and coconuts. The oranges matured once a year at the end of the rains, and were widely sold by a resident of Mpala, who acted as the representative of the mission. The other fruits were available on a more irregular and restricted basis. Bananas and papayas ripen throughout the year, and were regularly sold in local commerce. Older houses also had individual orange trees growing beside them, planted as seedlings provided by the mission.

Residents of Mpala lived not only by farming, but by fishing as well. The waters of Lake Tanganyika provided abundant fish for subsistence and for sale. The mackerel-like *mvolo* (*Luciolates stappersii*) was regularly caught in large numbers during the month of May, and the surplus smoked and sold to petty traders for transport and subsequent sale at Kalemie and elsewhere. It is this 'crop' which supplied the households of fishermen with their principal fund of cash for the year. The fund was usually spent on clothes for family members, as well as on fishing equipment such as nets, hooks and the like. The ongoing supply of consumables such as kerosene, salt and soap was maintained by women, who purchased these items with money earned by the brewing of corn and millet beer (*kibuku*), the distillation of manioc liquor (*rutuku*), or the sale of manioc, firewood and rice.

During the dry season, smelt-sized *dagaa* (*Stolothrissa tanganicae*) could be caught in great numbers by those fortunate enough to own a large dragnet. Such a net is roughly 60–100 feet or more in length, requires collective operation, and constitutes a considerable investment. The

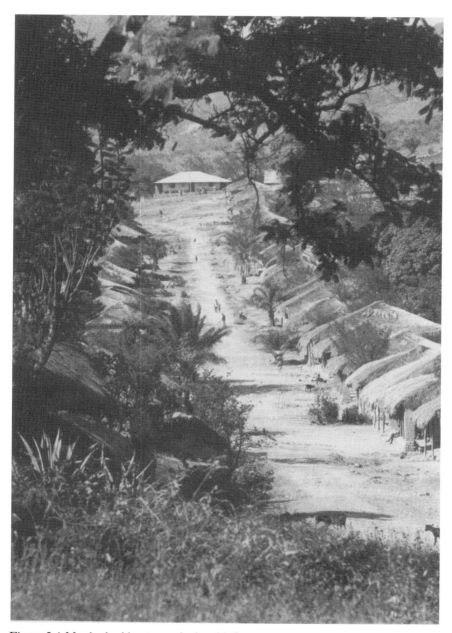

Figure I.4 Mpala, looking towards the chief's

catching, sun-drying and selling of these fish could form the basis of a personal fortune and a career in commerce. Conflict over such a net's use and profits figures prominently in one of the case histories presented below.

Even when it did not provide cash 'crops' of fish, Tanganyika served as a 'larder'. The small fish *tubunda* (perhaps *Bathybates vittatus*) could be caught by hand-net from the rocks along the shores, or by the hand-lines of little boys who fished in the afternoons. Rivers could be fished by individual men for the large *nsinga* catfish (perhaps *Dinopterus cummingtoni*), whose fat was much prized; or by groups of women using *butupa* (*Tephrosia vogelii* Hook. f.) fish poison.

Hunting, in contrast to fishing, was less important to the life of Mpala than it had been in the past. Older BaTabwa remember a time when people had to live in tight enclosures and could not leave the house at night because of leopard, and when herds of elephant regularly crossed the ridge an hour's walk above the village. At this time, both large and small game could be hunted easily, and the hunters' cult, the BaMbwela, was of importance.

At the time of my stay, however, almost all the game in the area was gone. The Belgian priests' method of hunting at night with headlamps (to provide meat for the large number of children in their charge as orphans and pupils), coupled with the technique of the Armée Nationale Congolaise, who, during the disruptions following Independence, machine-gunned whole herds from light planes, functioned gradually to diminish and finally to eliminate an animal population already decimated by the rinderpest murrain of the turn of the century. During my stay, only small antelope such as bushbuck and duiker were trapped in hunters' snares. Bushpig was occasionally caught as well.

Much hunting in the area was done by groups of BaMbote, some of whom are sedentary. These people sold to BaTabwa the meat they did not need themselves or exchanged it for manioc or salt. They also sold or traded other forest products such as firewood, honey and mushrooms.

Involvement in the money economy was well established, though this system of exchange was far from all-encompassing. Households made regular use of money to purchase manufactured goods such as salt, soap, kerosene and biomedicine. In addition, money was given in payment for some traditional services such as divination and certain treatments with local medicines. It was the means by which parts of the marriage relation were established and parts of death indemnities were paid. Money was also the medium of exchange for such goods as tobacco, dried corn and millet, beer, meat and fish. The prices of these were tied directly to those of essentials: salt, soap, kerosene and matches.

The area surrounding the village of Mpala is dominated by secondary grassland and Brachystegia woodland. The former consists of the long grasses and scrub which grow on and around fallow manioc fields. The latter comprises the relatively limited number of plants and trees which are able to survive the six-month dry season with its attendant burning of the bush. Most of the medicinal plants commonly employed by residents of Mpala derived from this kind of terrain. Others could be obtained from the rocky face of the bluffs overlooking Lake Tanganyika, or from near the water itself; and yet others derived from the *miuru* riverine forest, which follows the paths of small streams whose continuous moisture permits the more luxuriant growth of a greater variety of plants than may grow in the woodland.

Other medicines had to be brought from afar. The best place for obtaining the most renowned and the greatest variety of medicinal plants was the vicinity of the village of Kiobwe, some eight hours' walk into the interior from Mpala, near thicker forest. People travelling in the area for other reasons would often take advantage of their trip to bring back with them the dried root of a medicinal plant unobtainable in Mpala's environs.

This knowledge of (indeed, in certain instances, preference for) forest-found medicines coincided with the emphasis upon affecting animal substances (*vizimba*), to be discussed below. Together, they might be taken to indicate the relative stability of the relationship between pharmacological knowledge and its environment of origin. That is, people moved out of the forest and to the water relatively recently and there has been a corresponding change in the practicalities of making a living. Medical practice, however, continues to reflect a cultural emphasis on the forest and the things it provides.

The epidemiologic study of the incidence and prevalence of biomedically defined disease entities was not the purpose of this research. Rather, its aim was an understanding of Tabwa medical culture and its systematics, depicting, among other things, illness categories as defined by people themselves. However, I will briefly note here that the following were the major infectious and parasitic diseases in the community: measles, tuberculosis, polio, syphilis, gonorrhoea, mumps, malaria, intestinal parasites (askaris, hookworm, whipworm), schistosomiasis (both *S. haematombum* and *S. mansoni*), trichomonas vaginalis, ringworm and scabies.

Measles and diarrhoea were the principal causes of death in infancy and childhood. The former illness assumed epidemic proportions every four to five years. People said that measles had become more virulent since the elimination of smallpox through wholesale vaccination. During my stay, government agents came to Mpala once to vaccinate against smallpox, and twice to vaccinate the canine population against rabies. There was no vaccination against measles.

Such parasites as amoebas and filarial worms were absent. Medical assistants at Moba said they were not to be found in the area. Most communities employed the Lufuko or other streams as sources of drinking water, because the water was said to be colder and less brackish than that of the lake. Lake water, however, was used by those without the means to walk the distance to the river (about a mile from the village).

Pit latrines were in universal use, and a group of Mpala's judges inspected these annually, fining those whose latrines were in poor condition or were in need of overhaul. Most houses were made of sun-dried Kimberly brick, were large and reasonably airy, and had separate kitchens.

For people in Mpala, illness, like the life of which it is a part, is a whole, though multifaceted, experience consisting of several distinct but tightly interwoven levels or domains: the physiological, the social and the metaphysical. Significant disturbance in one means a corresponding disturbance in another; and, inversely, restoring the balance of one can mean restoration in all.

Like the phenomena it proposes to describe and examine, this study is also holistic and heterogeneous. It cannot be said to be organised around a single hypothesis or theoretical perspective; to be making a tightly unified argument in which the 'point' of medical practice lies elsewhere, with medical understanding taken as an allegory (Clifford 1986) for something else. Instead, the movement of the text is maintained within medical culture itself; going from the physiologic to the larger social plane; then returning to the microcosmic level of therapeutic practices and of medicinal substances themselves, and finally concluding with the metaphysical concerns and interventions to which therapeutic practices provide the gateway.

Each level is supported by a generalising language appropriate (indeed appropriated) to its features. Part I, 'The Defile of the Signifier', concludes where most ethnographies of medicine begin: that is, with a particular instance of illness, and the process of divination leading to cure. Earlier chapters place this in the supporting contexts of physiology, bodily processes and diagnostic and aetiologic possibilities, including options and preferences for types of divination. Taken as a whole, then Part I is almost complete in itself, and gives a view of the compositional dynamic made possible by the openness of the system and its numerous options for diagnosis and cure. In addition, it can be read in conjunction with Part II or Part III.

Part II, 'Generation of Identity, (Re)Production of History', is built around two detailed case studies, each of which is intended to give a sense of how significant illnesses have bearing on the progress of subjects' lives. The first case is of an individual, the second of a lineage group. Taking instances of sickness as the invariable of our study allows us to see more clearly the slippages and discrepancies between sickness and social dramas or conflict. That is, rather than seeing all problematic illness as, in effect, 'created' by the social or political affairs, we can, by looking at the illnesses, gain an understanding of how links to the social are made or unmade by people acting in the indeterminacy of a given moment. Inversely, seeing how illness is underdetermined by conflict also permits us accurately to construe how personal and immediate lineage histories grow out of the moments of concluding prompted by illness and other life crises. As with Part I, this part can be read on its own.

In contrast, Part III, 'Intervening in the Substantial Real', is perhaps best read in conjunction with at least the first three chapters of Part I. If it is to be read alone, the last three chapters of Part III will serve. Centred on therapies, Part III offers a construal of the qualities and the logic of the world which makes therapies 'true'. In this way it articulates the substantial reality in which the dimensioned body of Chapter I has its existence. From this, Part III reconsiders 'religion' and 'magic', redefining them as they may be more appropriately construed as continuous with (and indeed varieties of) therapeutic practices.

In writing I have tried to create an intermediate intellectual terrain on which the Tabwa medical culture and its open systematics can be understood and appreciated as such; i.e., as knowledge complete in its own right, not something subordinated to activities and interests of other social domains. In this way, I have tried to develop generalising languages which can be justified by their functions as a sort of 'transmitter' permitting dialogue between our understandings of life and death and those of the people with whom I lived for a number of years.

PART I
THE DEFILE OF THE SIGNIFIER

1

DIMENSIONS OF THE BODY

The body is not universal. It may be an object to which we can point, it may be humans' substantial being; and it may be one element of what is at stake in our mortality. Nevertheless, it is so culturally conditioned that the body translated must be the body transfigured. The body transposed is the body transformed.

The point in pausing to assert the ethnographically obvious is to draw attention to the power with which a biomedical model will have informed most readers' understanding of anatomy and of illness. There are two significant consequences of this.

The first is the presumption that other medical systems are wrong in their reference to physiological reality (or that their adequacy will one day be demonstrated in biomedically comprehensible terms). Their rightness is therefore to be located outside themselves, outside the terms they set (e.g., in their reference to the social or the political, for which they are taken as allegorical texts). The second presumption is that material reality apart from the body is itself universal; that the thingness of things and the wordness of words are the same everywhere; and, thus, that the realism of the therapy is poetic rather than practical, figurative rather than literal.

Here the ethnographer encounters a particularly thorny area. Inasmuch as the domain created by this differential is the discipline's home, we come already equipped with devices for negotiating it. 'Their' deficiency of understanding necessitates 'our' supplementary explanation, to create the equivalence (of culture, mind, being, value) that is ethnography's particular social product. This economy of supplementation, or of value added, is fundamental to the craft. It remains unchanging although the terms through which it is accomplished are regularly modified.

New terms reflect new emphases in explanation; new agreements regarding what will be taken seriously (and so explained) and what will be dismissed as unimportant (and so explained away). Concepts of magic and religion give way to ideas of symbol, ritual and metaphor as ethnographers find more refined ways of balancing identity and difference. Along the way we are continually subject to our particular occupational hazard: the exotic becomes the mundane to us.

In this study, I am attempting to take seriously Tabwa medicine as a whole. That is, I try to explain what it is, how it works and the qualities that reality must possess for Tabwa medicine to be as it is. I try not to explain things away. The new terms and understandings which develop from this commitment begin here, with the multidimensional body.

This is a body that unites in itself the material and the meaningful and does so in each of three domains: the physical, the physiological and the metaphysical. However, the lines along which distinctions are drawn are such that the body's multiple dimensions accord with none of these three and, instead, are best articulated as follows: the body as object (i.e., the body anatomised), the body as process, the body as responsive subject, and the body as site of physiological physics.

Through these, the body is united to, yet distinguished from, the substantial reality around it. Through it begins an approach to illness and therapy along revised terms of understanding.

BODY AS OBJECT

Although people have an idea of anatomy which includes internal organs as well as the labelling of body parts, anatomy does not figure significantly in the description of illness or, with certain exceptions, in pathology. Instead, organs and their activities (whether beneficial or detrimental) are discrete entities which do not significantly influence one another. As a consequence, pathological processes have the qualities of events or occurrences. Although the features of the body as object thus have bearing primarily in determining the means of administering bodily medicines,[1] in this discussion they form the necessary background to our understanding of the body's characteristics and of its multiple dimensions.

What follows is a structure-by-structure itemisation of the body's contents. Paraphrased from people's comments, definitions of organs include their functions and their malfunctions when these were described.[2]

Ubongo **(KS)**/*tonfuwe* **(KT)** – **'brain'.**[3] This lies within the head. It is white, like milk, but thick, like oil. Thought rests there. The brain lies inside a pocket, like plastic, which covers or encloses it. Blood vessels enter the pocket just a little and feed the brain. With head pain, the brain has overfilled the skull. After the pain starts, the brain comes down and eventually comes out the nose as mucus (*kamasi*).

Macho **(KS)**/*menso* **(KT)** – **'eyes'.** Inside each eye is the *kakisi*, a small lamp (*taa*), 'like a light bulb' (*kama vile amopule*), which lies behind the lens within the pupil. God put it there, to enable people to see. Without it, people are blind even though their eyes may appear normal. Blindness also occurs when *vidudu* ('insects') get into the eye and cover it with white material, like a spider's web. People with a *mududu* in their eyes can see only darkly (*gizagiza*).

Masikio **(KS)/*matuwi*** **(KT) – 'ears'.** Inside each ear is a little thing called the 'mother of the ear' (*mama ya sikio* (KS)/*nina kutuwi* (KT)) which enables one to hear. If something happens to this, one is deaf.

Kho **or *khoromeo*** **(KS)/*mkolomino*** **(KT) – 'oesophagus'.** This is a hole, but long, like a vein. Some people say there are two of them: one for water, and the other for food. It goes between the throat (*kapono*) and the stomach (*kifoto*). In the throat is the *kansonga bwali* ('epiglottis'). This 'catches' the *bukali* (manioc polenta) as it goes down.

Pumzi **(KS)/*mupuza*** **(KT) – 'lungs'.** These help with breathing. When a person has *mpika* ('dyspnoea'), his lungs are 'closed' (*pumzi inafunga*) or are 'heavy' (*zito*). Despite this association between lungs and breathing, many people indicate that air circulates freely in the chest, and no one visualises the lungs as the receptacle or vessel for the transfer of air.

Moyo **(KS)/*mutima*** **(KT) – 'heart'.** God himself put the heart in the body. It 'breathes' (*inapumua*). Its 'work' (*kazi*) is like that of a watch, or a watch's mainspring. It beats and beats. If blood enters it, it stops beating, causing death. If it begins to beat irregularly (*kucheza*, literally 'to play' or 'to dance') the blood dries up and the person will die. If you grasp a person by the wrist, you can feel the *sekond* ('pulse'). If you grasp it, and the blood is 'lying down' (*inalala*), the person will die. If you feel the *sekond* and it is pounding very rapidly, it is illness. The *sekond* is the same as the heart. The heart has no other function than to pulse. Ordinarily, it beats very slowly (*polepole*), but if you drink tea or coffee, hot things, it will increase its speed. Also, in the presence of a 'strong' (*ngu'vu*) illness, there is shallow breathing and the heart beats rapidly, perhaps because the air from breathing moves around it.

Kifoto **(KT) or *katonge*** **(KT) – 'crop' or 'stomach'.** This structure is called the *kifoto* by many, but some say the term *kifoto* applies only to this organ in birds ('it has a little hand-towel inside' (*essuie-mains*, i.e., membrane)). In humans and animals the structure is called *katonge*. It is very white. When a person eats, the food goes into this. When the food enters it, it swells, and the person feels full, satiated (*kushiba*). It is just a reserve where the food is stored, but it also grinds or pulverises the food (*kusaga, kukamua*); it transforms or turns it over (*inageuza*). One person said that the *kifoto/katonge* had three sections, in the most central of which was water, while food was in the next. Several people said that, from here, waste materials leave the body as urine (*mikojo*) and faeces (*mavi*). The *kitofu* appears inside the *kifoto* as a tiny dot; on the outside it is manifest as the navel. God put it there to close the abdomen.

Maini **(KS)/*mabu*** **(KT) – 'liver'.** This organ is a kinsman (*ndugu*) of the *moyo* ('heart') and the *safura* ('spleen'). All occupy one place and it is not possible for one of them to be located at a great distance from the others. It is a 'thing of blood' (*kitu cha damu*); it contains blood and sends blood to the heart, to which it is connected by a vein. Some people say that the function of the *maini* is to protect the heart, while others say that it has no specific function, but that 'it helps a little' (*anasaidia kidogokidogo*) and 'just sits in all its peace' (*anakaa tu na rha yake yote*). With reference to illness there is also disagreement. Some say that it is impossible for one to have an illness of the liver, while others say that, though the liver cannot become ill spontaneously, one can get an ulcer or lesion (*kidonda*) on it from drinking too much distilled liquor (*rutuku*).

***Nyongo* (KS)/*kansongwa* (KT) – 'gall bladder'.** This is a small, white or clear (*nyeupe*) organ or vessel (*chombo*) which lies near the liver. The liquid (*maji*) it contains is a bitter (*chungu*) poison (*sumu*). There is some division of opinion concerning the *nyongo*'s precise function. Some say that during digestion, it puts its liquid, drop by drop, into the stomach, to loosen (*kuregeza*) the food which the stomach contains. Others say that the *nyongo*'s only function is 'to care for the liver' (*kutunza maini*). Still others say that, when healthy, the *nyongo* does nothing at all. It just sits (*inakaa tu*), and breathes or pulses slightly (*inapumua kidogokidogo*).

In response to the consumption of tainted food, however, the *nyongo* becomes quite agitated. At this time, it makes one vomit a yellow substance with a bitter taste. This substance is *nyongo* itself ('bile'). From time to time, the *nyongo* may also spontaneously overfill, discharging its contents into the stomach by means of a vein uniting the two, and thereby causing nausea and vomiting. From the stomach this substance may move about the whole body, causing it to become hot or feverish. If the *nyongo* turns from transparent to dark, the person will soon die. In addition, the meat of an animal whose *nyongo* is black cannot be eaten, because the organ's poison has spread throughout the animal's body.

***Safura* (KS)/*masafuluwe* (KT) – 'spleen'.** This is a small organ which lies in the chest below the heart, side by side with the liver, on the left side, beneath the ribs and almost under the left arm itself. It is spongy in appearance, for which reason it is often called *mafafa* (KS) after the rubber ball of the same name. It is divided into two or perhaps almost three sections.

In health, the *safura* 'helps with breathing' (*anasaidia kwa kupumua*), releasing warm air into the body by means of the holes within it. In this process, it swells, and the swelling is manifested in the total organism as breathing. Some people say that it has the additional function of assisting with digestion, by permitting the food to enter the stomach little by little. One person suggested that the *safura* is the seat of hunger (*mwanzo wa njaa*).

The *safura* also has pathological functions. In certain illnesses such as *kimbeleka* ('infantile malaria'), it becomes quite large and 'sucks' (*kufionza*) the child's blood, making him anaemic (*kukosa damu*). At such times, one can see the *safura* sticking out, like a finger, in the abdomen below the ribs.

This pathological absorption of blood is also part of the illness *safura* ('dropsy'). In it, the person becomes so anaemic that eventually he has no blood at all, only water. The body becomes quite swollen from retention of it. (Though the illness appears to be named for the organ which causes it, the term *safura* also refers to the state of aqueousness itself – as when potatoes have been overcooked.)

Finally, the *safura* and/or the *bela* (see below) is also responsible for shortness of breath. When children have *kimbeleka*, for example, they often breathe shallowly, 'like a duck' (*kama vile bata*); and such breathing is due to the *safura* or *bela*, which is standing up.[4] Similarly, the *safura* may become erect when one is running, causing sharp pain in the side and difficult breathing during the time of exertion.

Bela (KT) – 'pancreas'. Many people do not completely differentiate the *bela* from the *safura*, and say that the two terms are synonymous. Others distinguish between them, describing the *bela* as a long organ approximately the width of a man's hand and the same length. It lies alongside and flush to the stomach, but behind this structure, between it and the back. The *bela*, it is said, is the *lumbeleka* itself, the very organ for which the childhood illness is named, and children are therefore forbidden to eat it. It appears that the *bela* is similar if not identical in function and pathology to the *safura* near which it lies.

Butumbo (KS)/malla (KT) – 'intestines'. This is the long 'stomach' into which the food passes as it comes from the *kifoto*. Its purpose is 'just to receive' (*inapokea tu*); it has no pathological function.

Fito (KS)/filo (KT) – 'kidneys'. These are two bean-shaped organs lying in the small of the back (*kiuno*). They have no known function.

Mfuko wa mikojo (KS)/kasusu (KT) – 'bladder'. This is the vessel (*chombo*) or organ into which urine passes before being eliminated from the body. It may also function pathologically, as during the illness named after it. In this, the patient drinks enormous amounts of water, urinates equally copious quantities, and becomes thin and weak. It is rare for a person stricken with this disease to live more than a year. There is no known cure.[5]

Ngozi (KS) or maongo (KS) – 'skin'. The skin, like the *safura*, has holes in it, and has a respiratory function. Air passes in and out of the holes at the base of body hairs (*mayonya*) with a rhythm as regular as that of a watch. For this reason, one must bathe every day. Should the holes become closed by dirt, one would develop fevers. Medicines applied to the skin enter the body through these holes, and perspiration comes out of them, bringing body wastes. The skin on the top is black, and has a small amount of blood in it. The skin underneath is white, and contains a greater amount of blood. The hide of an animal is thicker than that of a human being, and, for this reason, animals need not drink as much water as humans do. The contents of their stomachs may be drier than those of a human being with no ill effect.

Damu (KS)/mulopa (KT) – 'blood'. Though it is never described as an organ (*chombo*), blood is almost inevitably mentioned in discussions of body parts. In a state of health, blood moves to all parts of the body, though this movement is not related to the beating of the heart. Water from the food in the stomach mixes with blood and is thereby carried throughout the body, feeding it.

If the blood 'lies down' (*inalala*) or 'dries up' (*inakauka*), its deviation from the norm has an adverse effect on the body's condition. 'Paralysis' (*bulebe*) is the result of inactive blood, as the coldness of the limb and the tingling sensation experienced by patients indicate. 'Fever' (*homa*) can sometimes begin as 'chills' (*baridi*), which occur because cold air has entered the body through the pores and caused the blood to 'condense' (*kujifunga* – literally, 'to close itself'), withdrawing from the flesh its warmth. 'Anaemia' (*kukosa damu*) is a 'lack of blood' demonstrated by paleness of the palms and sallowness of complexion, and is often accompanied by weakness and lassitude. Finally, death results if the blood ceases moving altogether.

The comprehensiveness of this list is deceptive, for it is difficult to elicit descriptions of organs and their functions. People do not concern themselves overmuch with anatomy, and, in fact, many of my first attempts to understand the body were frustrated precisely because no one wished to indicate that she or he had an idea of human internal anatomy. People say that only a sorcerer, who could have butchered a person, could know for certain what the inside of a human body looks like. Nevertheless, people also say that the bodies of human beings and of animals are similar, and it was on this basis at least that some descriptions were finally offered.

If we take this barring seriously, we are pointed in the direction of the biomedically unthinkable, viz., a medicalisation of the body which is non-anatomical or even anti-anatomical in its foundations. Anatomy and anatomical functions are of medical significance in so far as they determine forms taken by therapeutic substances. Medicines are made in accordance with the capacities of the body to absorb them. Illnesses, however, exist in the dimension established by bodily processes, a dimension characterised and mediated by abstraction and miniaturisation.

THE PROCESSUAL BODY

Although they are situated in the body as object and are accessible to therapy through it, bodily processes escape and efface the body's anatomical dimension as such. Instead their most immediate location is the unseen but inferrable interior of the unanatomised body. An inner space of flexible dimensions and indefinite capacities, this body not only contains process, but is itself in process. It is as a processual body that a person is born, matures, grows old and – at any point in the sequence – may die.

Experience of the processual body thus inheres both in perceptible sensations and in observable circumstances. Through these, people confront the paradox that life is not entirely of the body, and is, in many respects, other than the body. The split here, between bodies and lives, becomes the slit through which can emerge the relationship between signification and medicalisation. With beginnings in anatomy and conclusions in personal/lineage history, the processual, unanatomised body is the effective foundation of Tabwa medical experience.

Miniaturisation I: Process in Bodies

For the purposes of this discussion, miniaturisation can be described as the device by which the processual is articulated in/on the body's anatomical dimension. Anatomical objects, eyes and ears have sight and hearing by virtue of smaller entities within them (p. 00). These are the sense itself, and they also articulate the difference between objective appearances and subjective experiences. Eyes which look normal but are blind, ears which seem normal but cannot hear, make unelidible the non-coincidence of subject and object, even at this, the level of structures where being is most objectifiable.

Miniaturisation also articulates bodily processes which are sensed though not seen. Thus, thirst (*kiuu*) derives from the heart, which has become dry because of the warm air surrounding it in the chest. Water loosens (*kuregeza*) the heart as well as the 'gall bladder' and the 'stomach'.

Similarly, the sensation of hunger (*njaa*) derives from the snake (*lombozoka* or *nzoka* (KT)/*nyoka* (KS)) that inhabits the abdomen of every human being. When this snake lacks food, it begins searching about inside, causing the growling of the stomach and the sensation of movement that one so often feels when hungry. This is the only internal sensation appropriate to the state of health. In illness, it is the standing, swelling, spitting or agitation of the snake which are responsible for a variety of syndromes whose symptoms include abdominal pain, vomiting and diarrhoea. Therapy of these illnesses is directed at the snake, whose return to a normal position or behaviour will automatically result in the cessation of symptoms.

People are not altogether clear regarding the exact location of this snake, whether it lives within the stomach and/or intestines or beside them; and there is a respect in which this vagueness is one of the generative capacities of the undissected body. By this I mean that inferences based upon what can be seen outside the body encounter no epistemological impediment which would block their application to circumstances within the body. Symptoms are interior events that are of the same order as external ones, creating the physiological translucency through which the meaningful and the medical can be united. The other two types of illness caused by *wadudu* (sing. *mududu*) demonstrate this.

In ordinary conversation, the term *mududu* is applied to worms and insects. However, the category also includes such animals as rats and snakes. People say that, in general, a *mududu* is any small creature which 'is not pleasing to the eyes' (*haipendezi na macho*), and their response, especially to snakes, reflects a combination of fear and loathing. Any snake which ventures into an area of human activity is immediately hunted and killed. My field guide to African snakes was quite a popular read, in the horribly titillating fashion of the gothic.

In addition to those of the abdomen, there are two other principal types of illness in which *wadudu* figure prominently. These are the various types of osteomyelitis (of finger, limb, or joint) and female reproductive disorders.

In general, people perceive inflammations of bones and joints as a consequence of a *mududu* which enters the limb or finger by unknown means, and then proceeds to burrow down until it reaches the bone, splitting it.[6] Where the *mududu* attacks the joint, a permanent disjuncture of the bones results, leaving the limb or digit useless. In the early stages of the illness before the swelling of the area is very far advanced, medicines are applied whose aim is to prevent the continued burrowing of the *mududu*. Should the illness have already progressed too far for simple reversal, other medicines are applied, whose aim is the encouragement of the opening of holes over the area, through which pus, and, ultimately the pieces of the bone or the *mududu* itself, are expelled. After the expulsion of these things, the lesions will heal in the manner of an ordinary infection. If unsupervised, the illness may take a less benign course, leading to death.

In addition to osteomyelitis, there are a number of female reproductive disorders, such as dysmenorrhoea, menorrhagia, repeated abortion and miscarriage, and repeated infant death, which are all due to the activities of another type of *mududu*. This is a snake particular to women, called the *kisumi*. People say that the *kisumi* is a snake or a mole or a snake with a mole's face and teeth. It is this creature which is also responsible for such congenital defects as harelips and birthmarks. Normally, the *kisumi* acts as guardian of the conceptus and protector of the foetus. It 'closes the path' (*inafunga njia*) of the woman, enclosing the 'strength of the man' (*ngu'vu ya mwanaume*) and thus permitting the onset of conception. As the baby grows, the *kisumi* lies alongside it; and post-partum pain is the *kisumi* moving about in the abdomen, seeking the warmth of its former companion.

As a pathological agent, the *kisumi* can be felt moving about in the abdomen, and causing the pains of dysmenorrhoea (*nkazi*). It may also scrape the interior of the uterus, and thus cause menorrhagia, abortion and miscarriage. Harelip is the result of the *kisumi*'s having eaten the infant's upper lip, while birthmarks derive from the *kisumi*'s blowing upon the child.

Further, at the time of parturition, the *kisumi* may blow upon the child's fontanelle, killing it; or the *kisumi* may retain the placenta, killing the mother. The *kisumi* may attempt escape from the woman's body, and either lie at the entrance to the vagina or actively move in a serpentine fashion, around the room. If it is not returned to its proper place, the woman will die.

Finally, by blowing upon the fontanelle, the *kisumi* may render a child 'healthy to the eyes only' (*na afia kwa macho tu*) and thus cause the repeated deaths of children for no apparent reason. As with the other *mududu*-derived illnesses, treatment is of the abnormal activities of the creature, not of the symptoms which these activities produce.

The idea that *wadudu* are pathological agents responsible for certain syndromes may be said to have a number of ramifications. In one respect, such miniaturisations convey the alienating aspect of an illness which has a fixed progress that is both other than the person's will and dangerous or debilitating to the person's body. Systematic deviation suggests the presence of another, alien consciousness which has aims of its own.

In another, more cosmological respect, the presence of *wadudu*, customary residents in the body and not always pathological agents, suggests an analogy between the unseen interior of the human abdomen and the unseen interiors of termitaries and mountains. Termitaries are known to be the habitations of snakes and small mammals. They are also sites where a number of medicinal trees and plants grow that are types of vegetation found nowhere else in Brachystegia woodland.

Like mountains, termitaries are associated with *ngulu*, spirits of the land which often take the forms of great snakes. One of these, *fwimina*, is particularly related to termitaries, heat and the dry season. Like the *kisumi*, *fwimina* is closely associated with sterility or temporary infertility, and like the *kisumi* as well, *ngulu* in general are as much agents of fruitfulness and abundance as of death and destruction.

Thus, the abdomen, like termitaries and mountains, is not a hollow space. Nor is it a solid devoid of dynamic content. Instead, such interior terrains are outwardly rounded, have transformative powers, precisely because they are filled with another kind of life.

Miniaturisation II: the Body as Process

In addition to containing processes as entities which though in it are other than it, the undissected body is definable as a process or as in process itself. This dimension of the body is most accessible when people speak of the relationship between body and life.

As process, 'life' (*uzima*) is identified with a number of different aspects of the physical person, though it is confined to none of these in particular. When asked, people say that life is everywhere in the body; but in conversation about specific organs or features, they will spontaneously comment that one or another of them is 'life itself' (*uzima mwenyewe*).

Among the items mentioned are blood, warmth, breath, the heart and the umbilical cord. Blood, people say, is the life of people and of animals. Without its active movement, creatures die. Sap is the blood of trees and plants, whose life is comparable to that of animals and people. Blood is like gasoline, in that it brings warmth or fire (*moto*) to the body just as gasoline brings heat to an engine.

Hence, warmth, too, is the life of people. If one goes to visit a critically ill person (*mugonjuwa hatari*), feels his limbs, and feels that they are cold, one knows the person is dying. 'If a person has cold in his body, it is the end' (*Kama ana baridi mu mwili, ni mwisho*).

Breath (*roho*) is also life. This is demonstrated during serious (*ngu'vu*) illness and critical (*hatari*) illness. In both cases, the patient breathes shallowly and irregularly. When he dies, his breath leaves his body. The KiSwahili term used for breath is also used for 'soul', 'will', the spiritual aspects of life, and even the heart itself. Dying is often referred to as 'cutting the breath' (*alikata roho*); and at least one person cited the absence of breath as a material entity in the body as a proof of the existence of God.

The heart is also identified with life, because when it stops beating, life also stops. In critical illness, irregular beating is indicative of impending death. In certain illnesses of the mind (e.g., *mubulibuli* and *wazimu*), the onset of the episode is marked by a 'splitting' of the heart or soul (*roho inapasuka*), which can then be felt to be beating wildly and irregularly as the patient sees spirits and persons who are not there.

Finally, the umbilical cord (*kitofu*) is identified with life because the infant's soul must traverse it at the moment of birth. At this time, the cord can be felt to be pulsing strongly in rhythm with the infant's own heartbeat. Cutting the cord too soon or improperly can result in death.

The identification with it of all these items emphasises life's dynamic quality. It is an *entity* which is a *process*, like fire or the regular ticking of a watch. Items associated with life are either qualities which pertain to it or material places where it happens. Indeed, the analogy between life and fire is underscored in the principles which govern transformations generally, and the fabrication of new entities in particular. Further, what we see when looking across the range of transformations is the respect in which miniaturisation not only captures abstract entities and inchoate processes for thought, but also makes them available for use in action.

Taken as a whole, fertility further illustrates this point. For BaTabwa, fertility is not an abstract potential which has existence apart from its active manifestation. *Kizazi*, the term for fertility, derives from the term *kuzaa*, 'to give birth', and *kizazi* more literally refers to 'birth' itself, as well as to the children who are its products. A woman who is neither pregnant nor nursing is therefore in some way infertile, or between fertile states.

After a birth, the placenta is buried within the room where the delivery has taken place. The women assisting dig a hole in the floor and place the organ in it, with the mother's side down and the infant's side up. As the earth is pushed in over the placenta, midwives are careful to hold up the umbilical cord, so that its tip is almost level with the floor when the work is completed. They are also always careful to announce what they are doing, and to call for witnesses. This is because the burial of the placenta in any other way results in a permanent 'cutting' (*kukata*) of the woman's fertility and is thus an act of sorcery. In its form, the burial of the placenta is like the setting out of a new seedling. The root and/or underground 'stem' of the new plant must be up if proper growth is to ensue.

The overall image of fertility is thus one of a series of births, represented by the placentae, which are strung together across time by means of the umbilical cords attached to each. A number of trees and grasses are propagated in this way. One of them, a grass called *kilaolao* (*Cyperus articulatus L.*), is used to treat the 'small dry season' (*kakipwa*), which is the temporary period of infertility lying between the birth of the last-born and the conception of the next. The tubers from which new offshoots grow resemble the rounded abdomen of pregnancy.

Consistent with the logic of this botanical objectification, ancestresses who give birth to large lineages may be referred to by the term *mama-zizi*, a term also applied to chickens or goats which give rise to large flocks or herds. *Zizi* comes from the word *muzizi*, meaning 'root', and connotes this method of propagation through the sending out of shoots, roots or runners from which new seedlings grow. This image of asexual propagation is especially relevant to matriliny, a social system in which pregnancy is a powerful attribute of the lineage itself, not of the strangers who marry into the group. Also, more abstractly, it is illustrative of time as realised in bodily processes and through their outcome.

At the dropping off of the infant's dried umbilical cord, the identification between the cord and life as process is again made manifest through the analogy of the root. The dropping off of the cord usually occurs five days after birth, and when it happens the child becomes a person whose death may be marked by open mourning; he is no longer a thing of 'only blood' (*damu tu*). At this time a ceremony (*kumurokea mtoto*, 'to illuminate the child') is performed in which the midwives who have assisted at the birth are cleansed by the infant (in what is his first truly 'human' act) of the 'darkness' (*giza*) which has been 'in their eyes' (*mumacho yao*) because of it. During the ceremony, the child is made to hold in its hand the dried umbilical cord which is then covered with manioc flour. After they have been cleansed by touching their foreheads to it, the midwives bury the cord, with the *kishina*, the end which was touching the infant, pointing east.

Shina is the term applied to a plant's stem or a tree's trunk, with branches attached and standing upright (*ki-* is the diminutive marker). The use of the word in this circumstance analogises again the processual relation of mother and child to that of tree and offshoot. The analogy, however, does not end here, with the structured depiction of a temporal relation. It is instead subsumed in a more complex and dynamic analogy which underlies the fabrication of certain oracular medicines.

When digging roots intended to have an oracular as well as a medicinal function, the Tabwa diviner/practitioner employs techniques and substances which make use of an homology between the medicines he is fabricating and the process of parturition itself. In such cases the diviner goes to the tree and selects a root which grows out from it in an easterly direction. He digs until he has exposed a length of root, and then spreads the western, trunk end of it with the red powder *nkula* (ground bark of the *mwenge* tree, probably *Pterocarpus tincturus*). The eastern end of the root is spread with *pemba* (kaolin). The middle section is then covered with dried grasses (*majani mulalia*), which are burnt. The root thus exposed and treated is then invoked, as are the diviner's *mizimu*; and the whole is left overnight. The next day, depending upon the nature of his dreams, the circumstances in which he finds the root, or other signs, the diviner is able to determine whether or not his treatment will be successful. If the response has been auspicious, he cuts out the middle section of the root and uses this in his preparation of medicinal formulae.

The marking of the western, trunk end of the root with *nkula* is analogous to the spilling of blood from the umbilical cord when it is cut after delivery, as well as to the rush of blood which follows the expulsion of the afterbirth. Women often say that it is not the child but the placenta which kills during and after parturition; and the minutes between the birth of the child and the placenta's expulsion are usually the most intense of the labour. In addition, the danger is double, for in cutting the umbilical cord the midwives risk the life of the child. Should the cord be severed before the child's soul has traversed it to reach his body, the infant will die. Thus, the mother's end of the umbilical cord is associated with the spilling of blood and the possible loss of life, with the past, with rupture and with closure. It is this association from which derives the darkness by which the midwives are affected until the purification ceremony five days later.

Opposite to this is the growing end of the root. Like the *kishina* of the infant, it has been spread with white powder and has auspicious connotations. Not the least of these is easterly direction, for the east is the place from which the dead are reborn, just as the west is the direction in which the living go after they die.

The analogy between parturition and certain oracular devices is thus clear. In both cases maturity, bloodshed and death are all identified quite literally with each other, with the west and with the colour red. Infancy, purity and life are all identified with the east and the colour white. In birth, the opposition is temporal, taking the form of states – one bodily (blood), the other fabricated (manioc flour) – from one to the other of which an irreversible transition is made. With oracles, on the other hand, the transition in time is structured into space and exists between poles which are both constructed (*nkula* and *pemba*). Rather than being a lived transition, the oracular device is a miniaturised realisation of the alternatives of life and death which exist in the situation. The powers invoked subsequently employ the device to make their commentary known.

Miniaturisation of the body as process works not only to realise processes or time in space, but also, inversely, to identify spatial orientations with processes. Here, there is a respect in which to be 'life-sized' is actually to be a small rendition of something even larger or more abstract than one's specific being. Such is the case in the identification of the body's orientation with that of trees.

People identify the body with the trunk of a tree and use for both the term *shina*.[7] This identification informs the approaches to the proper placing of human consciousness and also conditions the definitions of certain illnesses. Most prominent among these is the syndrome *mapituka*, in which the patient suffers vertigo sufficient to cause him to fall. *Mapituka* is also the name of a tree of any species which has fallen so that its roots are exposed. Infusions made of the roots of such a tree are used to treat this illness.

With a human being, as with a tree, falling is not the normal, healthy state. Like the roots of a tree, a person's feet should be (as we say) firmly planted on the ground. Falling in dreams is a premonition of death; and falling during a fight means one will be killed. Falling from dizziness or convulsions is a bad prognostic sign, indicating the onset of 'epilepsy' (*kifafa*), a potentially incurable illness. An upright stance, like that of a tree, means that one has a shadow (*kivuli*), the outward counterpart of one's soul. Opposed to this is the shadowless horizontality of death, and sorcerers are known to substitute leafless stalks of the banana tree for bodies of those whose souls they have stolen.

Analogies between the human head and the branches of trees are part of a larger association between the consciousness and verticality. Illnesses affecting consciousness (such as the convulsions of *negde* and *kifafa* or the headache of *mpungu*) and psychiatric disorders (*wazimu, mubulibuli*) emphasise the dangers of vertical space.

Similarly, in certain fertility medicines, twigs and branches or fruits which fall or are knocked from the tops of trees are made into infusions and drunk, or placed at the head of the bed to induce dreams of infants. People say that such dreams, which may also be of dead antecedents, frequently mark the onset of pregnancy. One older practitioner, Muleba, is of the opinion that the dead antecedent first enters a woman's head in dreams, and then descends to her abdomen as the conceptus.

Taken as a whole, therefore, what I am calling miniaturisation is the device through which some of the paradoxes of bodily being are articulated and objectified and so made available for action as well as thought. Identification of processes with things makes events into manipulable objects and thus founds the transposition of time into space. Inversely, the variations in scale which make a greater, more abstract entity accessible or visible in its smaller analogue also accord to that more ordinary thing exceptional weight. Space itself is thus neither neutral nor empty but is instead charged with diverse potentials.

BODY AS SUBJECT: THE HEEDING BODY

Consideration of sexual intercourse brings us to the dimension of the body where the life of the subject and the subject's life converge. This is the point at which bodily life can be risked or protected by the conscious choices of a thinking subject who nevertheless is vulnerable to transgressive desire.

It is the transformative potential of sex that forms the basis for this contradiction, and places intercourse in sharp contrast to digestion, the quintessential mundane process.[8] Where digestion always reduces something to nothing, intercourse is a potent force comparable to an agent in the physical sense, which can destroy as readily as it creates; and in any case always *does* something, even when its doing is annulled.

Illness and Sexual Intercourse

A number of illnesses which affect both children and adults are due to adulterous sexual intercourse or excessive conjugal sex. In the adultery-derived illness *mililo* ('fire'), an infant's head 'splits' (*kupasuka*) when it comes into contact with a parent (either mother or father) who has had adulterous sex and not taken care to cleanse herself or himself with medicines prior to approaching the child. Though he may have shown no signs of illness before, at the time of such splitting the child falls unconscious. His body becomes limp and cold, his eyes roll upwards, his pulse and heartbeat become rapid and weak, and without prompt medical intervention death rapidly ensues.

In the adult form of the syndrome, the wronged spouse becomes dizzy when the uncleansed, adulterous partner enters the house and/or comes into contact with her or him. Similarly, a woman in labour may suffer dizziness should her adulterous husband be within the house or outside it. If the adultery has been her own, the woman will become dizzy when she looks upon the blood spilled during parturition, or at the newborn baby. Even in normal circumstances, such dizziness is an ominous prognostic sign, a threat to normal consciousness and the life that goes with it. During labour, it is a sign of impending death.

With the illness *nsanga* ('mixing'), the infant and/or its mother will die on the spot if the adulterous partner of the father enters the house on the day the baby is born. The mother will die as soon as the two women see each other, while the child becomes ill the minute the partner crosses the threshold. After this first day, however, the mother is no longer affected; and the child is made ill only if the adulterous partner touches him. Such illness is due to the fact that the child has 'two mothers'. A similar form of *nsanga* derives from the adultery of the mother herself. Since the 'blood' that is the foetus contains a mix of the 'bloods' (i.e., semen) of a number of different men, labour will be difficult or fatal and the infant may be stillborn.

Excessive conjugal sex is also a cause of illness. *Kibende* can result from too much sexual contact during the last stages of pregnancy and the first months of the neonatal period. The child may be born with a fontanelle that is too large or one that is open. Cold wind enters through this aperture and thus reaches the abdomen, causing diarrhoea. *Kibende* may also be of spontaneous origin, and, in either case, is usually a relatively benign illness.

The illness *buse* affects older children who are nearer the age of weaning or just past it. During it, the child becomes thin and sometimes, his skin takes on a reddish cast. His bowel habits change as well. While he was sufficiently developed to know not to defecate in central areas of social activity, the child affected by *buse* inverts this behaviour and deliberately goes into the house to defecate.

Buse is caused by excessive sexual intercourse during the last stages of nursing. Such contact 'spoils' (*inaharibisha*) the mother's milk and thus gives rise to the illness. *Buse* may also be caused by excessive proximity of the child to its mother during her pregnancy with the infant that follows him. Should child and mother continue to sleep together at this time, the unborn infant will 'take the heat' (*kubeba vukuto yake*) of the older one, and thus cause *buse*.

Finally, sexual intercourse, both conjugal and adulterous, exacerbates certain illnesses. When a child is afflicted with measles (*suruba*) or 'smallpox' (*ndui*), his parents must abstain from all sexual contact. In addition, he may be visited only by those people who have 'slept cleanly' (*walilala safi*) or have 'slept only [on] one arm' (*walilala na mkono moja*), that is, those who have not had sexual contact with spouse or lover the night before. Visits by those who have had such sexual contact cause a worsening of the illness, which may result either in death or in a permanent disability such as blindness (of which there is great risk). People say that, in the old days, at the outbreak of a measles or smallpox epidemic, sexual intercourse would be forbidden to all residents within a village. However, in 'these Europeanised days' (*hizi siku za kizungu*) residents of households unaffected by the illness refuse to adhere to such rules. Many parents therefore lock their doors during the illness, and admit only those whom they know to be without spouses.

In addition, sexual intercourse of any kind is forbidden the patient during the treatment of 'epilepsy' (*kifafa*) and 'lunacy' (*wazimu*), and the therapeutic practitioner may also abstain from sex at this time. For the patient, sexual continence is but one of a number of taboos or restrictions (*mwiko* (KS)/ *vizila* (KT)) which obtain during treatment. Even when treatment is concluded, and the other *vizila* are lifted, one who has suffered from 'epilepsy' or 'lunacy' may never engage in adulterous sex. To do so would be to prompt recurrence of the illness.

Transformations and Sexual Intercourse

In contrast to its deleterious role in illness, sexual intercourse is a creative part of a number of other transformations. Most obvious among these are conception and pregnancy. People say that, at conception, the 'blood' of the man and that of the woman come together (*kupatana*, literally 'to get each other') to form what later develops into the foetus. The white 'blood' of the man forms the bones, while the red blood of the woman becomes the flesh.[9] It is through intercourse that the two are combined, and long ago it was thought that sexual contact had to be repeated throughout the pregnancy to ensure the development of a strong child. However, people say that in these days, they have often seen situations in which a healthy child is born to a woman who has been separated from her husband for the duration of the pregnancy; and so public opinion has been revised on this point.

Anywhere from a few weeks to several months after the birth of the infant the transformation called *kumusumbula mtoto* is undertaken. In their first act of intercourse after the birth of their child, parents sleep together with the baby between them before dawn and the infant's awakening. Opinions and practices vary as to whether or not coitus is interrupted. In either case, the parents, at the moment of climax or immediately afterwards, arise simultaneously to a sitting position, the father holding the baby by one arm, and the mother carrying on her shoulder a brand-new, unused carrying cloth. A small fire, the kindling for which has been laid out the night before, is lit in the bedroom with matches, and on it is placed a small pot containing an infusion of root medicines. Opinions vary again as to the type of medicine used, but the ones most commonly cited are those employed to enhance male potency. The infant is given some of the infusion to drink. In the remainder, the father soaks a small string or strip of cloth, which he then ties around the infant's waist. The parents then return with the baby to the bed for a short time, before finally arising for the day.[10]

This transformation may be enacted effectively by any married couple for any child, and people say that it was not unusual for a young couple ignorant of its methods to ask another couple to do it for them, in exchange for a small gift. If the transformation has been successful, the infant will cry just at the moment when the adults rise, but should the action fail the child will cry either prior to the appropriate moment, or not at all. Failure in the process of *kusumbula mtoto* results in the death of the child, either on the spot or during the following day. Should it succeed, however, it results in the 'maturing' of the child (*kukomesha*, literally, 'to cause to be mature').

Prior to this maturation, the child may be medically treated only by its own parents, or by those who have abstained from sexual intercourse. Medicine prepared by others (indeed, some people say all medicine) simply will have no effect in the body (*haisikiliki*, literally, 'is not heeded'), and cure will thus be impossible. After the ceremony, however, the infant body is susceptible to treatment with medicines. The medicated string tied around his waist protects the child from *kidonda tumbo*.[11]

The third transformative process in which sexual intercourse plays a part is the prophylactic treatment of *buse*.[12] When the child has reached an age at which the parents no longer feel obliged to restrict their sexual activity, they will undertake such treatment by first having sexual relations and then, without washing, urinating into a common pot. Quite early the following morning the parents take the pot and the child into the bush. There, the urine is mixed with either the soil of a termitary or the burnt bark of the *kalongwe* tree (*Dalbergia nitidula Bak.* sterile), charred for the purpose using a bundle of roof thatch ignited by matches.[13] The mixture is then applied to the child's legs, which are simultaneously massaged beginning at the ankles and working upwards to the loins.

Finally, incestuous sexual intercourse is central to the fabrication of magic substances meant to confer upon their owners good fortune and great wealth. Both the substances and the act essential to their activation are referred to as *kisoni*. To obtain such medicines, a person (usually described as a man) seeks out a diviner/practitioner who prepares for him a formula composed of plant substances (*miti* (KT)) and tiny portions of certain animals (*vizimba* (KT)).[14] The person then takes his medicines home and places them on or at the head of his bed. His partner may be his daughter or his sister. Their sexual intercourse must take place in the presence of the preparation, which is then returned to the practitioner for completion. As payment for her part in the medicine's creation, the partner has absolute veto power over the disposal of the wealth derived from it. The practice of *kisoni* is one kind of sorcery.

Summing up the range of values surrounding sexual intercourse reveals that sexuality is an ambiguous power whose meaning changes according to the structure of the circumstances in which it is found. Sexual potency is an amoral force. Uncontrolled, it is destructive. Contained, it can be used to transform. In itself it must always be something, it is a physical agent. Effective management of sex is therefore crucial.

Uncontrolled sexual intercourse is represented by adultery and excessive conjugal sex. In this sort of sexual relation, personal pleasure[15] is the aim. The result of such contact is a reduction in the bodily integrity of the person wronged.

With the infantile syndromes *mililo, kibende* and *nsanga* the child's head 'splits'. Such opening is a reversal of normal development, in which the fontanelles gradually grow closed during the first months of life. In addition, the hole constitutes a breach in the body's boundaries through which cold air passes to the detriment of health. In *kibende*, this lack of integrity results in diarrhoea, while in *mililo* and *nsanga*, shock rapidly followed by death is the consequence. With the illness *buse*, as described above, heat leaves the infant's body because excessive sexual intercourse has spoilt the mother's milk.

The dizziness which characterises the adult forms of *mililo* and *nsanga* can also be interpreted as a manifestation of a loss of bodily integrity. Dizziness or paraesthesia (*zunguzungu*) which is not true vertigo (*mapituka*) is one of the symptoms of *kidonda tumbo*. The dizziness is caused by an openness of the rectum and/or vagina which permits cold air to enter the body.

Adulterous sex and excessive conjugal sex, then, can be called uncontrolled because the pleasure is placed above the restraint imposed by social necessity. In such circumstances, coitus can have destructive, rather than creative, power. It precipitates illness by causing the reduction of bodily integrity, which, in turn, permits entities foreign to its interior (such as cold air or winds) to enter into the body and to alter pathologically the activities taking place there.

Within the context of marriage, the ambiguous power of sexual intercourse is controlled through simple containment. Mundane conjugal sex results in conception and pregnancy, but is controlled through abstinence in order for its creations to be brought to their most successful completion. Similarly, conjugal sex is controlled when it is actively detrimental to certain created transformations such as the medical treatment of the illnesses 'epilepsy' (*kifafa*), 'lunacy' (*wazimu*), 'smallpox' (*ndui*) and 'measles' (*suruba*), and such processes as beer- and oil-making and forging.

In all cases the 'slippery' (*uterezi*) nature of coitus, as well as its 'heat' (*vukuto*), short-circuit the process. Medicines cannot coalesce (*kupatana*, the term also used for the process of conception) in the presence of sex. Rather, the heat which it generates either adds to or detracts from the specific amount of warmth demanded by the transformation itself and results in beer which is sour, nuts which yield little oil, poor-quality iron, and the failure of medicines to guide an illness successfully through its more benign course.

Since, in a mundane marital setting, sexual intercourse is physiologically creative, but potentially destructive of certain fabrications and their results, married couples must strategically abstain from sexual contact in order to promote successful outcomes. Their capacity to work together to strike a balance between personal desires and necessary restraints is taken as a measure of their compatibility as people and of their achievement as spouses.

In its final, ceremonial context, sexual intercourse is placed entirely at the service of fabrication, and can be said not to have pleasure as a component. The power of sex is diverted, through the practice of coitus interruptus, to the creation of a new, culturally constituted entity or integrity. In the therapeutic maturation of the infant, *kumusumbula mtoto*, the child's body is separated from the heat of its parents' and others' sexual activity. The belt tied around its waist at this time separates the infant from the cold winds of *kidonda tumbo*. The baby is thus given bodily integrity; it receives its own cultural thermostat and, in the form of potency medicines, its own sexuality. It has become a culturally mature, new entity, a being amenable to medical treatment.

With the incestuous relations of *kisoni*, the power of sexual intercourse is directed towards the fabrication of a different sort of entity, viz., the medicines which will bring great wealth and good fortune to the incestuous pair. Finally, in the ceremony of *bupyani*[16] the inheritor of a deceased spouse's name spends the night and has intercourse with the widow(er), and thereby frees the latter to resume a normal life. Through this act of coitus the integrity of marriage, disrupted by death, is re-established to be continued or socially ended (by divorce) as the partners prefer.

In all these processes, then, sexual intercourse is managed not only through abstinence, but also through the interruption or ceremonial framing of the act itself. The power of coitus, potentially disintegrative in adultery, and ambiguous in mundane conjugal relations, becomes creative in the context of cultural transformations.

The ambiguous, transformative power of sex takes our thought in two complementary directions. The first of these concludes consideration of the body as subject by noting that sex always involves not two, but three. Although derived from the contact of two people, sex always has an impact on at least a third entity.

When that third entity is a person, the body responds to the presence of the illness not as a mechanical but as a 'heeding' organism. That is, the response of the wronged person's body is more akin to hearing or seeing than to a material reaction to contagion. In this respect, the body in itself can be said to meet the threshold of the status of the subject. It is capable of being entered into relations of reciprocity (albeit negatively constructed) without the conscious intervention of the person.[17] In the context of problematic illness, this capacity is a basis for the effectiveness of divination.

The second area towards which sexual intercourse directs our thought is the dimension of the body in which the subject is perceptible as an object whose physiological processes are entirely continuous with the physical processes in a wider world. Here, the principles of order conditioning what happens in the body are identical to those conditioning events outside it.

THE PHYSICS OF THE BODY

The systems we are accustomed to consider as fundamental to the order of ethnography take on a more powerful value when we consider them in the context of medical practice. Here, associations discerned by the ethnographer are not only, of course, consciously held and used by people themselves, but are also constitutive of the substantial world in which bodies have being and lives are placed at stake. Connections are real, so rules articulate the physical conditions which found and limit not just bodily transformations, but all others as well. What we see emerging from associative detail is the simpler set of underlying principles uniting and governing the physics of which physiology is part. Crucial to Tabwa medical practice are the principles connecting fire and cooling to life and death.

Fire

Connections in medical thinking among sexual intercourse, fire and transformations are suggested by the identifications outlined in the preceding section. Coitus must be kept away from those transformative processes (such as the manufacture of beer, oil and iron) which require for success a carefully controlled amount of heat. Intercourse is also incompatible with 'hot' illnesses, such as 'measles' (*suruba*) and 'smallpox' (*ndui*), the intensity of which it increases. The illness *buse* derives from the heat of the unborn foetus, the sudden absence of whose warmth is also responsible for both post-partum cramps (or pain) and post-partum depression.

The adultery-derived illnesses *mililo* and *nsanga* make the identification even more explicit.[18] The term *mililo* literally means 'fire' and, in addition, one of the principal herbal medicines used to treat the syndrome is an infusion made from the tree *kalilolilo* (*Indigofera emarginella* A. Rich). The same tree is also employed in the treatment of *kibende*[19] and a small branch of it, broken off along the road, is carried by some Tulunga diviners in the same hand as their *mikia* (sing. *mukia*) to prevent rainfall in the direction in which they are travelling.[20] In both its name and the method of its treatment, then, the illness *mililo* is connected to fire. Associations with the sun and with the prevention of rain further connect it to the dry season – fire on a larger, even cosmic, scale. Finally, female infertility, referred to as a 'little dry season' (*kakipwa*) and often caused by adultery, underscores this association between sexual contact and heat.

As described above, the term *nsanga* means 'mixing' and it refers both to the 'mixing' of sexual partners which occurs when a man's lover encounters his wife, and to the 'mixing' of the 'bloods' (*damu*, that is, semen) of multiple partners within the body of an adulterous woman. *Nsanga*, however, is also the term used to refer to the collection of foods communally cooked and eaten at funerals. Flour, fish, beans and other items are contributed by everyone in the community. They are all stored in one set of containers, and one set of pots is used for preparing the meal.

Nsango, near-homonym to the above, is the term applied to the mixture of herbal infusions drunk by the novice Tulunga practitioner at the time of his initiation. This puts him into a state of heightened consciousness, in which objects glitter as with an inner light. At this time, he is close to insanity (*wazimu*) and death.

As with *mililo*, then, the range of meanings associated with the term *nsanga* makes clear the identification between sexual intercourse and fire. Further analysis, however, reveals that, more than simply related terms, bodily warmth, coitus and fire are varied forms of one thing and the processes of burning, heating and cooling are governed by one set of principles whether outside the body or within it. Realised in different forms, each with slightly different characteristics, they are refracted realisations of a single process that people employ in various ways in medical practice.

In one objectification, the destructive homogenisation of fire is represented in the form of *majani mulalia*, grasses which have survived the previous dry season's burning of the bush. A bundle of such grass is ignited with matches and burnt on an exposed root as it is prepared to serve oracular as well as therapeutic functions. *Majani mulalia* may also be employed to cleanse a hearth ritually before therapeutic use is made of it. Should such grasses be lacking, thatch taken from over the door to a house – a place where 'all people pass' – can be substituted.[21]

By surviving the year's bush fire, *majani mulalia* come to objectify the 'everything' that is destroyed in wholesale burning. It is through this characteristic as well as through similarity of function that they are paradigmatically connected to the thatch grass under which 'everyone passes'.

Thatch, in its turn, is connected to a number of other objects past which 'all people' move. These are a root which crosses the road, a stump which stands alongside the road, and a tree which stands by the road and in whose shade travellers rest.

Such objects, people say, are passed by 'those with good souls and those with bad souls' (*baroho nzuri na baroho mbaya*), as well as by those who are pregnant (*bamimba*) and those who are not. Thieves and honest people alike may step over a root, traverse a stump, or rest in the shade of a roadside tree, eat sugarcane there and then continue their journey. From the vantage of such a point, one can clearly grasp in hand and in thought the totality of human experience as it has passed there – person by person and story by story, so to speak.

Majani mulalia, like their paradigmatic counterparts, objectify this experiential totalisation. The wholesale burning which they have survived is a temporal point – one year's time – which has passed them, and which has thus invested them with the 'everything' that the fire has destroyed. People say that when they are burnt on the medicinal root, *majani mulalia* 'mature' (*kukomesha*, to cause to become mature) it into an oracular and therapeutic device. In this process they can be said to impart to the root all of human experience. From this pool, the root as oracle selects that particular response which relates to the case at hand.

When they are burnt in a hearth, *majani mulalia* carry similar meaning, though the processual end to which they are used is different. In this case, the burning of the grasses constitutes a destruction of all immediate human histories which have previously unfolded. The hearth is thus cleansed (*kusafishwa*) of its past, and made ready for its therapeutic function.[22]

As the reductive homogenising power of uncontained, adulterous sexual intercourse corresponds to that of burning, so does the additive, creative, homogenising power of conjugal sex correspond to that of heating. People frequently refer to intercourse as 'joining together' (*kuungana*), and describe conception as the 'coalescence' (*kipatano*) of the 'bloods' (*damu*) of man and woman. In this process, a new entity – a child – is formed; and, people say, through this child and the household into which it is born, the *mizimu* (the dead antecedents) of each partner are joined into a new group.

The transformative counterpart of the contained power of conjugal sex is the process of heating, in which the destructiveness of burning is contained through the use of pots and of media such as water and oil.[23] In these, practitioners combine medical plants (*miti*) with other substances (*vizimba*), and blend them into a new entity, a medicine. By means of pots and media, the reductive effects of fire are limited, and the homogenisation of burning becomes the coalescence of heating, with creative results.

Cooling

The process of cooling complements those of burning and heating and can be said to have both active and passive senses. Extinguishing is the active aspect of cooling. It is objectified in a number of ways and has varying functions in medical practice.[24]

The illnesses 'measles' (*suruba*) and 'smallpox' (*ndui*) are 'hot' not only because of the high fevers with which they begin, but also because they are associated with land spirits (*pepo* (KS)/*ngulu* (KT)) whose punishment often took the form of epidemics of these, and which are associated with the sun and the dry season. In addition to showing the incompatibility with sexual intercourse noted above, these illnesses are also such that they must not be treated either with washes of cool medicinal water or by the application to the skin of medicines which have been burnt in a pot and ground to a powder.

Both of those therapeutic methods are directed at the 'extinguishing' (*kuzimisha*) of an illness, and with measles and smallpox each will result in the failure to appear on the body of the papules which are its culmination; their progress would be extinguished. This would short-circuit the more benign course of each disease, with the result that the illness would 'remain inside the body' (*inabakia mumwili*), and the liver would consequently be 'smashed to bits' (*inapondeka kabisa*). With 'measles', such a turn for the worse would be marked by explosive diarrhoea with bile-colored stools (a sign of the destruction of the liver), and rapidly ensuing death.

When anger combines with disease to produce a life-threatening illness occurrence, the extinguishing power of cool water has a role in circumstantial therapeutics. Anger (*asira*) or hidden grudges (*fitina*) are hot emotional states whose presence can cause or exacerbate sickness. When they are found to have such an effect, a *mutimbe* ceremony may be called for.

In this ceremony, a small rock or clod of earth is taken from over a door. It is heated on a fire around which are seated all the disputants in the social conflict relating to the problematic illness occurrence. As it heats, each person states all of his grudges and grievances. When all have concluded their confessions the rock or clod is removed from the fire and plunged, sizzling, into the cool water that has been placed in a new gourd. People say that as the rock cools so does everyone's anger. All parties drink of the solution and thus the conflict is resolved.

The rock selected from a place over the door objectifies exactly that same process. People say it is used because no matter how angry they may be, all persons must lower their heads to pass under the door frame when entering a house. To lower the head (*kuinama*) is to be humble, submissive and calm; a cool emotional state. Thus, the rock realises materially what the therapy does temporally; that is, it marks the precise point at which heads are lowered within a constraining framework and anger is transformed into calm and reconciliation.

The active sense of cooling is also realised in a particular transfigurative animal substance, the pelt of the melanistic serval (*nzima*) (*Felis serval*).[25] The cat's ability to conceal itself and its dark colour combine with its name to objectify the processes of blackening, cooling and extinguishing (*kuzima*, 'to be extinguished'). This is its 'meaning' (*maana*) when it is used as a *kizimba* in the preparation of transfigurative and transformative formulae. Used in the treatment of illness, the *kizimba* of the *nzima* works to restore the patient to the cool, unmarked state of health. Likewise, the same extinguishing capacity can also be employed improperly to destroy the hot states of pregnancy or the possession of a Bulumbu spirit, a use which would constitute sorcery.

In its active sense, then, the process of cooling is extinguishing, the dynamic opposite of the processes of heating and/or burning. Extinguishing reverses these processes themselves, and inverts their products, returning situations to the zero point from which they began. In contrast to this, the passive sense of cooling involves the elimination of fire itself, but with the retention of its products. This too has a significant place in medical practice, and is represented by ashes (*majifu*) and the ash heap (*kiziala*).

When Bulumbu possessing spirits or other *pepo* must be 'put in order' (*kutengeneza*), one of the necessary arrangements is the lighting of a new fire. This may be done with purchased matches or by the more traditional friction method. In either case, such a fire must not come into contact with water. If a chicken, killed in honour of the spirit, is to be cooked on it, the pot must be handled with care, so that the water does not drip onto the fire. In addition, the fire must not be extinguished with water, but must be poked apart with a stick (*kuchocheza*) and allowed to go out by itself. The ashes from such a fire are then carefully collected and buried, often with the unbroken bones of the sacrificed chicken. These practices assure that the association forged by the ignition of the fire is maintained, though the fire itself may no longer exist. Active extinguishing of the fire 'spoils' (*kuharibu* or *kuharibisha*) the spirit, rendering it powerless.

The processing of charring through which certain medicinal formulae are prepared is managed in a similar fashion. Ingredients, both plant (*miti*) and animal (*vizimba*), are combined in a pot, which is then placed on the fire. The substances are burnt to ash in the pot's dry heat. They are then removed from the fire, allowed to cool of themselves, and ground into a homogeneous black powder. This power is a new entity, a medicine compounded in accordance with the necessities of treatment, and thus the dry equivalent of an infusion. Though the process of cooling has eliminated the heat of the fire, it has not undone fire's effects. People say that such burning increases the strength of a given medicine. This option contrasts sharply with that of the Luba, in whose medical practice fire *reverses* the meaning of medicinal formulae (Burton 1961).

The *kiziala* or ash heap is identical to this but on a larger scale. It is the place where cooled domestic fires, in the form of ashes, are thrown, along with cooked foods which have spoilt without being eaten. It is the burial place of stillborn infants as well as of prematures and those who have died prior to the loss of the umbilical cord. Infants of this type are all referred to as *kaonde*. They are not human, but are 'just blood' (*damu tu*), 'life' itself but lacking the boundaries that would have made them persons. Their passing must not be mourned with wailing and songs.

Twins (*mapacha* (KS)/*bampundu* (KT)) are also buried in the ash heap. They, too, are not human, but are spirits who have left their residence in a mountain and entered the body of a woman to be born.

The death of both *kaonde* and *mapacha* is commonly referred to as a 'return' (*kurudi*) rather than as a 'departure' (*mwendo*) or as 'passing away' (*kufariki*), and it is this feature which accounts for their burial in the place of cooled fires. Having never lived as human beings, they have never been quite of this world. As a consequence, they do not fully undergo the extinguishing discontinuity that is death, and therefore are not buried in the customary burial ground.

After burial in the ash heap, the bodies of *kaonde* and twins may be disinterred and the bits and pieces employed as *vizimba* (sing. *kizimba*) in medicines and amulets fabricated by Tulunga practitioners. Such is also the possible disposition of *kapondo kanfitwa*, the charred remains of an outlaw (*kapondo*) who has been captured and burnt alive.[26] (The use of human relics of any sort is regarded by lay people as sorcery, and possession of them as necessary ingredients for the therapy of 'throwing the person in the bush' (*kumutupa mutu mupori*) is what makes Tulunga practitioners sorcerers *d'office*.)

The ash heap is also the burial ground for medicinal roots which have been employed in the fabrication of infusions and whose strength is spent. Such roots are never simply disposed of by patients or their families. Instead, they are set aside and returned at the end of the therapeutic relationship to the practitioner who provided them. He may then bury them in the ash heap, or leave them at the foot of a tree, deep in the bush.

Finally, clippings of hair taken from the heads of children who have been born of fertility medicines provided by a Tulunga practitioner are buried by him in the ash heap. The clipping of the hair is part of a ceremony which marks the end of the practitioner's role as therapist to the children's mother and as paediatrician to them; a role which can span more than a decade. As with the disposal of medicinal roots, the burial of the hair in the ash heap terminates a relationship (the 'fire') while preserving its transformed effect (the 'ashes').

What the above examples make clear, then, is that the passive sense of the process of cooling (like the containment of burning that is presupposed in heating) is the transforming power of fire, with fire's destructiveness removed. While active cooling is extinguishing, and constitutes the dynamic reversal of both process and product, passive cooling preserves the results of mixing and heating and thereby makes these available for subsequent use. The ash heap thus corresponds to such waste places as the crossroads, the ford of a stream, a root crossed by everyone, the door to a house, etc. All are places where everything is reduced to a kind of anonymity, which is also a pool of potential for the construction of new cultural entities, a site where processes are placed in abeyance.

Death

Just as the controlled heating that is conjugal sex results in the conception and fabrication of a new human being out of the coalescence of bloods of man and woman, so does deviation from that regulated amount of heat result in sickness (excessive heat, as in fever) and, ultimately, death (excessive cold). Death (*kifo*) is sometimes referred to as 'to be extinguished' (*kuzimishwa*), and in both its physiological and social aspects, death follows the same principles as the process of cooling.

People recognise a state of critical illness (*mugonjwa hatari*), in which a person lies between life and death.[27] They say that when a person is dangerously ill, his heart beats irregularly, and can be felt 'walking about' (*kutembea*) inside his chest. His breathing is also irregular and may be rapid and shallow. His pulse (*saa* or *sekond*, literally 'clock' or 'second') is weak and rapid, and is perhaps perceptible only in the upper arm or at the neck. Importantly, his limbs are cold to the touch.

Such coldness (*baridi*) is due to the fact that the blood is no longer circulating properly, a condition which also characterises paralysis of the limbs (*kupoza*). Blood (*damu*) is warmth (*vukuto*) and is also the physiological life (*uzima*) of a person. The cessation of its movement about the body is coincidental with other danger signals. When it finally stops circulating altogether, cold enters the body, and the person dies, his soul (*roho*, also meaning breath) leaving his body through the top of his head (*katikati ya kichwa* (KS)/*luboziabozia* (KT).

After death, the soul of the deceased travels to Kibawa, an underground cave or cavern lying to the southwest. In it dwell the souls of all the dead save sorcerers,[28] and from this common pool, as from the ash heap, individual *mizimu* (i.e., beneficent dead) return to the world of the living in two different forms.

The first of these, *msambwa*, is a propitious spirit which guides and protects the living. Though derived from the ranks of more ordinary *mizimu*, it distinguishes itself from these by repeatedly causing illness or misfortune. As a consequence, a small shrine is created,[29] which is, people say, both the residence of the spirit and the *msambwa* itself. Through this, the dead antecedent receives the special attention she desires.

The second form in which the dead return to the world of the living is as a new child, born to a kinswoman. People make the analogy between the womb and the grave, saying that the condition of the individual is the same in each, viz., she or he is not visible to the eyes (*haonekani kwa macho*).[30] In addition, the appearance of a dead antecedent in dreams frequently marks the onset of pregnancy, and is thought by some older people to be the point at which that same antecedent enters the woman's body to be reborn.

In either case, what happens is that the dead are plucked from their more anonymous condition by the living, on whom they are dependent.[31] In a form that is a modification of that which they were in life, they return to the world of living, and are incorporated in the creation or fabrication of new beings, human and non-human.

HEALTH, ILLNESS AND DEATH

When asked to define the condition of health, people usually describe it as a state in which one 'feels nothing' (*hasikii kitu*) except hunger (*njaa*). The healthy person goes about his affairs as usual, and sleeps a dreamless sleep.[32]

Indeed, the absence of detailed discussion and of a group of specific prophylactic practices initially makes it difficult to develop any precise conceptualisation of the states of health and illness as abstracted from particular instances. It is only through a consideration of ideas relating to anatomy and sexuality that features of the two emerge as such.

Anatomically, the state of health is characterised by the smooth and regular functioning of the dynamic organs of the body. The heart (*moyo*) beats regularly, 'like a clock' (*kama saa*), and breathing (*kumpumua*) is accomplished by the spleen (*safura*) and lungs (*pumzi*). In the digestive process, food is stored in the stomach (*kifoto*), then mixed with small amounts of bile (*nyongo*). It is then subjected to squeezing (*kufiyanga*) and grinding (*kusaga*) in the intestines (*butumbo*), during which time the liquid nourishment (*maji mazuri*, literally 'good water') is extracted and carried by the blood to the parts of the body. Liquid and solid wastes are eliminated as urine (*mikojo*) and faeces (*mavi*).

A healthy body has a well-balanced relation to its environment, external and internal. Its apertures of anus, vagina, fontanelles, and pores are closed to the winds (*pepo*) of the outside world, and thereby protect it from cold.[33] Likewise, the healthy body is unaffected by the heat of conjugal sexual intercourse. The inhabitants of its internal environment, in their turn, are orderly. Neither the *lombozoka* of the stomach nor the *kisumi* of the uterus move about improperly or scratch the body's interior.

In illness, the situation is reversed. Organs such as the 'spleen' and 'gall bladder' may function improperly, causing anaemia and digestive malfunction, respectively. Cold winds may enter the body though its various orifices, and diarrhoea or dizziness result. Illness also renders the body vulnerable to the effects of sexual intercourse, the presence of which can cause an already critical condition to worsen. Finally, the inhabitants of the body, normally contributors to its ongoing balance, themselves become disorderly; standing, swelling, spitting, scratching and moving about instead of lying still.

The state of health, with its bodily integrity, is thus a dynamic one, notwithstanding the fact that it is negatively represented as the absence of symptoms. In health, forces and beings of potentially pathological nature are kept in their proper places; and an overall balance is maintained between the extremes of hot and cold. In illness, on the other hand, bodily integrity breaks down, and nature, in the forms of winds and 'insects' (*wadudu*), becomes the governor of human physiological functioning. The body is no longer balanced between hot and cold states, but, pushed by an illness that does not 'hear' or 'feel' (*kusikia*) medicines, the body swings from the extreme 'heat' (*vukuto*) of high fever (*homa kali*) to the extreme cold of the circulatory failure that characterises critical illness (*ugonjuwa hatari*) and, ultimately, death.

For all that illness is opposed to health, however, people nevertheless accept its necessity as part of their grudging acceptance of death as a part of life. It is said that even the 'people of long ago' (*watu wa zamani*) died, though not so frequently as people do now.[34] When I tried to offer Katambwa, an elderly friend, reassurance during the course of his treatment for tuberculosis, he responded to my consolation with a question, 'Have you ever seen a thing which did not die?' (*Umekwisha kuona kitu kisikufa?*). He went on to say that even the grasses died and turned brown and were burnt each year, after which they sprouted anew. He too would die, he continued. 'We are all facing the same hole in the ground' (*Siwote tunaangalia mushimu*).

Indeed, it is distaste for the suffering of illness and the fear of the loss that is death which are the principal devices by which one's motivation to conform to society's rules is renewed. People say that arrogance (*kiburi*), which causes one to treat others with rudeness and injuriousness, reflects a belief on the actor's part that he will never have need of another, that he will never need to borrow money, that should his children fall ill he will be able to treat them successfully alone, that he himself will never be sick.

This same arrogance, they say, leads people to neglect their *mizimu*. As Kalulu, in a hilarious and highly theatrical enactment of these principles, described them: when you are well, you say you have no money to buy a chicken for your *mizimu*, when really, you're saving it all for beer. You refuse to go to a diviner, saying divination is nonsense and thievery. But when you're sick, you're scared. You tremble all over and break out in a cold sweat. When they ask if they should go to divine for you, you hastily nod; and when they return and tell you a chicken must be killed to your mother's brother, without hesitation you reply that there's three *zaires* in your suitcase under the bed. You pray to your God (*Mungu wako*) for recovery, swearing that you'll always remember your *mizimu* if they just let you get well, this time. But, as soon as you are better, you forget them. This is why *mizimu* send illness. They say, 'Look at that one! Look at his arrogance! Well, he'll see', and one is stricken.

It is thus the mortal necessities derived from the realities of sickness and death which underpin the moral order informing social rules. It is these which give its sometimes onerous obligations meaning. One is not only held steadfastly to one's duty by threat of death, but society as a whole can be seen as existing in the dialectic between dissolution and (re)organisation (through the powers of sexual intercourse and fire).

Sex and fire are the manipulable forms in medical thought in which the abstract principles governing transformation are objectified. The unboundedness that is fire's capacity to destroy, to reduce different things to the same state, is matched by the unboundedness of adultery, which mixes those who should be kept apart and results in the dissolution of boundaries on a physiological level.

Inversely, conjugally contained sexual intercourse, like the culturally controlled use of fire, results in the fabrication of new entities – both human and medicinal. In the hands of responsible, well-meaning individuals, sexual intercourse becomes the very tool by which dissolution is reorganised. Social identities are pulled from the anonymity of death and given new life in the namesakes of the deceased.

Similarly, the ash heap (*kiziala*) is the source of some of Tabwa medicine's most powerful components, human *vizimba*. The relics of certain persons, disposed of in this waste place, are removed from it, and through the controlled fire that is heating can be reorganised into life-saving medicines. Human beings can thus be said to employ both sexual intercourse and fire in their active containment of dissolution through a reorganisation of its products.

In the cases of responsible persons, this reorganising ability is employed only for the benefit of the social group as a whole. With sorcerers, however, such is not the situation. The tools of sexual intercourse and of fire are basically amoral, and may be used for any end one might wish. Sorcerers employ them to contain death, not from a motive that is essentially modulated and balanced, but from one by which they themselves become totally free from the threat of dissolution while others become totally subject to it.

Through incest, sorcerers divert sexual intercourse from its mundane purposes of reproduction and pleasure, and employ its powers to fabricate *erisi*, medicinal amulets whose strength and meanings (*maana*) are such that the sorcerers must never die. Very powerful practitioners (*wafumu*), sorcerers *d'office*, are said to be incapable of dying unless ceremonially relieved of their medicinally derived capability. People say that when word arrives that a well-known sorcerer (*mulozi*) is dead they are astonished to hear the news and ask themselves how he could have died whose sorcery (*bulozi*) was so powerful. One would have thought he would live forever.

As they make themselves fairly invulnerable to death, and thus take on alarmingly superhuman qualities, so do sorcerers by the same act reduce other human beings to the status of 'meat' or 'animals' (*nyama*). Famous (or notorious) hunters were said to have numerous devices by which they never failed to be successful. One technique was to kill a kinsman and use that person's soul to drive game toward the sorcerer-hunter. He would see his mother's brother astride the buffalo which came within shooting range. Another method was to shoot the *tracks* of animals encountered in the bush. As the smoke from the firing cleared, an animal would be found lying dead, while, in town, the pregnancy of a kinswoman would 'be toppled' (*kubomoka*).

In addition, sorcerers eat human flesh, which they magically exhume from the grave the night after burial. During several sorcery cases occurring in Mpala, stories circulated reporting the sorcerers' comments on the flavour and texture of the meat deriving from various body parts.

Finally, people who are chronically ill, and who suffer repeated episodes of severe illness followed by partial remission, may be termed *wabovu*. The literal meaning of the word is 'rotten' or 'unsound', and when it becomes a person's condition (*hali yake*), his case is considered hopeless. Kin, and even the patient himself, will wash their hands of the situation, saying that the person is now 'just meat' (*ni nyama tu*). The sorcerers are said to have marked such a person for slaughter in the way human beings hobble a goat the day before a celebration. Even if an *mbovu* person moves to another village, he will not recover, for the sorcerers there will only see that he is marked and so pursue him in their turn.

By refusing to submit to the death which is everyone's lot, then, the sorcerer distorts the alternation of dissolution and reorganisation which is humanity's mortal limit. The sorcerer employs both the components of medicines (*miti* or plant substances and *vizimba* or animal and human substances) and the transformative processes (heating and sex) by which they are created, but he does so towards the end of raising himself perpetually above death while keeping others perpetually subject to it. In so doing, he gives death a particularly hideous aspect. He makes it absurd by making it selective.

2

THE DISORDER OF THINGS I: DIAGNOSTIC CATEGORIES AND THE CLASSIFICATION OF ILLNESS

As a process, diagnosis mediates between emergent physiological events, deviations from the norm experienced by the subjects as their own, and the knowledge the subjects (and others) can have of what these deviations are and what outcomes they imply. Crucial to its effectiveness and authenticating its relationship to cure is the localising effect inherent in diagnosis (Canguilhem 1991) considered as the application, however tentatively or hypothetically, of any diagnostic category to any physiologic state.

This chapter is intended to convey some understanding of how diagnostic categories are held in mind and are used to make the experience of sickness (Young 1982) accessible to knowledge and intervention. This includes consideration of the criteria by which the categories are clustered together or are classified into larger groups.

What we will see is a system whose features reflect the sociability and sociality of illness and sickness. Rather than an enclosed, completed taxonomy within the confines of which every illness has place, the diagnostic categories people use are actually the starting points of or building blocks for a constructivist approach to knowledgeable intervention. This is to say that, while everyone may share the same elements from which diagnoses may be made and therapies initiated, each person can have a slightly different view of how categories fit together, and, therefore, of how the illness can be best progressed to cure. All of this is quite apart from the basic variations in individual views about the salience or relevance of specific symptoms to any particular diagnosis whatsoever. As elsewhere (Last 1981), what initially appears as a lack of system on closer inspection turns out to be a system oriented towards the proliferation of possibilities, open to the individuation of events.

In addition, diagnostic categories establish the grounding set of conditions in terms of which herbal treatments are undertaken and maintained, even which divination is also sought. Their designations also condition, though do not determine, the criteria by which people can decide whether or not a particular instance of being sick is problematic and requires divinatory insight. Thus, diagnosis also serves as the objectivising architecture, structuring and informing the move towards divination. In this sense, diagnostic categories define not only deviation itself, but also the possibility of over- or under-reacting to instances of illness.

Hence, as instruments for the production of knowledge from and through experience, diagnostic categories provide the complement to divination. One makes illness available to/for knowledge, the other makes illness accessible as intelligence (Chapter 3). Together they constitute the methodological devices by and through which an unintelligible sickness passes as it undergoes the transition/transformation from the incoherent and indecipherable to the communicative and, hopefully, the cured. Together they underwrite a therapeutic efficacy that is also a defile of signification.

DIAGNOSTIC CATEGORIES

Diagnostic categories comprise the 206 different terms which are used to refer both to aspects of being sick and to illness entities. It is in and through the use of these terms that illness is made accessible to and for knowledge. Illness terms also refer to the categories by which disparate sensations and/or diverse symptoms are localised, and which form the basic units of diagnosis and, therefore, of treatment.

In this discussion a diagnostic category is a 'conceptual entity which classifies particular illnesses, symptomatic or pathogenic components of illness, or stages of illness' (Frake 1961: 115). A diagnostic category thus links the *illness occurrence* that is a specific instance of being sick to the broader set of possibilities and impossibilities that constitute its medical context.

People use illness terms to reply to the questions 'What do you feel?' (*unasikia nini?*), 'Which illness is this?' (*huu ni ugonjwa gani?*) and 'What do they say this is?' (*wanasemaje juu na ugonjwa huu?*). To facilitate our understanding, the illness entities to which these terms refer may be divided into two types. The first we can regard as primary. These are diagnostic categories whose internal relations make them correspond roughly to the 'symptoms' of biomedicine. They are the terms in which people spontaneously announce what they feel; and they are the terms always used to reply to the question 'What do you feel?'

The other type of illness entity is constituted by the combination of primary diagnostic categories with one another and with other, sometimes non-physiological, features. The internal relation among these corresponds roughly to that of the 'syndromes' of biomedicine, and we can, for the sake of clarity, regard these as secondary.

Primary Diagnostic Categories

Terms referring to primary illness entities number some twenty-six of the total, and are the simplest terms in which deviations from health may be described. Table 2.1 sets them out.

The presence of any one of these types of deviation is sufficient to constitute an instance of being sick (Young 1982), and even mild

Table 2.1 Primary diagnostic categories

Local term[a]	English
baridi	'chills'
homa	'fever'
kikohozi	'cough'
kuendesha tumbo	'diarrhoea'
uzaifu/kuregea	'feebleness'/'weakness'
kufaa/kuvimba	'swelling' (localised or generalised)
kukosa damu	'anaemia'
kulomoka/kutapika	'retching'/'vomiting'
roho kunyonga	'nausea'
kusofu/kusofeka	'weight loss'
maumizo/kuchochomea	'pain'/'stinging'
kuwasha	'itching'
kuzimia	'fainting'
mafua	'chest and nasal congestion'
ngazi	'tingling and numbness'
nsepensepe	'hiccups'
roho kupapa	'palpitations of the heart'
roho nyeusi	'lack of appetite'
tumbo kufungwa	'constipation'
tumbo kunyonga	'lower abdominal cramps'
tumbo kupanda	'feeling of abdominal distension'
usaa	'pus'
vidonda	'lesions'
zunguzungu	'dizziness' and/or 'paraesthesia'
damu	'bleeding'
maongo tu yote	'malaise'

[a] 'Local terms' in this table are in KiSwahili, the language most frequently spoken in the area. English terms in quotes are glosses.

manifestations of any of the above are worthy of comment. Someone simply saying that s/he feels one can cause discussion of the person's state of health, regardless of whether or not this prevents her/him from fulfilling normal responsibilities.

Complementarily, deviation from a normal physiological state *must* fall into one of these categories if it is to be considered illness. Deviations such as baldness (*kipara*), crippledness (*kilema*), blindness (*kipofu*) and pregnancy (*mimba*) are not considered to be illness as such. Such states are referred to as 'conditions' (*hali*), and people distinguish 'conditions' from 'illnesses' (*magonjwa*) on the grounds that persons characterised by the former feel no physiologic pain. Victims of blindness and crippledness are said to feel pain 'only in their souls, when they think of where they might be if they were not blind or crippled'. Conditions such as old age and menstruation, however, are referred to as 'illness' because of the aches, pains and increasing disability which characterise the former, and the bleeding which characterises the latter.

Certain categories, such as 'nymphomania' (*nkunde*, an illness of women only) and 'hiccups' (*nsepensepe*) occupy a hazily defined area. People class these as illness only on the functional basis that they are treated with medicines.

All abnormal bodily sensations are given social existence through the use of these basic terms. Though each such term is sufficient to label a single instance of being sick, the description of a given illness occurrence may require the use of more than one. Since the group of primary diagnostic categories contains only one contrasting pair ('diarrhoea'/'constipation'), terms may be combined and recombined to produce a description that fits whatever illness occurrence is at hand. Thus, primary diagnostic categories provide the basis for one level of generative capacity in the diagnostic system as a whole. In seeing over five hundred individuals who had over six hundred different instances of illness, I never encountered one which people thought defied description through the use of these primary terms.

In contrast to many secondary terms, primary illnesses are fundamentally without progression. That is, their categories define deviations from health which either exist or do not exist. Though a given symptom or set of symptoms may be preceded and/or followed by others, there is nothing in the categorical definition which connects them, forming them into a meaningful sequence, the 'progress' characteristic of syndromes. Similarly, no reference is made, by the use of these categories, to events or circumstances which lie outside of the body itself. Treatment aims at the simple reversal of these deviations, and not at the guidance of the illness through a particular course which is deemed appropriate.

Finally, primary illness terms tend to form the pool from which presenting complaints are drawn. They are more often and most easily offered in response to the question 'What do you feel?' and people tend to describe any illness through the use of them, even though the particular combination of symptoms may also have another name.

Secondary Diagnostic Categories

Though people themselves make no formal distinction between primary and secondary diagnostic categories, and regard all such entities as kinds of illness, analytic distinction can be made on the basis of the kinds of criterion utilised in the formation of the secondary type, as well as on the manner in which they are used. Numbering some 180 of the total, secondary categories employ criteria which take into account a variety of different aspects of the illness entity and its situation. These are as follows:

1. *Physiological.* These are the deviations from bodily health outlined above, i.e., primary diagnostic categories. To this may be added specifications as to physical location, when necessary.
2. *Social.* Some secondary diagnostic categories include specifications as

to the age and sex of the patient. Others also include criteria relating to the circumstances which preceded the onset of the illness.

3. *Pathological*. Secondary diagnostic categories may include reference to or definitions of the internal events which are presumed to underlie the external manifestations of the illness (its symptoms).

4. *Prognostic*. Certain secondary diagnostic categories also include information on the possible alternative courses the illness may take, including whether or not it will end in death.

5. *Aetiological*. Although divination is the privileged domain for the discovery of particular aetiologies, it is important to recognise that the secondary diagnostic categories may also refer to the social sources or origins of an illness. Inversely and as significantly, some categories may specifically foreclose reference to a particular aetiological agent.

While primary diagnostic categories may be applied by any individual to a given illness occurrence, and, indeed, seem to be the very terms in which illness is perceived and perception described, the application of secondary illness terms to a given instance of being sick can be a matter involving some speculation. This is usually collectively conducted. A number of people — family members, neighbours and friends — may be called upon to give opinions as to what the illness might be. In some cases the judgement of a specialist is required for final 'recognition' (*utambuwa*). Due to the increased amount of interpretation involved, and the greater degree of uncertainty, terms for secondary diagnostic categories tend to be hidden, or latent, in descriptions built from primary terms. They are not so readily or frequently offered, but can be elicited by the questions 'What do they say this is?' or 'What illness is this?' They won't come up in response to the questions 'What do you feel?' or 'What do you think this is?'; and in fact people invariably reply to the latter question with 'I don't know.'

As a group, secondary diagnostic categories show a greater degree of internal contrast than primary categories. More than one term may be applied to a given instance of illness only if the symptoms manifested by the illness have widely differing privileges and/or sites of appearance. An example of this would be the coexistence of *upele* ('itching skin eruptions') with *nkulo* ('chest disease') and/or *nkamba* ('headache', sometimes 'temporal arteritis'). If the symptoms are not so widely dispersed, only one term may be applied, in the process of elimination that is differential diagnosis.

In some instances, treatment of syndromes is aimed at the successful completion of the more benign of the illness's possible courses, rather than at simple reversal of the symptoms. Examples of these would be *suruba* ('measles') and *luisia* ('osteomyelitis of the finger').

Secondary category terms cannot be employed to generate new descriptions of illness occurrences. Deviations from health which do not meet all the requirements for classification under a particular category may fall 'between' categories, as it were. In such a case, people will say they do not know or cannot identify what illness a person has, and will employ only primary diagnostic categories to describe the symptoms.

Finally, while the names of primary illness entities are mainly descriptive, the names of secondary entities may be suggestive. The feature of the illness on which the suggestive name is based may be either physiological or social.

The relationship between primary diagnostic categories and secondary ones is easily seen through the examination of two symptoms and the numerous syndromes in which these play a part. Deviations from health which take the basic forms of 'diarrhoea' (*kuendesha*) and/or 'vomiting' (*kutapika*) are regarded as instances of illness. Each can be fatal. In the absence of further qualifying characteristics, illness occurrences consisting of one or both of these symptoms would be classed in the primary diagnostic categories bearing their names and would be treated.

However, when these symptoms appear in conjunction with certain other characteristics, illness occurrences manifesting them must be classed in one of a number of different secondary diagnostic categories. These areas follow:

1. Kibende
Symptoms: Diarrhoea with watery faeces.
Social criteria: Occurs only in neonates and infants of a few months of age.
Pathology: This illness is caused by the improper opening of the *kibende* or anterior fontanelle. The 'openness' of this area is indicated by its failure to pulse in rhythm with the infant's heartbeat. The open area in the head permits cold air to enter the abdomen, and diarrhoea results.
Treatment: Consists of the application to the fontanelle of castor oil, onto which is sprinkled powdered bark of one or more types of tree, and/or scrapings from the bottom of a mortar.
Prognosis: This is usually a mild illness, but it can be fatal if it is particularly acute or remains unchecked.
Aetiology: Variable. Openness of the head may be caused by too much conjugal sexual intercourse during the last stages of pregnancy. Many instances of this illness, however, are of insignificant aetiology.

2. Mililo
Symptoms: Infantile syndrome consists of diarrhoea and/or shock of acute onset. Adult syndrome consists of dizziness.
Social criteria: Infantile syndrome occurs in neonates, infants and toddlers. Adult syndrome affects women during parturition.
Pathology: In the infantile syndrome, pathology is most explicit. The child's head 'splits' (*kupasuka*) (or the fontanelle 'reopens') from the top of the

skull to the centre of the forehead. This opening is indicated by lack of pulsation and/or by sinking of the area. The pathology of the adult form is less clear.

Prognosis: In both forms the prognosis is grave, with the illness usually terminating rapidly in death.

Treatment: Adult syndrome is treated by an infusion made from the trees *kibunga* (*Temnocalyx obovata (N. E. Br.)* Robyns) and *kalilolilo* (*Indigofera emarginella* A. Rich.) with which the eyes of the patient are washed. Infantile syndrome treatment consists of application of *kalilolilo* to the top of the head, among other techniques.

Aetiology: Cause of the illness is adultery of the father/husband of the household. Should he enter the house after adulterous intercourse without first having cleansed himself medicinally, the infantile syndrome and milder forms of the adult syndrome result. The most acute forms of the adult syndrome, occurring during parturition, may arise even without close proximity of husband and wife.

3. Kasesa

Symptoms: Diarrhoea which is accompanied by severe cramps or which consists of bloody stools, or stools which are almost entirely blood.

Social criteria: May occur in persons of any age or sex.

Pathology: The abdomen of every human being contains a snake. This illness is caused by the snake's scratching about inside, causing pain and/or lesions, which bleed.

Prognosis: This is a serious illness, but it can be cured.

Treatment: Consists of medicines used as enemas and as infusions which are drunk.

Aetiology: Variable. Some cases may have mundane causes, such as the eating of green mangoes with salt. Other cases may require divination to determine the precise origins of the illness.

4. Lukunga

Symptoms: Diarrhoea of watery, milky stools, progressing to diarrhoea and vomiting of the same milky substance. A further diagnostic sign is the presence of two or three small white papules on the palate.

Social criteria: Occurs only in neonates and infants.

Pathology: Diarrhoea is caused by the 'splitting' of the infant's head down through the palate. The white papules are indicative of the possibility of the occurrence of such splitting, and their presence alone is sufficient to precipitate treatment.

Prognosis: If treatment is begun promptly, preferably before the onset of diarrhoea, or very shortly thereafter, prognosis is quite good. If, however, the illness has already progressed to the stage of vomiting, the outlook is grave.

Treatment: Consists of the preparation of a medicine, which has been burnt and mixed with salt. This formula is then applied to the palate, to the skull at the widow's peak and the nape of the neck, and, sometimes, to the palms of the hands and soles of the feet.

Aetiology: Variable. This is normally a mild, congenital illness, but divination would be made into cases which did not respond to customary treatment. This illness has only recently arrived in the area around Mpala. People there say that children born before and just around the time of Independence grew up without ever having it. *Lukunga* is said to have come from the BaLuba of the Kasai. People living near the Zambian border say they have never seen or heard of it.

5. Lombozoka

Symptoms: Abdominal pain followed by diarrhoea and vomiting.

Social criteria: Occurs in persons of any age and sex.

Pathology: This illness is caused by the agitation or the swelling of the snake in the stomach, a situation which is itself provoked by consumption of foods which the snake dislikes or which have spoiled. It may also occur spontaneously.

Prognosis: Unless it is of exceptional intensity or duration, this is not considered a very serious illness.

Treatment: No specific treatment is given.

Aetiology: Variable. Divination would not ordinarily be undertaken for this. The name of the illness is the name of the snake.

6. Tutumbilia

Symptoms: Vomiting which persists after the stomach has been emptied. The vomitus itself consists of bile in which are mixed small 'bundles' (*tufulushi*) of mucus.

Social criteria: Occurs in persons of any age and sex.

Pathology: This illness occurs when the snake in the stomach spits. The small particles of mucus are the snake's saliva and from this the illness derives its name.

Prognosis: This is considered to be a minor illness.

Treatment: No specific treatment.

Aetiology: Variable. Divination would not ordinarily be undertaken for this illness.

In addition to the illnesses outlined above, there are also other types of sickness which include these symptoms and might be classed as syndromes, but which lack a definite illness name. These are as follows:

1. *Diarrhoea of infants due to eruption of first teeth*. If the child's parents have seen the teeth beginning to emerge, it is not uncommon for them simply

to endure the diarrhoea, providing there are no other symptoms, such as loss of appetite, excessive crying, etc. This is because it is believed that the diarrhoea will not respond to treatment, but will spontaneously cease when the tooth has fully erupted.

2. *Absence of a kapokelela (KT kasonga) bwali.* Diarrhoea of infants may be caused by the absence at birth of the *kapokelela bwali* (literally 'that which receives *bukali*'). This is an organ which lies very far down in the throat and which is not generally visible, if the infant is not crying. Structurally, it corresponds to the epiglottis of biomedicine. Its absence may also cause chronic thinness in a newborn. Both symptoms are due to the fact that the throat is 'just a hole' (*shimu tu*), permitting foods to pass too rapidly into the body. Only a lay specialist or other experienced person may make the definitive diagnosis. Treatment is directed towards the growth of the *kapokelela bukali*, and not towards the direct reversal of the diarrhoea as such.

3. *Vomiting of bile without mucus.* This is caused by the swelling of the snake in the stomach, or by the snake's standing up and touching the 'gall bladder' (*nyongo* (KS) or *kansongwa* (KT)). This contact causes the 'gall bladder' to spill too much 'bile' into the stomach, and vomiting of the substance results. The 'gall bladder' may also spontaneously overfill, with the same result.

4. *Simple vomiting.* This is caused by the consumption of undetectably spoiled foods, which soil the stomach.

The above discussion makes clear the relation of primary to secondary diagnostic categories. In all cases the classification of a given illness occurrence into one of the secondary categories presupposes consideration either of features of the illness situation which lie beyond the symptoms themselves, or of physiological characteristics which modify the primary symptoms. In all cases, as well, the syndrome name, and, therefore, its application to a given illness occurrence, carries with it presumptions about the pathology of the illness, as well as its prognosis.

The fixity of relation between pathology and syndrome means that it is the cause of the illness rather than the symptom which informs treatment. Therapy of an illness such as *kibende* makes clear that the cause of the diarrhoea is being treated as such. The diarrhoea itself is only a symptom which will stop spontaneously, once the infant's head is properly closed. The illness *mililo* provides another example. In it, two different types of symptom occurring in two different categories of human being are both called by the same syndrome name, because the aetiology of both is the same and the pathologies of both are fundamentally identical.

Diagnostic categories, then, provide the terms fundamental to the perception of being sick and to the recognition of the illness a person has. The symptoms of the primary categories are illnesses in themselves. They also constitute the physiological criteria of the secondary categories, or syndromes, which often include non-physiological characteristics as well.

The complexity of syndromes which combine social, anatomical and physical circumstances into a single entity demonstrates that although illnesses may be *in* the body they are not exactly *of* the body in any simple sense. Instead, physiology is such that there is a continuity between the body's inside and its outside, so that symptoms are events like any others; positive presences which are not absences of normal organ functions. In this respect, diagnostic categories contribute to the transfiguring structure through which the body as responsive object becomes the body as communicative subject, a transition completed in the resort to divination.

CLASSIFICATION OF DIAGNOSTIC CATEGORIES

Diagnosis is the identification or, as people themselves would say, the 'recognition' (*utambuwa*) of a specific illness occurrence, a particular instance of being sick. It is an analytic process whose aim is the elimination of all diagnostic categories other than the one most relevant to the particular sickness at hand. In contrast to this, classification of diagnostic categories into larger groups or contexts is a process of synthesis. Illnesses are grouped together on the basis of shared traits and those features which are not common to a number of categories are ignored. As a result, classificatory criteria tend to give a less complete picture of any given illness entity than do diagnostic criteria, whose value lies in the greater elaboration of detail.

In addition, the two processes have rather different contexts of appearance. Diagnosis is explicit behaviour which can be observed whenever one is in the presence of particular illness occurrences. People readily set about it when they are prompted by the presence of symptoms (or by the ignorance of the ethnographer).

Classification, on the other hand, refers to the conceptual construction connecting illness entities. It is not so easily observable, it operates independently of specific instances of being sick, and it includes reference to entities people may not themselves ever have seen. It is one area in which the systematics that make medical knowledge are demonstrable, but to discover them, it is necessary to employ techniques designed specifically to elicit classificatory principles.

My first forum for the learning of illness terms was the tri-weekly dispensary which I ran in my house. I would first ask people what they felt (*unasikia nini?*), and after noting their description of their symptoms, I would then ask if their illness had a name, or if anyone had been able to 'recognise' (*kutambua*) it. On this basis, I formed initial descriptions of disease categories, which I then confirmed or elaborated through conversations with other people.

When I had a substantial, though still incomplete, listing of illness terms,

I made a set of index cards on each of which was written the name of one diagnostic category. Included in the set were terms referring to such deviations as baldness, sneezing, blindness and so forth.

Working with a small set of people, selected to represent different types of medical knowledge,[1] I asked each person to group together those diseases which were 'kin' (*ndugu*). As we went through the process together, I obtained a verifying description from each person, and we kept our groupings in mind by putting the cards of related illnesses in one group. When people classed a new illness entity with others, I asked them to tell me the reasons for their choice. When the classification of entities was complete, I asked them to tell me the similarity (*ufwanano*) among all members of the group, and if there was one illness in the group which might be its prototype or model (*mfano*).[2] Finally, I asked people if the groups thus obtained might be combined into even larger groupings, and, if so, the basis upon which this might be done.

TYPES OF CLASSIFICATION CRITERIA

In the classification of illness entities into various groupings people employ several different kinds of criterion.[3] The two types most frequently used were morphological and existential. With morphological classification, people group together all diseases which have a similar appearance, or which are symptomatically similar. Existential criteria underlie the formation of groupings composed of illnesses which have similar sites of appearance in the body, and/or which tend either to appear simultaneously or to develop into one another. While existentially related illnesses tend also to be morphologically similar, such similarity is not the reason why these diseases 'go together' (*kufuatana*).

Other classificatory criteria include pathology, prognosis, and method of treatment. However, these criteria are secondary to the others in that they are less frequently and less consistently used. In addition they are almost always employed to subdivide further a larger grouping which has been established on the basis of morphological or existential criteria.

Aetiology, the ultimate, social cause of an illness, is significant in its absence as a criterion of classification. For example, despite the fact that there are some illnesses which are strongly associated with sorcery (e.g., 'tuberculosis,' 'leprosy,' 'insanity,' 'severe mastitis'), the association was never used as the basis for the formation of a group. This is due to the slightly different contexts of thought in which aetiological and other criteria appear.

The formation of diagnostic categories and the placement of these into wider groupings involves the consideration of the general aspects of illness entities. In this context, illnesses are impersonal, physiological entities, whose features remain unchanged regardless of the identity of the particular individual in whose body they appear. Knowledge of the source of an illness is not necessary to the process of identification of the occurrence as such. Aetiology is of significance precisely at the point at which the impersonal characteristics of the illness become united to the uniquely personal circumstances of the individual afflicted; that is, at the point where divination becomes necessary.

Morphological Criteria

The use of morphological criteria as a basis for the classification of illness entities is best illustrated in the large grouping of skin diseases. This group is particularly suited to morphological classification because it presents a large number of illnesses which have the same site of appearance (the surface of the body),[4] and which are clearly visible.

Table 2.2 is designed to show the criteria by which people group together various skin diseases.[5] Thus, *kibukulo* ('goitre,' no. 14) is a skin disease characterised by a swelling which does not split and emit pus as part of its progress/treatment. It is treated by application of medicine to the outside of the swelling. In these respects, it is identical to *tuzulu* (no. 15), 'the appearance of small swellings (bubo; enlarged lymph glands) in the neck', which is prodromal to *kabongila* ('sleeping sickness'). *Kibukulo* is also more similar to *masankutwi* ('mumps', no. 11), from which it differs only in method of treatment, than it is to *kapopo* ('osteomyelitis', primarily of the jaw, no. 22), or *suruba* ('measles,' no. 28), from which it differs in a larger number of respects.

As an inspection of Table 2.2 shows, the largest subgroupings of skin diseases are distinguished according to the form taken by the lesions themselves; whether they remain flat and are not raised above the surface of the skin (i.e., the 'macules' of biomedicine), whether they are larger, localised swellings (corresponding in size, if not always in form, to the 'nodules' of biomedicine), or whether they are small, raised eruptions (the 'papules' of biomedicine). The category of 'macules' is further subdivided on the basis of location. Illnesses considered by people to be identical in form are nevertheless given different names according to whether they appear on the head or on the body.

The category *vivimbo*, 'large swellings', is further classified according to the forms of the swellings themselves. The subcategory 'blisters' is set off from other types of swelling because such lesions are localised in the upper part of the skin and contain water rather than pus. They are, as people put it, 'like a burn' (*mfano wa moto*).

Swellings which are not blisters are subdivided according to the progress of the illnesses themselves. In the first subgrouping of this category are included all those swellings which do not split and emit pus as part of their progress and/or treatment. These illnesses are further classified on the basis of whether or not they are medically treated.

Table 2.2 Classificationof skin diseases

Diagnostic categories	Criteria for groups and subgroups					
1. *visebula/matole* – 'ringworm of the scalp'					Head	Non-swelling macules
2. *imba* – 'dandruff'						
3. *kibakula* – 'ringworm of the body'					Body	
4. *lubandu*						
5. *tulanzi* – 'body dandruff leading to leprosy', 'macular tuberculoid lesions'						
6. *ukoma* – 'leprosy'						
7. *mabobela*	Blisters				Large swellings – *vivimbo*	Swellings
8. *moto wa mungu*						
9. *piakusu* – 'chafing', 'heat rash'						
10. *nyungu-nyungu**						
11. *masankutwi* – 'mumps'			Area is not / does not split	Nodules		
12. *kipombolo* – 'bruise'						
13. *muntekia*						
14. *kibukulo* – 'goitre'						
15. *tuzulu/milungu* – 'lymphatic swellings in neck, prodromal to sleeping sickness'						
16. *kaputensungu* – 'small, shallow boil'	Boils	Lesser forms	Area split(s) – emits pus			
17. *kipute/jipu* – 'boil'						
18. *pumbumapute*						
19. *kimeni* – 'large boil', 'diphtheria'						
20. *mumenapabe*						
21. *luisia/kesi* – 'osteomylitis of the finger'	*madidu*	Greater forms				
22. *kapopo* – 'osteomylitis'						
23. *kapindi* – 'osteomylitis of the joint, particularly the shoulder'						
24. *kamanu* – 'mastitis'						
25. *maaya* – 'abscess'						
26. *lionde* – 'septicaemia/bacteremia'						
27. *ntete/kitete* – 'chicken pox', 'alastrim', 'final papules of measles'					Fever	Papules – *chunuku*
28. *suruba/katuta* – 'measles'					Deadly	
29. *ndui/kabola* – 'smallpox' (a) *bulezi* – millet-sized, invariably fatal (b) *masaka* – sorghum-sized, frequently fatal (c) *mihindi* – corn-sized, rarely fatal						
30. *bukuta*			No discharge	Itching	No fever	
31. *pese*						
32. *masoli* – 'urticaria, hives'						
33. *upele*						
34. *lunanu*			Discharge			
35. *nyngu-nyungu**						
36. *kaswende* – 'syphilis, secondary lesions'						
37. *kisengula* – 'syphilis, tertiary lesions'						
38. *visokoto* – 'yaws'			No discharge	Non-itching		
39. *ntonge* – 'lesions of yaws on soles of feet'						
40. *tunkuli* – 'yaws'						
41. *vzibula* – 'yaws'			Discharge			
42. *kulaulwa*						
43. *bwingilizi* – 'neonatal milia'						
44. *chunuku*						

The second subgrouping includes all illnesses which follow the pattern of boils (*jipu* (KS)/*kipute* (KT)) in that localised swelling, followed by the spontaneous or induced splitting of the skin with emission or extrusion of pus, constitutes the normal progress of the illness. This group is next subdivided according to the 'size' (*ukubwa*) of the illness, a term which includes not only the size of the area affected, but also the seriousness of the prognosis.

In the normal course of events, the lesser forms (boils) are minor illnesses which are cured in only a couple of weeks and which leave no permanent disability beyond, perhaps, a scar.[6] They are subgrouped on the basis of size, depth, number and location.

In contrast to boils, however, even the most minor of the greater forms may take weeks, if not months, to cure, and leaves permanent disability. With osteomyelitis, the cartilage attached to the limb is usually destroyed, and, if the illness completes its classic progress, the bone itself splits. After recovery, the affected digit or limb is useless, and there may be permanent disfigurement, especially in *kapopo* (no. 22) of the jaw. Mastitis (*kamanu*, no. 24) usually takes several months to cure, and often results in the suppression of lactation in the affected breast, either permanently or for the duration of the particular lactation period.

The great resemblance in progress among these types of illness is reflected in their common classification under the general term *mududu*. The two illnesses which are not so classified, *maaya* ('abscess', no. 25) and *lionde* ('septicaemia', no. 26), differ from the others in form, but are, if anything, more serious than they. It is to these that the *mududu* illnesses may progress, if they are not properly treated, and the prognosis for both is quite grave. Only an exceptional practitioner would undertake treatment, and only an especially fortunate patient would survive.

Chunuku, 'papules', are distinguished from the other types of swelling because of their small size (that of a pinhead, approximately). Included in this group is a subcategory of those illnesses which begin with fever, such as *suruba* ('measles', no. 28), *ndui* ('smallpox', no. 29), and *ntete* (possibly 'chicken pox', no. 27). The first two are quite deadly, and, hence, are set off from the last. However, the presence of fever indicates that the illness begins in the abdomen, and only later comes out to the skin.

With the exception of *kaswende* ('syphilis', no. 36), all other illnesses characterised by papules are considered to be superficial diseases affecting the skin only. These are formed into subgroupings first according to whether or not they itch, and then according to whether or not their course includes the discharge of water or pus.

A comparison of the classification of skin diseases with the descriptions of these same illnesses would demonstrate the differences between the two types of process. The first concerns the means by which illness entities might be associated with/differentiated from one another as abstractions, while the second is a means by which a specific instance of illness can be recognised, identified, understood, and treated. With classification, groupings of diagnostic categories are made on the basis of the size, form, progress and prognosis of the lesions. These characteristics are sufficient to determine which skin diseases are alike. However, they are not sufficient to describe a given illness entity fully or to recognise (*kutambuwa*, i.e., diagnose) a given illness occurrence.

Thus 'measles' (*suruba*, no. 28) and 'smallpox' (*ndui*, no. 29) are identical from the classificatory point of view, both being characterised by high fever, appearance of papules, and poor prognosis. They are nevertheless differentially diagnosed on the basis of features which are not relevant to classification. 'Measles' begins with fever, accompanied by cough. The absence of the cough indicates that the illness may not be 'measles' but 'smallpox'. Further, the lesions of 'smallpox' appear primarily on the face and trunk, whereas those of 'measles' must appear all over the body, if the patient is to be cured. 'Smallpox' is further subdivided on the basis of the size of the papules, which are the size of millet (*bulezi*, the miliary papules of biomedicine), sorghum (*masaka*) or corn (*mihindi*). The prognosis is best with the last type, and the disease will always terminate fatally in the case of the first.

Existential Criteria

Existential classification of diagnostic categories is the formation of groupings of illnesses not only (or not even) on the basis of morphological similarity, but also on the basis of the developmental relations among the diseases. The group of chest diseases provides a good example of this type of classification.

Figure 2.1 shows the developmental relations among the types of respiratory disease. Each illness entity is in some sense terminal in that it may be followed by cure, or may remain chronic, without progressing to another illness. However, it may also take an alternative course, in which it develops into another illness (indicated by arrows); which illness may itself then be terminal or progressive.

Thus, *kilimi* ('hyperextended uvula') may be a terminal illness, either being followed by cure or becoming chronic; or it may progress to *kikohozi* ('cough') and *mafua* ('chest and nasal congestion').

Kikohozi may succeed *kilimi*, or may begin spontaneously, without previous complaint or perception of *kilimi*. However, even when *kikohozi* begins spontaneously, *kilimi* is presumed to be present, as the extension of the uvula is said to cause itching (*kuwasha*) in the throat and thus prompt coughing.

Mbavu ('rib pain') never occurs spontaneously, but appears only as a

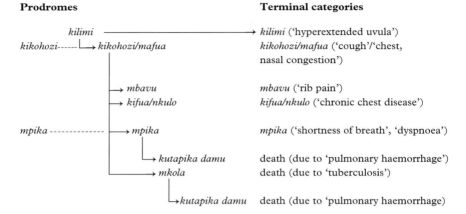

Figure 2.1 Developmental relations among types of respiratory disease

consequence of coughing. Though it may be treated separately, it will nevertheless spontaneously subside when coughing decreases. If *kikohozi* persists, it may become *kifua* ('chest disease'), a chronic illness. *Mpika* ('shortness of breath' or 'dyspnoea') may follow either *kikohozi* or *kifua* or may appear spontaneously.

Kutapika damu ('severe pulmonary haemorrhage' or 'severe haemoptysis') may not appear spontaneously. It is always preceeded by *kifua*, and is of acute onset and extremely poor prognosis. A person may survive such bleeding only once or twice, and a person who has experienced it is therefore considered to be doomed. Even should he live beyond the first episode, people say that he will probably not live out the year, and it is just a matter of waiting until the next, fatal episode occurs.

If *kifua* does not remain chronic, or give rise to an episode of *kutapika damu*, it may yet progress to *mkola* ('tuberculosis'), another fatal terminal disease. *Mkola* is practically incurable. European medicines have no effect upon it, and even the most skilled of traditional practitioners has little chance of success. A person suffering from *mkola* may either die a lingering death or succumb suddenly to an episode of *kutapika damu*.

While the above discussion presents the developmental relations among abstract, separable illness entities, what actually occurs 'on the ground' is the reclassification of a particular illness occurrence in which the various diagnostic categories appear as stages. Table 2.3 illustrates this by showing the symptomatic relations among the types of respiratory disease.

The significant symptom in the illness *kilimi* is the extension of the uvula itself. The throat may or may not be inflamed (in cases I saw, it was), but this is irrelevant to diagnosis.

Table 2.3 Symptomatic relations among types of respiratory disease

Disease	Symptomatic relations
kilimi	Extension of uvula
kikohozi/mafua	Extension of uvula/cough/chest, nasal congestion
mbavu	Cough/chest, nasal congestion/rib pain
kifua/nkulo	Chronic cough/dyspnoea (mpika)/extension of uvula
mkola	Chronic cough/dyspnoea (mpika)/thinness/coughing of blood
kutapika damu	Chronic cough/dyspnoea (mpika)/pulmonary haemorrhage

As mentioned above, it is the extension of the uvula which causes itching (*kuwasha*) in the throat, and thus prompts coughing (*kikohozi*), with attendant chest and nasal congestion (*mafua*). *Kikohozi* may occur spontaneously, and people may seek treatment and be cured of it without active reference being made to the presence of *kilimi*. However, when they discuss the cause of coughing, people invariably mention extension of the uvula.

When the cough and chest congestion of *kikohozi–mafua* is accompanied by pain in the lower ribs, the illness is referred to as *mbavu*. This term also may be used to label rib pain alone, and *mbavu*[7] is treated with techniques and medicines which are different from those used to cure *kikohozi*. Nevertheless, people insist on the point that *mbavu* never occurs except in conjunction with *kikohozi*, and treatment of the former must be in addition to treatment of the latter.

If the cough of *kikohozi* continues for a prolonged period, the illness may be rediagnosed as *kifua* ('chronic chest disease'). The cough may be unproductive, or may result in sputum, either clear or white. It is accompanied by difficult breathing (*mpika*) and weakness (*kuregea*). This is a chronic illness, which grows worse at the new and full moons, with relatively complete remission during the intervening periods; a feature which is characteristic of all chronic illnesses. People say that prognosis is better if *kifua* has begun early in one's life. Individuals whose illness begins in adulthood are much more likely to develop *mkola* or *kutapika damu*.

As with *kikohozi*, though it may not be one of the explicit symptoms, *kilimi* may nevertheless be thought to underlie 'chronic chest disease'. Cutting the uvula may be one of the series of treatments of *kifua* attempted. This is done by passing a small loop of thread around the structure, extending it, and then cutting it with a razor blade. Specialists in this type of treatment live to the north of Mpala, around Kalemie. Other treatments of *kifua* do not involve the uvula, but focus on the chest itself, seen as the seat of the disorder.

Individuals suffering from *kifua* will have some discomfort and limited disability due to their illness. They will not, however, become thin; and loss of weight (*kusofeka, kusofu*) is one of the critical signs that the illness has become *mkola*. The coughing of blood is another perhaps more important sign. Though people say that thinness alone is sufficient to diagnose *mkola*, they nevertheless also say that when a person begins to cough blood 'it is *mkola* itself' (*ni mkola mwenyewe*), indicating by their tone of voice that the diagnosis was somehow more equivocal before.

This equivocation is itself of some significance, for it derives not only from the vague nature of the symptoms involved, but also from the social meaning of the diagnostic category. To say that a person has *mkola* is tantamount to pronouncing him as good as dead, and people, including practitioners hesitate to do this. I have seen and heard of cases in which the person was not only thin, but was also coughing blood, and was yet not said to have *mkola*. In one such case, the practitioner still had hope of effecting cure; while in another case the diagnosis *mkola* was not made by the practitioner until bad feeling had developed between her and the patient's family, leading to a temporary rupture of active social relations.

Kutapika damu, though a diagnostic category, is not an illness state, as such. Rather, it is an acute episode in or complication of a more chronic condition, whether *kifua* or *mkola*. Both of the latter illnesses are necessary prodromes to *kutapika damu*, which therefore may be said to include chronic cough and difficult breathing as some of the symptomatic characteristics by which it is defined. However, it appears to be the bleeding which alone is diagnostic.

Haemorrhage begins without warning. The person may 'vomit' (*kutapika*) a quantity of blood ranging from a glassful to more than a basinful, despite the fact that only moments before he or she appeared perfectly normal (within the limits of the chronic illness). In one instance of this, a woman who had been diagnosed years before (at the hospital) as having asthma had been to visit the new baby of a relative one Sunday morning. Upon returning home, she had abruptly begun to bleed and was dead within an hour. People said that this is characteristic of *kutapika damu*, and that had she survived this incident, it would not have been for very long.

Awareness of the others to which a given illness may be developmentally related is important to treatment. Experienced practitioners say that during therapy, they attempt not only to treat the symptoms at hand, but also to bear in mind the other, more serious illnesses which may occur should early treatment be unsuccessful. As one of them aptly stated it, the idea is to move ahead of the illness, and put a barrier across its path, so that it makes no progress.

The foregoing discussion and illustrations have demonstrated the methods and criteria people employ in the classification of illness. Though other criteria, such as pathology, prognosis, and method of treatment may be used, the primary ones are morphological (i.e., having to do with the form, whether physical or symptomatic, of the illness) and existential (i.e., having to do with the occurrence of the illness). Though the examples discussed showed an almost exclusive use of one type of classification or the other, the two are not mutually exclusive, and many groupings show the use of both.

DIFFERENCES IN CLASSIFICATION

Though the kinds of criterion people used were always the same and the characteristics attributed to the diagnostic categories themselves varied little, there was nevertheless some variation in the contents of groupings put together by different people. A re-examination of skin diseases illustrates both the differences and the reasons for them.

In Table 2.4 are presented the three different classifications given me and, in the last column, the classification used in Table 2.2, which is a composite drawn from systematic classifications, as well as general observations. What one finds in comparing all four columns is that there is a central core of illnesses about the classification of which everyone is certain. Then, there are a number of illnesses which display some of the characteristics of a given subgrouping, but not others. Classification of these, rather anomalous illness entities shows a greater degree of variation. If the former are a type of 'kin' association, the latter may be thought of as a sort of 'kith' – the imagery evokes for us clusters and varied types of affiliation, with gaps between.

Group III was formed round the diagnostic category 'boil' (*jipu* (KS)/ *kipute* (KT)). That is, after having formed their groups, or when in the process of forming them, people consistently cited 'boils' as the archetype (*mfano*) of the category, and used the term to refer to the group as a whole. Significant features of this illness are localised swelling, followed by rupture (spontaneous or induced) and emission of pus, after which healing occurs. As the swelling 'ripens' (*kuivia*) it fluctuates in response to light digital pressure, and eventually shows a place where it is to be incised (the 'eye' or *jicho*).

Everyone was in agreement that Group IIIb should be classed as boils (viz., *kaputensungu*, *kipute*, *pumbumapute*, *kimeni*, *mumenapabe*). These display all the features of a boil, and, as noted in Table 2.2, the differing names given to them refer to such things as size, location, number, etc. Other types of localised swelling, however, do not completely follow the progress of boils,[8] and their proper classification was more problematic.

Kilimamboka (Column 1) and Luvunzo (Column 3) included in Group IIIa such illnesses as 'mumps' (*musankutwi*), 'bruises' (*kibombolo*) 'goitre' (*kibukulo*) and 'lymphatic swelling in response to localised infection' (*muntekia*), because they all swell in the fashion of boils. Since none of them splits or emits pus, however, they were nevertheless subdivided from the archetypal group.

Table 2.4 Differential classification of diagnostic categories

Kilimamboka	Mumbyoto	Luvunzo/Kalulu	Composite
Group I			
visebula/matole	visebula/matole	visebula/matole	visebula/matole
imba		imba	imba
kibakula[a]	kibakula[a]	kibakula[a]	libakula[a]
lubandu	lubandu[1]	lubandu[2]	lubandu
	imba		
tulanzi[b]	tulanzi[b]	tulanzi[b]	tulanzi[b]
ukoma[b]	ukoma[b]	ukoma[b]	ukoma[b]
Group II: 'blisters'			
mfano wa moto			
mabobela	mabobela	mabobela	mabobela
moto wa mungu	moto wa mungu	moto wa mungu	moto wa mungu
piakusu		piakusu	piakusu
		nyungu-nyungu	nyungu-nyungu
Group IIIa: 'swellings'			
masankutwi[c]	[d]	masankutwi	masankutwi
kibombolo		kibombolo	kibombolo
linsonkela			
lona			
muntekia		muntekia	muntekia
		mbawe	
		kibukulo	kibukulo[5]
			tuzulu/milungu[f]
Group IIIb: 'boils'			
kaputensungu	kaputensungu	kaputensungu	kaputensungu
kipute	kipute	kipute	kipute
pumbumapute	[g]	pumbumapute	pumbumapute
kimeni	kimeni	kimeni	kimeni
mumenapabe	mumenapabe	mumenapabe	mumenapabe
kamanu	kamanu		
kibukulo	kibukulo		
	linsonkela[h]		
	lionde[i]		
Group IV: 'insects'			
luisia/kesi	luisia/kesi		luisia/kesi
kapopo	kapopo	kapopo	kapopo
kapindi	kapindi	kapindi	kapindi
		kamanu	kamanu
maaya			maaya
lionde			lionde
vilungu[j]			
bumbolela[k]	bumbolela[l]		
	imbwa[l]		
	mulambo[l]		

Kilimamboka	Mumbyoto	Luvunzo/Kalulu	Composite
Group V: 'Eruptions'			
ntete/kitete[m]			ntete/kitete
suruba/katuta[n]			suruba/katuta
ndui/kabola			
			bukuta
pese	pese	pese	pese
masoli	masoli	masoli	masoli
upele	upele	upele	upele
lunanu	lunanu	lunanu	lunanu
nyungu-nyungu	nyungu-nyungu	nyungu-nyungu[o]	nyungu-nyungu
[p]	kaswende	kaswende[q]	kaswende
	kisengula	kisengula[q]	kisengula
	visokoto	visokoto[r]	visokoto
	ntonge	ntonge[r]	ntonge
	tunkuli	tunkuli[r]	tunkuli
	kizibula	kizibula[r]	kizibula
kulaulwa	kulaulwa	kulaulwa[s]	kulaulwa
bwingilizi	bwingilizi[n]	bwingilizi	bwingilizi
		chunuku	chunuku
		lusonkela	

[a] The cluster of categories from *kibakula* down to *ukoma* were classed together first because of the morphological similarity of *lubandu* and *imba* to *tulanzi*, and then becasue of *tulanzi*'s ontological relations to *ukoma*, into which it develops.

[b] *Tulanzi* and *ukoma* were classed with a group of incurable illnesses.

[c] All categories in this group were classed together because none is treated; all are self-limiting disorders.

[d] *Masankutwi* ('mumps') was not classed here, but was classed as anomalous because of the transience of the illness, the nature of the swelling, its location, and accompanying symptms (sore throat, difficulty swallowing, etc.).

[e] *Kibukulo* ('goitre') was classed in Group IIIb by Kilimamboka, and was declared by Mumbyoto to be anomalous because the swelling neither causes pain nor emits pus.

[f] *Tuzulu/milungu* ('bubonic prodrome to sleeping sickness') was classed in Group V by Kilimamboka, and was classed as anomalous by Mumbyoto because the swellings were not incised.

[g] This diagnostic category was unknown to Mumbyoto.

[h] *Lusonkela* ('stye') was classed here by Mumbyoto because 'if it appeared on the thigh, it could be called *kaputensungu*' ('small, shallow boil').

[i] *Lionde* (or *maaya*, 'abscess') was classed here by Mumbyoto because of the resemblance between it and *mumenapabe*. The only difference between the two is that one is soft and the other is not.

[j] *Vilungu* ('lymphatic swellings of sleeping sickness') was classed here by Kilimamboka because of its resemblance to *maaya*.

[k] This was classed with *mududu* because it may develop into it.

[l] *Bumbolela*, *imbwa* and *mulambo* were put by Luvunzo and Mumbyoto into an altogether separate category of their own because of the similarity among them of their pain and their method of acquisition.

[m] These illnesses were classed together, but because of their 'fierceness' (*ukali*, i.e. virulence) and the fever accompanying them, they were somewhat separated from the other class of skin illnesses clustered below.

[n] Classed by Mumbyoto with other childhood diseases.

[o] This was also classed with *moto wa mungu* because both take the form of blisters.

[p] *Kaswende* and *kisengula* were classed by Kilimamboka with *sofisi* ('gonorrhoea' and *kitinda mimba* ('female, internal gonorrhoea').

[q] This was also classed with *sofisi* ('gonorrhoea') and in a group of illnesses affecting fertility.

[r] Also classed with incurable illnesses.

[s] Also classed with lesions.

In contrast to this, Mumbyoto (Column 2) applied his categorical specifications more absolutely. 'Mumps' and 'goitre' were said by him to be anomalous; the former because it is an illness which spontaneously remits after only four days, and the latter because there is neither pain nor emission of pus during its course. *Muntekia* he classed with lesions, because the swelling of lymph nodes usually occurs in conjunction with infected cuts, ulcers and the like. Finally, Mumbyoto included 'stye' (*linsonkela*)[9] in his Group IIIb because of its resemblance to 'boils.' He said that despite the fact that this illness is not treated, if it were to appear on the thigh, it would be called *kaputensungu* ('small, shallow boil'), and thus deserved to be classed with its kin.

In the case of Group III (a and b), then, people were confronted with a cluster of illnesses about the classification of which they were quite certain, and then others whose proper category was less clear. In response to this, two of them modified their criteria of classification somewhat, separating some of the characteristics of boils (i.e., swelling), from others (i.e., rupture and emission of pus), and adding other criteria where necessary (i.e., treated or not treated with medicines). One continued to adhere rather firmly to the whole cluster of features, classifying in other categories those illnesses which were anomalous.

The discrepancies in classification of Group V present a rather different picture. The anomalous illnesses of Group III were unusual in that they did not match all the characteristics of boils. However, they did not display features which might easily lead one to classify them in any other category, either. With Group V, on the other hand, illnesses which were not a part of the core group were different precisely because there was some other feature about them that made their classification elsewhere seem appropriate.

Group V is that of 'eruptions'. The archetype of this group is *upele*; a skin disease characterised by itching papules, which later become water-filled vesicles. As with Group III, there was a core of illnesses which everyone classified in the same way, subdividing them according to prodrome (viz., those that begin with fever), presence or absence of discharge, etc., as discussed above.

The problematic illnesses in this group were those that had other distinctive features, in addition to those of morphology. Thus, Kilimamboka (Column 1) classed the 'secondary' and 'tertiary lesions of syphilis' (*kaswende, kisengula*) with 'gonorrhoea' (*sofisi*) and 'female, internal gonorrhoea' (*kitinda mimba*), because all of these are contagious venereal diseases. He also put in this group the various types of 'secondary' and tertiary lesions of yaws' (i.e., *visokoto, ntonge, tunkuli, kizibula*) because these are identical in form to the lesions of 'syphilis'.

Mumbyoto (Column 2) classed the lesions of 'syphilis' in the 'eruptions' category, but put those of 'yaws' in a separate class of their own. Luvunzo and Kalulu (Column 3) classed 'syphilis' with 'gonorrhoea', in a group of reproductive disorders. *Visokoto*, the most debilitating of the lesions of 'yaws', they classed in a group of incurable, or almost incurable, illnesses. The milder form of 'yaws' they classed with the group of 'eruptions'.

Finally, while the others classed the tiny papules of 'neonatal miliary impetigo' (*bwingilizi*) with eruptions, Mumbyoto considered these to be a variety of childhood illness and classed them with other infantile diseases. In addition, 'stye' (*lusonkela*) was classed as a non-itching eruption by Luvunzo and Kalulu, in contrast to the classification made by Kilimamoka and Mumbyoto.

Differences in classification, then, reveal the strategies of reasoning through which groupings are formed. In the case of skin diseases, each subgroup was organised around a specific illness, which was held to be the archetype (*mfano*) of the category. The cluster (or succession) of symptoms displayed by this illness was the criterion for membership in the group. People were in accord regarding the classification of a core of illnesses which met all significant criteria (i.e., which closely resembled the archetypal diagnostic category) much as there might be certainty about membership of a core group of kin. Discrepancies occurred in the classification of those illnesses which did not display all significant features, and those illnesses which had other characteristics which might cause them to be better classified in other groups. Like kith, they could be identified by their affinity to a variety of different clusters of 'kin'. Although further or statistically larger study would perhaps reveal a system in which certain strategies or criteria are considered to be more useful than others in the resolution of doubtful cases, it is likely that the very discrepancies themselves contribute to the proliferation of therapeutic possibilities.

The corpus of diagnostic categories is the significant conceptual ground constitutive of illness as a bodily event. Through it illness is defined and perceived, and therapeutic alternatives are considered. Yet it is important to bear in mind that the system itself is not taxonomic, nor do the rules of its use press towards taxonomic completion.

Despite agreement on its core, there can be significant variation in the classification of those of a group's illness entities whose features place them at its periphery. The debatability of diagnosis thus exists not only at the level of matching illness occurrences to categories, but also at the level of matching categories among themselves. At the moment of 'recognition' (*utambua*), these variations form one basis for the proliferation, rather than the narrowing, of therapeutic possibilities. The pattern of proliferating opinions, punctuated by intermittent consensus, is fundamental to the operation of medical knowledge, and, indeed, to the maintenance of hope.

Recognising a particular illness occurrence has to do with determining which of its attributes is most salient, and to which broader category it may attach. An outline, so to speak, is drawn around and so localises events, bodily and extra-bodily, in a process of discernment which brings forth the entity otherwise obscured in the resistant indivisibility of life. Treatment may thus be seen as an engagement in identification which is not so much a labelling as an evocation, a process consistent and continuous with the more abstract evocations of divination.

3

THE DISORDER OF THINGS II: AETIOLOGY OF DISEASE AND THE PROCESS OF DIVINATION

AETIOLOGY

Although we think of medical systems primarily in terms of what they do – that is, in terms of the therapeutic action they make possible, the other of their significant functions, bonded to the first, is the kind of thing they make it possible, through their use, to *say*. Placing aetiology in the context of narrative makes clear the respects in which a given approach to the body and to diagnosis establishes its corresponding discursive economy. By this, I mean to refer not just to the type of narrative that may be credited or taken as warrantable, but also to the type of entity that is accorded agency in that narrative, and, further, the kind of agency it is accorded.

In biomedicine, questions of aetiology are answered in the same biological or physiological terms as questions of pathology. Aetiology refers to the cause of the disease as a deviation in the normal functioning of physiologic processes. Explanations have to do with *how* people, in general, come to present a specific constellation of systemic phenomena. Although 'silenced' at the level of dialogue, the biomedical body can nevertheless be made to 'speak', to participate however passively in the production of narratives about itself. The physiological closure of the biomedical body is balanced by the continuing refinement of technologies by which information about that body can be more accurately and more easily retrieved.

In contrast to this, and in a manner consistent with the definition of illness as an occurrence which is more in the body than of it, aetiology in Tabwa medicine refers not to the cause of the disease as such, but to the cause of the *particular illness occurrence*. This is taken to be the bodily form of a particular event; the unintelligible version of a message meant to be realised in speech. Explanations thus have to do with *why* so-and-so, a unique individual, became ill at a specific point in time; and as with an accident or with the weather, the reasons lie not within the occurrence, but outside it. Questions of aetiology must be answered in social-historical terms, not in biological or physiological ones.

In this aetiological perspective, illness becomes an important sub-category of a more general class of misfortunes which includes bad accidents, continually strained relations with one's friends and neighbours, and lack of success in hunting, fishing, farming, beer brewing and commerce. Divination is the only means by which may be discovered the causes of occurrences such as these.

Though in theory every instance of illness must have an aetiology, people do not concern themselves with the causes of minor diseases. When I asked Kalwele, a friend and Tulunga practitioner, if one would divine into the cause of *kibakula* ('ringworm of the scalp'), he gave me a rather jaundiced look and dryly asked, 'Would you divine for lice?' If pressed, people will say that such illnesses 'come from God'. By this is meant that they are part of the normal course of human events; and it is said that children who do not suffer occasional, transient fevers will not have the 'strength of the blood' (*ngu'vu ya damu*) which will enable them to grow into healthy adults.

Questions of aetiology do arise, however, with reference to illness occurrences which display one or more of three characteristics that make them problematic. These are:

1. Unresponsiveness to medical treatment. An illness which fails 'to heed' (*kusikia*) herbal medicines may become problematic even though it is not particularly disabling.
2. Unintelligibility. An illness which cannot be classified into one of the secondary diagnostic categories may prompt aetiologic questioning.
3. Dangerousness. An illness, whether acute or chronic, is always problematic when it poses a threat to life or is particularly disabling.

People summarise these characteristics more poetically when they speak of what motivates one to divine. They say that one sees how one's counterpart (*mwenzako*) suffers, how he gets no sleep at night, how he feels his entire body; and so one goes to divine, that he might be comfortable and sleep well.

Recourse to divination is *always* made for those illnesses which are dangerous. Divination would also be the appropriate response to an illness which displayed a combination of the first two problematising features. However, with illnesses which manifest only one of these, social and financial factors strongly influence the choice to divine and the timing of divination.

Diagnosis, literally 'recognition', of illnesses of the problematic type(s) outlined above must include a recognition of their non-physiological sources if treatment based upon the diagnosis is to be effective. Without such recognition, medicines will not be 'felt or heeded' (*kusikilika*) in the body, and cure will be impossible. Inversely, cure is the ultimate proof that the illness truly has been recognised. The recovery of the patient relies not only upon the correct classification of the problematic illness into the proper diagnostic category, but also upon correct analysis of the occurrence as part of a set or sequence of social circumstances or events.

Apart from God (*Mungu*), there are three types of aetiology, each of which represents a different sort of discontinuity between the patient or members of his family and the social environment. Each is associated with certain precipitating events and with a particular prognosis, the two of which place the occurrence in a historical context. Each type of aetiology is treated by a specific circumstantial therapy whose aim is not the direct relief of symptoms as such, but is rather the restoration of proper relations in social life. Each type of aetiology gives to the illness occurrences attributed to it a different meaning. The three types are as follows.

Mizimu/Mipasi

Mizimu are those of a person's dead kin who act as benefactors, and to whom the person expected to appeal in times of misfortune. S/he is also expected to remember them with small gifts of money or beer when things go well. As people say, these antecedents are not many and are not far removed, genealogically, from the person her/himself. They are usually mother (and mother's sisters, also called mother), mother's brother, mother's mother, mother's mother's brother, father, and siblings of the person. Illnesses derived from these are punishments for breaches in intra-familial obligations to the living and the dead. In theory, no illness derived from them may be fatal.

Pepo

Pepo are a group of non-human beings whose arrival in the area is relatively recent. Unlike *mizimu*, *pepo* are spirits who have never been human. There are possessing and non-possessing types, the former of which first arrived during the thirties, while the latter arrived as late as the forties and fifties.[1] *Pepo* are sent by *mizimu* to confer some specific benefit, such as fertility, knowledge of medicines, hunting and fishing skills, etc. They also confer general protection and well-being. Illnesses deriving from them are either devices meant to prompt the establishment of a shrine, or punishment for breaches of intrafamilial and/or spiritual obligations. Like *mizimu*, *pepo* usually do not kill through illness. However, they may do so if their wishes and warnings are ignored.

Vibanda and *Walozi*

Vibanda are avenging ghosts of those who may be, but are not necessarily, kin of the patient. Revenge may be sought by one who has been murdered through the sorcery of the patient or members of his family; by a kinsman who has himself been so murdered and whose death has not been properly acted upon by the family; by one whose spouse has remarried without first having been inherited by a kinsman and thus properly cleansed; and by an infant or child who (as a ghost) has been transferred to a household other than its natal home through the adultery of one of its parents. *Walozi* are sorcerers whose jealousy of the well-being of others, or whose bitterness over conflicts with them, causes them to employ medicines which kill or disable through illness.

Illnesses derived from *vibanda* or *walozi* are very dangerous and represent the complete social incompatibility of two or more persons. If proper steps are not taken, these illnesses will inevitably be fatal. Illnesses derived from sorcery are especially significant because of the presumed relentlessness of the force which underlies them.

A complete aetiological explanation of a given illness occurrence must take into account two factors in addition to the various types of aetiology outlined above. These are the personal and social history of the patient; and the seriousness and, sometimes, the form of the illness itself. The function of divination is the formulation of such an explanation, one whose plausibility is evaluated partly in terms of the extent to which the three factors are properly coordinated.

DIVINATION: DESCRIPTION
Types of Divination

The three principal types of divination practised by lakeside Batabwa are *kashekesheke*, Tulunga and Bulumbu. *Kashekesheke* is said to be the oldest type, though it is also the least spectacular. Tulunga, a newer method, is also indigenous to the area and is the most highly regarded of the three. Bulumbu is one of the varieties of *pepo* which came to the area in the thirties. It now seems to have displaced *kashekesheke* as the more ordinary type of divination – the divination of first recourse.

While a number of different varieties of *kashekesheke* divination have been described to me, I have seen only one, and know of only one practitioner who lives and works in the area of Mpala. This man, Mukupa, employs a medicine-filled *inchia* (Grimm's duiker, *Sylvicapra grimmia*)[2] horn which he places in the middle of a dried, hollowed-out gourd held in the palm of his hand. Other medicines, rubbed at the time of his initiation into small incisions (*machanjo*) made at his temples, on his forehead, and between his thumbs and forefingers, enable him to see the causes of illnesses in dreams. After having such dreams, Mukupa is prepared for the actual session in which he questions his apparatus, and through it the family, about the aetiology of the illness occurrence. As questions are put to it, the horn moves about the gourd, indicating a negative response. When a positive response is reached, the horn stands upright in the centre of the gourd.

Though different in the specific devices they employ, all types of *kashekesheke* use the same structure of response. Free movement is negative, while sticking or stopping is positive. Divination using axe heads spun on

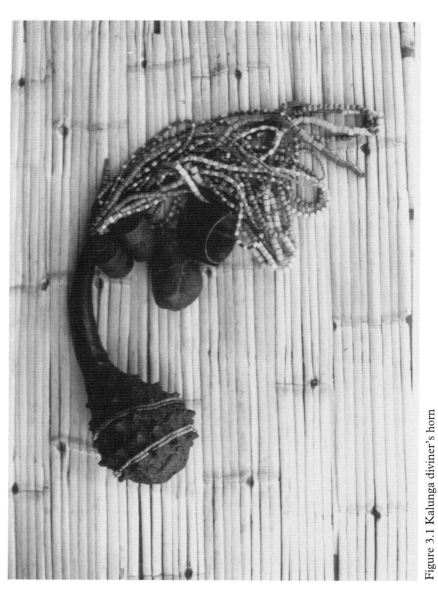

Figure 3.1 Kalunga diviner's horn

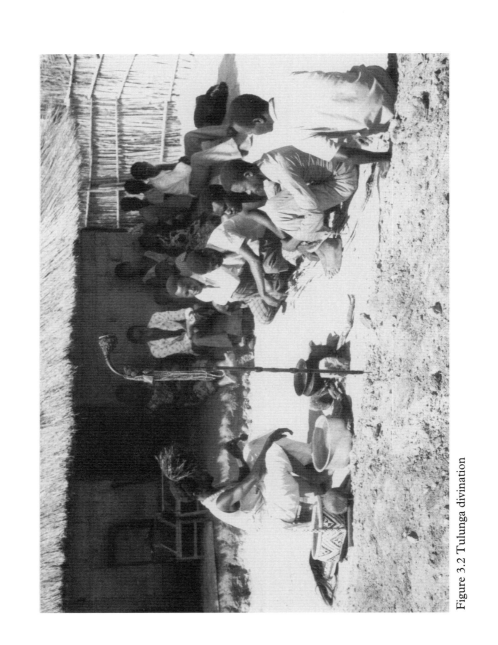

Figure 3.2 Tulunga divination

the ground, objects which slide down strings, and objects rubbed on a board are all known. Similar types of oracles called by the same name have been described among the Luba (Burton 1961: 65).

With Tulunga, as with *kashekesheke*, medicines rubbed into incisions on the head and hands enable the diviner to receive in dreams whatever beings (human or non-human) are causing the illness occurrence he is to diagnose. A medicine-filled *swala* horn (Bohor reedbuck, *Redunca redunca*), kept at the head of the bed while sleeping, confers these same powers and also offers protection against the fiercer of the aetiological agents (such as *vibanda*), who, in their vengefulness, may kill the diviner himself. The horn, with its powers, is the *kalunga* from which this group of diviners derives its name.

The morning after having conclusively dreamt of the cause of the illness, the Tulunga diviner meets with the family, at either his house or theirs, and uses boiling water as the oracular device through which he presents the case. His *kalunga* is balanced upon a carved cane, which has been set upright in the ground by means of a spike. Water freshly drawn from lake or river is put in a clay cooking pot (provided by the family). The pot is put on the fire, and the opposing sides of the brim are rubbed with *nkula* (red, powdered bark of the *mwenge* tree, possibly *Pterocarpus tincturus*, also called *mukula* and *mukulungu*) and *pemba* (kaolin), respectively. As the water heats, a medicine-filled *lukusu* seed is placed in it. When it is boiling the diviner poses a question and plunges his hand into the water in order to withdraw the seed. When the response of the oracle is negative, the seed is easily removed. When the response is positive, either the seed sticks to the bottom of the pot, or the diviner senses the water as hot; the seed is withdrawn using a small drinking gourd.

With Bulumbu divination, dreaming may or may not be practised prior to the divination session. In either case, at the time of the session itself, the diviner's assistant, the *kitobo* or *kapamba*, enters the room or house of the Bulumbu spirit, calls it by shaking its ceremonial rattles and then leaves. Shortly thereafter, the diviner shows signs of impending possession,[3] and enters the room to assume both the garb and the identity of his divinatory spirit. It is the spirit which then poses questions about the illness and makes the final aetiological pronouncement.

Process of Divination

The types of divination are thus quite different from one another in terms of the devices which each employs. Various factors may influence the selection of a particular type of divination and of a given diviner. However, the progress of a divination itself is similar for all these.

When selecting a type of divination, people make their choice through a consideration of several different factors. Among these is the nature of the illness itself. Its seriousness, as measured by the suffering of the patient and/

or by the threat it poses to life, will influence the type of divination sought.

In addition, the patient's and his family's general assessment of the social situation surrounding the illness also has bearing upon the selection of a diviner. While the illness may not itself pose an immediate threat to life, such a threat may exist in the environment in the form of open conflicts or unspoken but suspected grudges. The presence of such breaches affects the perception of the seriousness of the illness and thereby influences choice of divinatory method.

In general Bulumbu and *kashekesheke* diviners constitute the first line of defence. Their diagnoses are sought for minor illnesses which seem to take an unduly long time to remit, chronic or recurrent minor ailments, and non-threatening illnesses of children. Neither type of divination is thought to be as accurate as Tulunga, and both are less expensive, costing 20–30 *makuta* instead of 50–100 or 180 *makuta*, the price for Tulunga divination. Bulumbu diviners are also said to have a decided tendency to attribute all illnesses to *mizimu* or to *pepo*, and to ignore *vibanda* and *walozi* when making their diagnoses. This is attributed to the fact that Bulumbu gain supplementary income from the arrangement of *pepo* and that, in any case, they are powerless against the more deadly type of causative agent.

Tulunga diviners, therefore, tend to be sought in cases where the illness itself is more life-threatening, or where the family wishes to take into consideration all possible aetiological sources. Tulunga may also be called to give a second opinion, to confirm or deny a previous diagnosis made by another kind of diviner.

While the type of divination sought is influenced by the general factors outlined above. the selection of the particular practitioner of any type is influenced by more mundane features of the situation. Among these are the relative fame of a diviner, his proximity, availability, fees, and so forth. For an important divination, the family may try to select an individual to whom they are relatively unknown; that is, someone who comes from another community, or a person who has not divined for them before. The person's ignorance of them and of their history becomes the device by which the family create conditions meant to underwrite the divination's truth.

Once the diviner has been selected, the process of divination is begun by 'sending the arrow' (*kupeleka mshale*). The arrow is a one-*likuta* coin, which has replaced the real arrowhead which was traditionally employed. It is placed upon the ground and invoked by the individuals into whose social circumstances the divination is to be made (for instance, by the patient or his agent in the case of adults, or by the parents in the case of a child, and by those close relatives who may also be concerned in either case). In the invocation are cited all possible causes of the illness, such as adultery, breach of intrafamilial obligations, negligence of obligations to a spirit, sorcery, etc. After its citation, each possible aetiology is instructed to present itself to the diviner if it is indeed that which is causing the illness. At the conclusion of the invocation, the arrow is lightly spat upon.

When the arrow has been properly invoked by all concerned parties, it is taken to the diviner's home, or presented to him or to his agent as they are encountered elsewhere (for example, passing on the road). In all cases, a one-word statement of the reason for the divination may be stated at this time (such as illness, bad dreams, or poor luck), but more information than this is never given.

With Bulumbu, the arrow is presented to the *kitobo* or *kapamba* and not to the diviner himself. The *kitobo* then places it upon or within the *mputo* basket, which is the divining spirit's residence. With *kashekesheke* or Tulunga, the arrow may be given to the diviner himself or to a member of his household. It is not passed from hand to hand, but is first placed upon the ground from whence it is taken up and placed at the head of the diviner's bed, for dreaming upon.

In those cases where dreaming is to be done prior to the session, the diviner prepares himself and the situation by invoking his medicines or his spirits, and by invoking his own dead antecedents, so that these may help him receive quickly a coherent dream of the cause of the illness (and sometimes also of its diagnostic category). Dreaming is done at night, and a number of diviners make it a practice to sleep apart from their spouses at this time. Bulumbu diviners sleep in the rooms of their spirits, and Tulunga sleep with their horns at the head of the bed. Tulunga and *kashekesheke* diviners may also smoke dried leaf medicines mixed with tobacco before sleeping. The subsequent dream will not only show to the diviner the category of the illness's cause (whether *mizimu, pepo, kibanda* or *mulozi*), but will also reveal to him the specific events which provoked the causative agent.

After the diviner has had a conclusive dream (that is, the next day or the day after), the session is held at the home of either the patient or the diviner, in either the morning or the afternoon. Those present as witnesses usually include representatives of both affinal sides of the family, as well as friends whose counsel is valued. The patient himself need not be present, but the presence of older kin is advisable, as the cause of the illness may be an event or affair of which the patient or younger kin know nothing.

During the session, the diviner will go through a list of all possible aetiologic agents. Ideally, and in those cases where the diviner has a hypothesis fairly clearly formed in his own mind, he will rhetorically ask questions about and eliminate certain possibilities, using his dream as the basis for his analysis, and his oracle as confirmation of it. He may also ask general questions of the family, and in those cases where the diviner is less certain, this may almost take the form of a diagnostic checklist. It is customary during this phase for the family to conceal some aspects of the information and to distort others, as a means of testing the diviner's accuracy.

Once the first series of questions has been run through, the diviner presents his hypothesis. This may be very sketchy, taking the form of a parable, or of a minimally structured representation of the situation such as one would see in a dream (for example, two women, the older of whom is pursuing the younger, or a snake looking down into a room from the wall above, etc.). The diviner is not expected to know all the details, and it is at this point that the family supply the necessary information by thinking about how the situational structure applies to them and by remembering the episode of their history to which it might refer. It is inappropriate for the family to attempt to deceive the diviner at this stage, although they may and do refuse hypotheses which they cannot honestly find to be applicable to themselves.

This is both the climax and the conclusion of the session. During this stage, as people produce their shares of the information, the family usually discuss among themselves the meanings and implications of the hypothesis that has been offered. They also discuss among themselves and with the diviner the course of action appropriate to their situation, should the diviner's definition of that situation be accepted. This course of action includes the circumstantial therapy which corresponds to the particular type of aetiology discovered.

When discussion has finished, the diviner is paid for his work. If they are not in complete agreement with him, the family will be tactful nevertheless and their most critical analyses of the diagnosis will not be made until later, in private discussions. In cases of uncertainty, or at the diviner's suggestion, an oracular beer may be brewed. This is corn and millet beer, which differs from ordinary beer (*kibuku*) only in that it is invoked at the first stage of brewing, when the grains are soaked. Dedicated (*kupupa*) to the dead antecedent named by the diviner, the outcome of the brewing constitutes a communication from that kinsman. Potent beer confirms the aetiologic diagnosis. Beer which spoils disproves it.

If they are dissatisfied with the results, the family may call upon another diviner. If they are satisfied, they will turn their attention to the ways and means by which the necessary circumstantial therapy may be undertaken. This includes consideration of such practical problems as price, cost and availability of ingredients, availability of necessary family members, and the willingness of those people and of the patient to undertake the therapy, etc. As with the selection of the diviner and type of divination, the seriousness of the illness itself influences the decision: the more dangerously ill the patient, the more likely the family to make great efforts to arrange with speed for the appropriate therapy.

The diviner who made the diagnosis is frequently asked to undertake the circumstantial therapy, but this need not be so, and another practitioner may be selected. Similarly, the diviner, if he is also a herbalist, may be asked to treat the patient, or the family may continue herbal therapy with another practitioner. Whatever the course selected, the ultimate proof of the divination is the cure of the patient, and an accurate divination (of all but illnesses caused by sorcery) should result in an amelioration of the patient's condition beginning not too long after the divination is made.

DIVINATION: ANALYSIS

The complex moment of social drama that is divination cannot be fully understood unless it is analysed from several different points of view. The functional perspective reveals the role which divination plays in the unfolding of the crises which occur in ongoing social relations. A psychosocial perspective reveals the role which divination can operate to bring into harmony people's inner states and outward, social circumstances. Finally an examination of the field and function of speech and language in divination draws attention to the juncture between the body as subject and the body subjected to events that are the expressions of the desires of an other.

Functional Perspective

People liken the diviner (*mfumu*) to the clinical technician. As the clinician uses his microscope to detect the presence of parasites not visible to the naked eye, so the diviner employs his extraordinary powers of perception to see into the social circumstances surrounding an illness and to give them definition. Though they say that the *mfumu* reveals aetiologic agents which would otherwise be unknowable, people also say that he renders 'intelligible' (*kujulikana*) a given illness occurrence. In this respect, divination is the logically consistent extension of the discernment that is diagnosis.

Inasmuch as illnesses for which people seek divination are those which are problematic, they are illnesses which are extraordinary, both in terms of the disruption they create in the lives of patients and of their families, and in terms of the questions to which they give rise. In the invocation which is the most meaningful part of 'sending the arrow', concerned individuals have listed all aetiologies of which they can conceive. Though these possible causes have been stated in general categorical terms, the persons making the statements may also have specifically in mind various historic episodes or incidents that might have provoked one of the possible agents. They do not, however, have a clear idea *which* of these is responsible for the specific illness occurrence at hand.

In divining, the *mfumu*'s dreams enable him to select from among the various possibilities whose relative importance is uncertain. He presents a hypothesis that organises a combination of factors, and thus establishes priorities which make some events and circumstances more significant than others. The *mfumu* tells laypeople which part of their recent social history is sound and which is sense, and thereby provides them with a structure, a meaning, about which they may make specific decisions.

As they discuss the results of divination, the family are not only considering those past events now seen to be of special significance, they are also determining action for the immediate future. The correspondence between aetiologic agent and circumstantial therapy means that each actor can surmise what his role will be, should the diviner's hypothesis be accepted. The family's final judgement of the divination thus consists of an evaluation not only of the internal logic of the diagnosis, but also of the appropriateness of the future interactions implicit within it.

What thus becomes apparent is the potentially critical role of divination in social dramas, those intermittent periods and processes of crisis in ongoing social process. Divination is a moment of consultation and conscious reflection, and can be the point at which the choice between breach and reconciliation is made. Tabwa diviners are aware of this, and frequently speak of themselves as arbiters of disputes and maintainers of proper social order. They are, as Kalwele put it, like judges (*bazuzi*), and their function is the arbitration (*mamzi*) of disputes. In fact, the judges of the local court frequently refer to diviners cases they consider to be too delicate to be handled by the law (such as sorcery accusations involving members of a single lineage group).

Diviners resident within a community are especially scrupulous in this regard, and take care to render decisions which serve to uphold well-known rules. Mumbyoto, for example, has said that he tries to avoid attributing illness to sorcery, because this only leads to trouble. Even when he recognises that there is a sorcerer in the family, he will not say so. Instead, he will tell the other family members that the illnesses are due to *mizimu* who are angered at the way in which one of their descendants is being treated by his kin. To them, he will recommend resolution of internal conflicts and reconciliation of family members. He will then speak to the sorcerer privately, telling this person that he and his activities have been recognised.

Laypeople are also aware of the scrupulousness of local diviners. It is a truism almost amounting to a joke that they will rarely cite sorcery as a cause of illness; and, even if they do, they will not name the sorcerer responsible. For this reason, local practitioners are somewhat suspect as frauds, and itinerant diviners frequently enjoy great popularity when they first arrive in a given area. They have nothing to lose by openly citing sorcery and naming names, and initially are seen to be very truthful and to have great power. Eventually, however, the disruptive effects of their divinations are felt within the community, and they come to be regarded as imposters, whose only aim is making money.

Psychosocial Perspective

In his article on Bantu magico-religious thought (1971: 178), Luc de Heusch comments that such systems 'are situated at the hinge between psychology and sociology, at the point of the spirit where ... systems of communication are built'. As a practice, divination is the gateway to both 'magic' and 'religion'. It is the practical, social counterpart of de Heusch's spiritual point; the hinge between the covert consciousness of individuals and the overt features of social circumstances.

Illnesses which raise questions about aetiology are those which have divided an individual from his social environment, or which have given that division a concrete, physiological form. While the sociological aspect of this discontinuity is depicted in the three types of aetiological agent, no significant divination would be complete if it did not include a fairly detailed examination and summation of the specific circumstances which surrounded the particular agents' actions. These circumstances include the feelings, attitudes and behaviour of the patient and those close to him.

People use a number of terms to refer to emotional or subjective states. Of these, the most commonly used are *uruma* (pity or compassion), *asira* (anger or hate), *wivu* (envy, or the most profound aversion possible for another human being), *woga* (fear), *haya* (shame, timidity), *furaha* (joy) and *uchungu* (bitterness, grief). These constitute the broadest markings-out of emotional terrain.

The two emotions which figure most prominently in the unfolding of illness occurrences are *uruma* and *asira*. *Uruma* is the emotion of nurturance. It is what prompts people to share food with one another. It is the emotion which makes a mother give in to her child's crying, and tend to nurse him beyond weaning age. It is the feeling which is appropriate to relations of kinship and friendship; and it is the emotion which prompts people to care for each other in illness, no matter how disgusting or frightening the illness might be. *Woga* in the illness setting is an adjunct of *uruma*. It is the combination of pity and of the fear of death which prompts people to seek divination, and to settle the differences which divination might reveal.

Asira is the will to destroy. It is the opposite of *uruma*, and it lies at the heart of conflict. *Asira* is clearly manifest in the refusal of nurturance, and is closely related to *wivu*, the active desire and effort that a person should die, into which it may also develop. It is a feeling which contradicts relations of kinship and friendship, and it is allied to sorcery and curses. If a person is ill, the presence of *asira* in his soul or the souls (*roho*) of those near him is, in itself, sufficient to make the illness worse. In addition, *asira* may indirectly cause illness by creating an atmosphere in the household or village into which sorcerers may easily enter and under cover of which they may freely practise.

The situation at the time of divination is one in which individuals have become divided from one another in ways which may be subtle or open. People may have secret anger, ranging from hurt feelings to grudges, which prevents them from communicating honestly and openly, despite the fact that superficial contact and interaction are maintained. Or they may actually have quarrelled, permitting *asira* to replace *uruma* completely within the familial group.

All of the types of aetiology, even the most minor, can be related to such divisions. *Mizimu* and *pepo* punish intrafamilial quarrelling with illness. Dead antecedents (*mizimu*) respond either to the quarrel itself or to the complaints voiced afterward by one or another party to the dispute.[4] *Pepo* are similarly responsive, though their punishment is a general reaction to the wrong as such, rather than a defence of the wronged party. *Vibanda* (avenging ghosts) derive from earlier quarrels, and punish destruction with destruction. Finally, sorcerers not only operate through and because of *asira*, but are pleased by its presence, and take advantage of it to work their evil deeds.

Thus, at the time of divination, discrepancies between the overt state of social relations and the covert state of emotional affairs are brought to light. The socially determined, circumstantial therapies necessary to proper treatment depend upon a reopening of appropriate lines of communication, the restoration of a union between the overt and the hidden aspects of social being. People must confess their grievances and resolve their differences, so that the invocation for the ceremony will be accepted by the *mizimu* and so that the atmosphere will be closed to incursions by sorcerers. Each of these is a precondition essential to success.

In this way, through the process of divination, a kind of psychosocial therapy which is also a kind of learning can be said to take place. It is not a treatment aimed at adapting the individual, in and over the long term, to his general environment. Rather, it is a therapy directed at the whole family group, whether members of the patient's own lineage, or his affines. Its aim is the more immediate one of resolving conflicts on both the social and the emotional levels. It employs the pity and fear caused by illness as its motive forces, and the rules of social order as its guidelines. Its contribution to life as lived is the greater knowledge people gain of one another.

Field and Function of Speech in the Body as Subject

Our understanding of divination is further enriched by an analysis which takes as its key the roles of speech and silence in the constitution of being. Problematic illness can be described as a set of circumstances in which alienation exists on a number of different levels. Physiologically, the ill person is alienated from his body, whose capacities no longer meet the demands of his will. Socially, there may be alienation in the relationships among family, neighbours or others. Certainly, the questions surrounding problematic illness suggest or provoke alienation where none may have actively existed before, if only because the resistance of the illness indicates that someone in the environment is alienated from the subject. Spiritually, there may be alienation between the patient (or those responsible for him) and his (or their) *mizimu*.

Thus, where there should be 'silence', in the featureless condition of health, there is instead expression in the form of the symptoms felt by the patient. Inversely, and at a corresponding point in social life, what should be plain speaking has been replaced by reticence. The aim of divination is to give voice to the latter, and, by this deciphering, to efface the former.

In the context of medical practice, this is more than an ethnographic commonplace. Here, it is the gateway to grasping the absolute importance of the field and function of speech as constitutive of being-as-identity in a setting where there is no other significant kind of being in the world. As such, speech is the objective correlative of death in abeyance; that is, through divination, speech is the abeyance of death itself, at least in theory.

People make reference in a number of different ways to the physiological alternatives present during incapacitating illness. Sick people who nevertheless continue to fulfil some of their obligations (such as working in their fields) will say 'I do this by the strength of my soul' (*Nafanya hii ya ngu'vu ya roho yangu*), or 'I tighten my soul' (*Nakaza roho yangu*). Similarly, a person who is completely incapacitated by illness, one who has given up work or who is no longer able to attend to his own bodily needs without help, will be said to be 'without self-control' or 'self-mastery' (*hajiwezi*). All of these phrases express the battle between the willing mind and the unable body. Where in health, determination can be deed, in problematic illness, the division between the two is always more or less evident.[5]

Social alienation may be described as lying between the person and those around him. On this model, the problematic subjectivities at issue are those of the others, whose anger is not directly accessible. Concealed by the silent veil characteristic of grudges or jealousy, the motives of these subjects are not open to modification. Indeed, by this very concealment, they are preserved from change, whether induced (as in conflict resolution) or spontaneous (as in the emergence of the pity likely to arise as a result of interaction).

Spirits, when alienated, actually move closer to the person. Far from having abandoned him, they are said to have in fact 'come near' (*wanamukaribia* or *wanamujongea*). When he is in proper relation to them, a person's *mizimu* and/or *pepo* will communicate with him in speech, either through the special consciousness of dreams or in the incarnated consciousness of possession. Should a person fail to respond to such communication (usually an instruction), the *mizimu/pepo* will cease to speak to him, and will makes its wishes known through illness. The patient will not dream of them, and cannot recover until their wishes have been articulated through divination. People say that *mizimu/pepo* employ illness in this way when they have seen that a person 'has no ears' (*hana masikio*) to hear their speech.

In both KiSwahili and KiTabwa one term (*kusikia* (KS), *kuuwa* (KT)) is used to mean 'to feel', 'to hear', 'to understand', and 'to heed'. In problematic illness, then, the heeding body is actively heeding the will of an other. While in health person 'feels nothing' (*hasikii kitu*) other than hunger (the only bodily sensation appropriate to health), in illness the perception of symptoms prevails. The body as subject, an entity at the threshold of language and its reciprocities, becomes the body subjected; constrained to express, through inappropriate sensations, a subjectivity that is both other to and alienated from the patient or his kin. Divination intervenes to decipher an unintelligible message, and the effectiveness of such decipherment is underwritten by a relationship between speech and being which spans the length and breadth of life.

Speech is associated with continuity over time. The KiTabwa term *kubanga* means both 'to speak to' and 'to interact with'. The east, the auspicious direction from which the dead return to be reborn, is *kabanga*. Their return or the onset of pregnancy is frequently heralded in the dreams through which they communicate with the living.

Speech is identified with life, with the transition to integrated from disintegrative being. An infant's first cry proves that its soul has passed into its body from the placenta (*kitanda cha mtoto*), the child's organic counterpart. The placenta is an object which is simultaneously 'the child himself' (*mtoto mwenyewe*) and a thing that is 'just blood' (*damu tu*) or 'just filth' (*uchafu tu*), destined first to be abandoned by the infant, and then buried by the midwives and left to rot. Though still less than a person, the infant who has cried has made his first step into human existence. Later, in the process of *kumusumbula mtoto*, the infant is 'matured' (*kukomweshwa*) so that his body may be impermeable to the consequences of adults' sexual intercourse and be susceptible of treatment with medicines. His cry after the process marks its success, the fortunate completion of another dangerous passage. Should the process be unsuccessful, the infant's failure to cry indicates his impending death.

Speech is also a significant element in the superhuman overcoming of conventional death. *Wafumu* (diviners) and members of the secret society Bulindu are said to have consumed so many medicines to preserve themselves that they cannot die a natural death. Without the performance by other adepts of a process which undoes the medicines (*kushindula*), such persons will physically rot while still speaking coherently. The graphic realism people use when describing this situation presents the striking image of a body devastated by putrefaction, stench and maggots, from which continues to flow the thin, clear stream of the human voice; pyrrhic victory over death.

Speech, then, constitutes all that is cultural (artefactual), conscious and continuous. It is associated with the transcendence of that which can be projected or imagined over that which is; with the transcendence of becoming over being. In each of the areas outlined above, speech has been the means by which the actual state is dynamically connected to a potential, presently non-existent, or imperfectly perceptible one. The association of such transcendence with speech is underscored in descriptions of prophetic dreams, which, like all dreams, have a verbal and a visual element. When subsequent events prove the truth of a dream, people say the circumstances of the dream have 'been completed' (*kutimilika*). What has become and now is has filled the outline set by what was dreamt.[6]

Problematic illness thus may be seen as the reverse of this state. Disintegrative being transcends integrated becoming. Speech, the stuff of which humanity is made, ceases, and is replaced by an unintelligible communication which has the threatening form of bodily symptoms. In so far as one can decipher the symptoms and articulate the history which surrounds them, in so far as one can make of these an intelligible narrative, one can set free the body of the patient, making possible his cure. Such restoration is the task of the diviner.

The diviner conducts his work by interposing his consciousness in each of the areas in which alienation has disrupted appropriate relations. He is unrelated to all parties, human and non-human, who are involved in the illness situation, and employs a consciousness which resembles but also differs from both human and non-human consciousness. By the time of divination, the diviner has communicated with the *mizimu*, *pepo*, *walozi* and *vibanda* who may be responsible for the illness, but who are unwilling to speak. The diviner puts into words the expression muffled in the heeding body, translating its aetiological, sociological, psychological and physiological aspects into rule-conditioned messages. His hypothesis makes possible the restoration of proper social and spiritual distances, by promoting the airing of grudges and the performance of appropriate circumstantial therapies.

The diviner and the process of divination can thus restore the supremacy of integrity and speech over disintegration and symptoms. They can thereby provide an outline for the restoration of the body to health, its normal, 'silent' or featureless condition. However, as in any medical system, it is actually the body itself which has the last word.

4

THE DEFILE OF THE SIGNIFIER:
FROM SYMPTOM TO LIFE HISTORY

While illnesses may be general, it is actually individuals who get sick, and it is here, in the lived experience of particular persons, that the ill body's communicative capacities contribute to a process of personal historisation. In problematic illness, the body-as-subject becomes the body subjected to the will of an other whose identity and motives must be discovered through divination if the patient is to be cured.

In the context of divination and the new understandings it creates, the body thus becomes a defile through which signification passes, an opening onto agents and aspects or areas of life which, though unseen, nevertheless have been exerting a powerful effect on events. Even if the illness is cured, in this role as defile, the body thus plays an active part in the development of what may turn out to have been a turning point in people's lives. Such a point is one at which the past events to which the illness is related come to be recognised and assimilated into the present moment, but newly recast into the roles they will have to play if the future is to be as people would wish.

The illness of Kaputa's daughter, Malaika, in 1977 served such a purpose for Kaputa and Kalwa, his wife. Describing it will allow us to see not only how illness intervenes in life histories, but how the body-as-subject actively participates in the process of historisation.

KAPUTA'S DAUGHTER'S ILLNESS

Early in 1977, Kaputa's daughter Malaika,[1] then nearly three years old, developed two swellings on the back of her head. These fluctuated when touched, then emitted pus, and finally became lesions which would not heal. I attempted treatment with penicillin, and the lesions decreased in size only to return anew. Creams, ointments and antibiotic washes all failed, as did the traditional medicines prepared by members of Kaputa's family. Despite our combined efforts, the lesions continued to discharge water and pus and to itch.

While the persistence of the lesions was vexing, they were not considered to be life-threatening; Kaputa and his wife, Kalwa, did not feel that curing them was a pressing goal. In March, a sister of Kalwa's and her child died at

Kala, Kalwa's birthplace, and Kalwa left Mpala with Malaika to attend the funeral.

They were gone a month, and when she returned, Kalwa said that her own relatives had attempted to treat Malaika with a series of penicillin injections, but that this had availed them nothing. They had then tried traditional medicines, but these hadn't been successful either.

Every morning, Kalwa would press the swellings to force out the pus, and then would sprinkle powdered plant medicine on them, but as of May–June 1977 the lesions remained unchanged. At this time, Kaputa remarked that, since the lesions had now endured almost six months, he and Kalwa were beginning to think that they ought to divine into the cause of the illness, but that they hadn't the money to pay for the divination.

A few days later we tried again to treat the swellings, this time using some newly acquired tetracycline capsules. After five days of this treatment, the pus and swelling stopped. The medication ran out shortly afterwards, but, even in its absence only water was discharged, and by the end of the month the lesions were healed, though hair had not yet begun to grow in these areas.

Just as these lesions were beginning to heal, however, Malaika began to have other symptoms. Every morning upon awaking, she would scratch, and swellings would then appear all over her body, sometimes including her face or the area around her eyes. The swellings would disappear after half an hour or so, but the itching would remain. These symptoms are those of the illness *masoli*, whose characteristics conform to those of the Western category 'urticaria' or 'hives.'

I suspected these to be symptomatic of bilharziasis, and suggested that Kalwa take Malaika to the dispensary for tests. Kalwa took her, but the nurse said he was not testing that day and the next day he left for Moba, site of the district office and hospital, located some thirty miles to the south of Mpala.

While he was away, Malaika began having extremely high nocturnal fevers (*homa kali*) accompanied by mild convulsions like *petit mal* seizures (*kustuka-stuka*). The fevers declined during the day although her temperature was never normal. Treatment with chloroquine (as of malaria) resulted in some remission, but this was followed by the return of high fever. During this time, the itching and transient swelling continued as before.

We all decided that Malaika and her mother should go with Allen and me to Kalemie for treatment at the hospital there. However, due to the gasoline shortage that accompanied the Shaba war of 1977, we could not get away as planned and, in the meantime, the temporary remission of her illness ended. Early in July (3 or 4 July), her fever became so high that her parents sat up all night watching over her. Her skin was burning hot, and she had repeated *petit mal* seizures.

Still convinced that the illness was bilharziasis, I suggested next that

Kaputa ask the newly returned nurse if he did not have some ambilhar (niridazole) tablets, despite the fact that he was not officially practising medicine. The nurse had none, and not unreasonably Kaputa was unwilling to scrape some pills together by asking other people in the village if they didn't have a few extra tablets.

Two days after the onset of this second set of fevers (Wednesday 6 July 1977) someone came to the house where Kaputa was working with me[2] to tell him that Malaika had been stricken with 'convulsions' (*ndege*). He left immediately. When he returned, he said he had found that she had not had a complete attack of *ndege*. Instead, she had been shuddering with violent *petit mal* seizures, and his mother had successfully controlled them by throwing medicines over Malaika with a broom (*kumusampula*).

I asked Kaputa if he and Kalwa had considered going for divination (*maaguzo*). He replied that they had been thinking of doing this, but had no money to pay for it. When I offered to advance him the money from his salary, he said he'd think about it. Shortly afterward he said he would borrow the money from our cook, Mupila, his classificatory brother-in-law.

Kaputa said he chose to arrange the matter this way because he still had a number of large debts around Mpala which he hoped to pay off with his salary. If he continually borrowed against it, there would be nothing left and after my final departure from Mpala (then imminent) everyone would mock him for having such debts when he had previously been so well off. Ever since they had been working together, he and Mupila had been close friends. One zaire would not matter between them; Mupila would not mind if he was not paid even though Kaputa's other creditors might be.

On the evening of Thursday 7 July, Kaputa prepared the arrow, and dropped it off at the diviner's on his way to the house. The diviner had not been home at the time, however, so Kaputa had to return the next day to have him set the time for the divination.

That same afternoon, Kaputa located some traders who were in Mpala waiting for dried fish, and who were selling ambilhar at three zaires for ten pills. He found this price (30 k the tablet)[3] to be terribly expensive (it was three times the 1976 price), but it was better than the other prices we'd heard (250 k the tablet); and it was the only source. I advanced Kaputa the three zaires, he purchased the medicine that evening, and began administering it according to the instructions that night.

The next day he came to work without having stopped at the diviner's. I was disappointed to hear that Malaika's fever and convulsions had been just the same, despite the niridazole. Kaputa planned to stop by the diviner's on his way home at noon, and to let me know immediately if the time set for the session was to be that afternoon. He laughed when I suggested that it might be better, in any case, to wait until the next day, because the illness might subside and then one's attitude might be different. He said that while he agreed that one's attitude towards the divination would be different, he nevertheless wished to go ahead with it as rapidly as possible.

That evening Kaputa came to the house to say that the diviner had set 10:30 or 11:00 a.m. the following morning as the time for the session to take place. Kalwa arrived shortly thereafter, bringing their daughter. The baby's rectal temperature was 39.5°C (103.1°F), and her mother said it was characteristic of Malaika's daytime condition, though her temperature was usually much higher at night. At this time, I gave her chloroquine to reduce the possibility of inflammation, and gave her mother mild antihistamines to give Malaika, in conjunction with the niridazole beginning the next day.

Commentary

The above description of the symptoms which led up to and surrounded the divination into Malaika's illness demonstrates the equivocal relationship between problematic illness and aetiological questioning that was considered in its general form in the previous chapter. The two lesions which constituted the initial illness occurrence were not life-threatening and so did not prompt divinatory investigation. It was not until their six-month resistance to treatment made them incongruous that Kaputa and Kalwa began to consider looking into their aetiology. Similarly, the itching and transient swelling of *masoli* were not in themselves sufficient cause to divine, notwithstanding the fact that this illness dovetailed with its predecessor. In both instances, other considerations took precedence over the imperatives of treatment.

In contrast, high fever, especially accompanied by passing convulsions, is a potential threat to life; and when it occurred, it prompted Kaputa and Kalwa to sit up all night watching their daughter. Confronted by this threat to his daughter's life, Kaputa rose to meet the demands of the situation, borrowing the money needed for the divination, locating the necessary medication and obtaining the money with which to buy it.

Once made, the decision to divine began to be sustained on its own momentum. Kaputa and Kalwa meant to go to the diviner regardless of a remission in the illness; and we all awaited his pronouncement with a certain tense expectancy.

THE DIVINER AND THE ARROW

At the same time as he started attempting to raise the money for a divination, Kaputa began to give thought to the particular diviner he would engage. They had already been several times to a local Bulumbu practitioner, a woman who lived just up the street from me. When new, her spirit had been quite 'hot' (*moto*), and people had travelled great distances to consult her. By this time, however, she had had her spirit for a number of years. Her clientele had dwindled and seemed to consist mostly of neighbourhood people seeking insights into relatively minor illnesses and misfortunes. Kaputa said he preferred to divine into this illness with someone else because numerous divinations with a person who knew one tended to result in the repeated emergence of a few problems, so that the real cause of the trouble might not be apparent.

At the time he said this Kaputa also said that he thought of calling upon another Bulumbu practitioner, also a woman, who lived in a different section of Mpala and with whom he had never before divined. Ultimately, however, he went to the husband of my next-door neighbour's older sister, who has also lived nearby and was a Kalunga. Kaputa said he chose him because Tulunga diviners are usually more accurate than Bulumbu and because he had never before been to this particular person, who came from the interior.

Having decided upon the diviner, Kaputa and Kalwa prepared the 'arrow' (*mshale*) they sent to him by placing it on the ground between them and invoking (*kulandila*) it. Later that same afternoon, Kaputa described their invocations as having been as follows.

Kaputa himself spoke first, saying:

> This is to say, arrow, I put you here below, on the ground, for the sake of having the illness of the child examined. In brief, this is to say that all matters are obliged (*vinapashwa*) to be visible before the diviner. If it is that I ... my wickedness in my actions, I am able to commit adultery (*kufanya usherati*) in the village and when I come home, I bring it to the child and cause her to be susceptible in this way the *mufumu* is obliged to see all.
>
> Or, another time, I am able to carry off the belongings of another person. Then, he becomes very concerned, he says that, 'Good, that (thing) that was only mine (*ile ilibakia tu kyangu*); we will look well in his house (*tutaangalia vizuri*) [i.e., we will take our revenge upon the members of his household].' The *mfumu* is obliged to see all of this.
>
> Or if it is the *mizimu* of the grandmothers, or my *mikalaye* spirits. Or Bulumbu. If it is that I am one who has divination, then I refuse, I don't have it arranged because of my youth. In this way the children are available. They say, the grandmothers, 'Ah, you see his arrogance. He likes youth more than he likes looking after us. Therefore, we will see by means of his children.' All of these things are obliged to be visible before the *mfumu*.
>
> Or father, if it is able to come from father's side. Or mother, if she is able to say, 'Children, they don't hear me. Therefore let me cause evil to enter into Kaputa's house, thus he will have deaths of his children (*watoto wamufwie* [literally 'they are dying to him']). Thus, another time, he will be be able to inquire, to recognise that we are his parents.' Truly, all, the *mfumu* is obliged to examine.

After making this invocation, Kaputa spat upon the arrow. Kalwa then made her speech, which Kaputa cited as being the following:

> This is to say, arrow, I put you here. If it is my wickedness (*ubaya wangu*), me the wife, if it is that I have committed adultery and then hidden it from my husband. Now, me, I walk about in a wicked way, I go, I bring badness into the house, all these things likewise must go to the *mfumu* that he examine them. Or if it comes out of the statements of our family in the village. Every time there is trouble you then walk around, you think 'Ah, these kinsmen of mine, they don't do right by me. I come here with my husband, and he also, he afflicts me. It is better to die.' Now there, instead of your death, the child is seized. All, the *mfumu* is obliged to look into. Or if it comes from my grandmothers, or *mizimu*, or *mikalaye*, when I, I am unable, I don't look after them well, and take care of all their things, the *mfumu* is obliged to see. Nothing more.

At the end of her invocation, Kalwa, too, had spat upon the arrow. Kaputa then took it up from where it lay and went with it to the diviner's. Arriving there, he threw the arrow to the ground, telling the diviner's wife that the affair was 'illness' (*ugonjuwa*), and specifying nothing more. She picked it up and said she would give it to her husband.

Commentary

During the days preceding the divination, as well as at other times, Kaputa talked about various aspects of his life. Sometimes his narratives were in response to specific questions of mine. More often, however, they were his part of the general conversations about life that passed between us as we worked. It was the problematic situations in his life that gave form to the invocation spoken by Kaputa when he prepared the arrow. As he made his statement, he was noting in outline all the conflicts and difficulties active in his life, his social field at that time. Among these were the following.

Theft

In the weeks immediately preceding the divination, Kaputa had been involved in a conflict about his newly purchased house and the lot on which it stood. In the early part of the year, after a series of disturbing incidents had been attributed by a diviner[4] to the notorious sorcerer living opposite them, he and Kalwa had been forced to move away from the house of Kaputa's father.

After some difficulty they found a new place, and purchased it for 51 zaires. The owner was a young man who had built the house himself, but who had no wife and preferred money to property. He said he would build himself another house when he was ready. At the time of purchase, two copies of the receipt had been made and the money had changed hands before a witness.

Shortly after Kalwa and Kaputa moved in, however, the relatives of the young man came to them claiming the house as their own. They told Kaputa that he must move out and seek the return of his money because the house and land belonged to their family and they wished to have them available for whoever else should need them.

Kaputa consulted with his own elder kinsman, with me and with the head of his section of Mpala. Everyone agreed that this claim was unfounded and that he ought not to move. If the family had helped with the building of the house and so claimed rights in it, they would do better to make their demands of their kinsman and to leave Kaputa out of it.

At the family's instigation the case was heard by the head of the section, with the nature of the conflict and its results being reported to Chief Mpala himself. The judgement went against them at both places, and for a time the matter was left at that.

A week before the divination, however, the conflict had burst out anew. One of the young man's sisters had become drunk and had gone to Kaputa's house. Standing before it, she had reviled Kalwa, saying that the latter would be thrown out of the house by Kaputa and that another woman would be moved into it. She also threatened Kalwa's pregnancy, saying that she didn't know but that failure to move might result in Kalwa's death in labour or the stillbirth of the child.

This matter, too, was brought before the section head, who determined to render no final judgement until after the birth of the expected baby. In the interim the hostile family were to consider themselves responsible for the pregnancy and were to bring medicines to guide it to a successful conclusion.

In Mpala, it is well known that thievery alone is sufficient to cause illness. The hostile feelings and statements of victims arouse their *mizimu* and so can cause misfortune or sickness to fall upon the thief or members of his household. Kaputa was not a thief but was considered by the family to be illegitimately possessed of something that was rightfully theirs. In addition to the bad atmosphere this hostility of theirs created, in which their *mizimu* might mistakenly attack Kaputa or his family, such tension was also inducive of sorcery. The family themselves might resort to it, as their threats implied; or an outside sorcerer might overhear such threats and use them as a social camouflage under which to work. Though Kalwa said she was unafraid, Kaputa expressed concern about the possibility of sorcery.

Mizimu/Bulumbu

Several earlier divinations had revealed Kaputa to have a Bulumbu spirit. This spirit had been his mother's, and had been a divining spirit. At first it had been quite powerful, but, as is usually the case, it had gradually weakened and had finally abandoned Kaputa's mother altogether. Rather than fake her divinations, she had given up her practice.

Sometime after this, Kaputa began to suffer an ongoing series of minor misfortunes, including bad luck, illness, and the like.[5] At each divination it was said that these were due to his mother's spirit, which wished to come to Kaputa that he continue his mother's practice. Each time, however, Kaputa refused to have the ceremony by which the spirit could be arranged. Bulumbu, he said, was nothing but trouble. The arrangement of a *pepo*, far from ending one's difficulty, was really only the beginning. He preferred the freedoms of his youth to the complications a spirit would make in his life. Nevertheless, Kaputa confided to me that sooner or later, the spirit would have to be 'put in order' (*kutengenezwa*). Thus, when he cited spiritual affairs in his invocation of the arrow, Kaputa may well have been referring, at least in part, to this spirit.

Family life
Intrafamilial relations were among the most problematic elements in Kaputa's life, and had been especially troublesome in the months prior to the divination. It was mostly 'matters of the family' (*mambo ya kijamaa*) that made Kaputa reluctant to live in Mpala, and this reluctance was the reason why he had never owned a house there or made a field.

He felt generally bitter at his kinsmen because none of them, not a mother's brother or anyone else, had ever tried to help him, although people had helped his siblings. During his childhood, while he was in school, the teachers had noticed he was very bright. They said he should continue his studies at the boarding school at Moba and ultimately become a teacher.

At that time the fee for the boarding school was something like 1,500 Congo francs a year, and there was no way possible for Kaputa's family to raise such a sum. However, one of the local priests had confidence in Kaputa and thought he should have the opportunity. He said that he himself would pay the school fees if Kaputa's family could get together the plates, bedding and clothing he would need during the academic year. Though Kaputa's mother has several sisters and one brother, the family decided they would not be able to assemble these things, and so his studies ceased.

There was another child, however, for whom the effort was made. This was the last born of one of Kaputa's mother's siblings; and because of the family's support he completed his studies. Unfortunately, after becoming a teacher, this man concluded that the heavy demands of his kinsmen on his slender resources would prove too much, and, according to Kaputa, he therefore turned to drink, spending every spare *likuta* on beer.

To the general sense of alienation deriving from this past incident, Kaputa could also add specific, present grievances. His father had recently been ill, with an incapacitating swelling of the leg and foot. During this illness he had complained several times about his children's supposed neglect of him. In addition, Kaputa pointed out the well-known fact that, when his mother was drunk, she went around her section of Mpala shouting to the world at large that it was worthless to give birth to boy children. (She had five boys and one girl.) At these times she would argue that boys grow up and forget one, and only girls take care of their parents. Better, she would conclude, not to give birth at all than to have only boys.

Such repudiation by a parent of a child is a possible source of illness. Though much weaker than this, it nevertheless resembles the curse (*laana* (KT)) by which *mizimu* are called upon by a parent to blight the life of his child. Kaputa said that everyone would tell his mother she ought not speak in such a way. They would remind her that in so doing she was 'selling her children' (*kuuzisha watoto wake*) – in effect surrendering them to any passing sorcerer who might overhear her, and use her withdrawal of parental protection as a cover under which to operate. Despite these warnings, however, Kaputa's mother persisted in this behaviour when drunk.

Other factors
In addition to the several problems outlined above, Kaputa and Kalwa had a number of other difficulties in their past history. They had been married quite young – when they themselves were 'just children' (*watoto tu*) – and early in their marriage Kaputa had left Mpala to go work in the Filtisaf textile mills in Kalemie. At this time, Kalwa had been pregnant with their first child.

Kaputa's intention had been to arrange everything and then to send for his wife and child. However, he was never able to do this and by the time he next returned to the village, the previously unborn child was walking. In addition, during the two years that Kaputa was away, Kalwa had moved back to Kala and had taken up with another man.

Kaputa's family wanted him to divorce her because of her adultery, but he felt that his wife's involvement was due to her loneliness and he decided to take Kalwa with him when he returned to Kalemie. There he would see the true nature of her character, and would decide whether to divorce or stay with her.

So, they went to Kalemie and while there they had their second child. During this same period, in response to an unspecified incident, a divination was made which revealed that Kalwa's former lover had made medicines to kill Kaputa or cause him to be stricken with *wazimu* ('lunacy') if he stayed with his wife. In addition, Kalwa's mother herself came down with *wazimu*. These events caused Kaputa's family to increase their insistence that the two divorce, but Kaputa reiterated his determination to stay with Kalwa.

Finally, life in Kalemie became too difficult. Kaputa's salary was insufficient to make ends meet and he saw that it would be better if they all returned to the village. Kalwa preceded him, returning with the children, who were now three in number. She went to Kala, and Kaputa followed. After a time, they moved to Mpala.

When I met them in 1975 the first two children had died. The third, a son, was about five years of age and Malaika was about six months old. Kalwa's previous adultery in itself, as well as the bad feeling resulting from it, could have had something to do with the illness for which divination was being made in 1977. In addition, the spirit of either of the two dead children might also have been responsible.

As the above discussion indicates, then, Kaputa and Kalwa were involved in a number of complex and difficult social situations during and around the time of their daughter's illness. Any one of these might have been the specific circumstance from which derived the aetiologic agent responsible for the recurring illness episodes, but the couple had no way of knowing which. Further, it was entirely possible that the illness was derived from an altogether different situation, one to which neither parent had given any thought. It is characteristic of problematic illness that it prompts such a questioning of life in general by those responsible for the well-being of the patient. However, only a diviner may make a clear determination.

Though his awareness of his circumstances may have informed the details of the invocation cited by Kaputa, the general form of *kulandila* is also fixed by convention. Adultery, theft, and negligence of *mizimu* all must be commanded to present themselves to the diviner if in fact they are the cause(s) of illness. Whether or not one has committed any of these acts is insignificant. Indeed, one's very willingness to withstand divinatory inspection is proof of one's innocence and/or of one's altruistic concern for the patient's welfare.

THE DIVINATION

The divination itself took place at 11:00 a.m. on Saturday 9 July 1977, at the home of the diviner. In attendance were Kaputa, Kalwa and I. Though his parents lived in Mpala, Kaputa had not asked them to attend the session. He said that as no one can expect his parents to be around forever, it is suitable for one to begin taking care of oneself as soon as possible. Kalwa's relatives all live in villages too far away to come for such a matter.[6]

The night before the session, Malaika's fever had risen sharply at around 1:00 a.m. It had remained high, and she had had mild seizures until dawn. During the morning, though her temperature was lower, she had remained feverish.

When we arrived at the diviner's house, we found him and his wife alone in the enclosed yard behind the building. She was pounding manioc, and he was splitting *matete* reeds, to make a mat. Kalwa was not there, and Kaputa went off to get her. I sat on a chair in the yard, while the diviner prepared things. He took a few sticks of kindling from the woodpile, and a tuft from the grass fencing that ran around the side of the house itself. While Kaputa was gone, neither of them said anything to me, and as I sat, I wondered why they should – since, when you wait in a doctor's office, you're not expected to make light conversation with the receptionist or with the doctor himself.

Shortly afterwards, Kaputa returned with Kalwa. The diviner immediately sent her to the lake to draw water in a metal pot, and, while she was gone, he selected a clay pot from among those lying, inverted, in the corner of the yard.

He had previously arranged the kindling and a couple of stones on the porch that ran around the side of the house, and he now started to light the fire, using matches. As he did so, he asked me if I didn't have a lighter to sell. He had lost his, and this business of buying matches all the time was a great nuisance.

Kalwa returned with the water, but the fire wouldn't light. The last couple of matches were spent on it; others were sent for and used without success. Just as it began to look as if the fire, as the diviner put it, was 'refusing' (inakataa), it lit. He put the clay pot on the fire,[7] then went and got a small valise which contained his divining equipment.

When the fire had been going a while, he poured some of the water from the metal pot into the clay one, and set the metal pot down beside him. He took nkula (mwenge bark) and put a small dot to the right- and left-hand sides of the pot. He took pemba (kaolin) and put this on the top and bottom edges of the rim.[8] He put some nkula on the centre of his forehead.[9] He then lit a cigarette and smoked a bit. Finally, he called us to come near for the divination.

Steam[10] was rising from the pot as he removed his shirt, dropping it around his waist, so he sat only in his undershirt. He had taken out his medicated nsuko gourd,[11] and put that on the ground to his left. In his left hand, he held a rattle. On his lap, to his left, lay his mukia, the medicated, magical antelope or steer tail which protects the diviner from harm. Its handle was completely covered by a decoration of braided copper wire.

During this first part of the divination, the diviner said nothing to us. He did not even look at us. Shaking his rattle one long time without interruption, he looked into the nsuko and dropped the medicine-filled lukusu seed into the hot water. He reached in and retrieved it, only to drop it in again. Again he removed it. He did this a good number of times, while we all sat watching him and saying nothing.

He would shake the rattle in a long continuous shake, then drop the seed into and retrieve it from the boiling water several times before using the rattle again. From time to time he would shake his head as he looked into the nsuko; and sometimes he would squint as if trying to see more clearly the images inside.[12]

Finally, after about five minutes, he turned to us and said, 'Elders (*wazee*), I give you a parable (*mfano*).'[13] The story he told went like this:

> There was a man who was a great hunter. He had children. One day he went to the forest and dug several pits for trapping animals. He told his children that he had dug these so that they would be able to get food. He said that they were always to go together to the bush to get animals from the pit. They were to take animals from one pit only; and were not to look into the other.[14] He who did so would fall in and suffer the consequences.
>
> The children did as they were told, at first. Then one day, one of them was mistaken. He looked into the hole where he was not supposed to and, seeing the darkness there, fell in.
>
> The other child went back to the village and told their father. The father reminded him of what he had said. Together, they went to the second pit, removed the animal, took it home and ate it, leaving the unfortunate sibling to die.

After telling us this, diviner went back to his examination of the case, dropping the *lukusu* seed into the water and withdrawing it. He then went and got a gourd, with which he would remove the seed if he could not take it out with his hand.

Finally, he began to speak. He asked Kalwa, 'What about this quarrel in the house?' She sat for a minute and then said there was none. He replied that he saw one, then said it was on Kaputa's side. He said, 'I see a woman whose husband has died. She has not been inherited, but another man enters the house. There is a third man who comes, and these two fight each other, and the woman is also beaten. Who is it?'

Kaputa repeated the circumstances back to the diviner, to confirm them. He then asked aloud, 'Who is it that has lost her husband?' He said there was no one he knew of who was like this in his family. The diviner looked at Kaputa and Kalwa, and they both tried to think of who it could be. Kaputa, perhaps partly to show that he was not resisting, asked Kalwa to help him think of the identity of the person. But they came up with nothing.

After a minute, the diviner turned back to his oracle, and asked if the quarrel came 'from the side of the husband'. He dropped the seed into the water and pulled it out with his hand. No. He looked at Kaputa and said, 'You don't have anything.' Simultaneously with this statement, he threw the seed at Kaputa. Not startled, Kaputa immediately retrieved the seed and handed it back to him.[15]

The diviner then asked the oracle if the quarrel came from Kalwa's side. He could not retrieve the seed from the water, and drew it out with the gourd. Yes. He asked her who it was in her family who had lost her husband. Kalwa didn't answer, but I could see the veins at the base of her neck pounding.

Kaputa then said that Kalwa's mother's husband had died. Kalwa pursued this, saying that her father had, indeed, died, while she was in Kalemie. However, her mother had been inherited, and if there had been trouble about the inheritance, Kalwa knew nothing of it, because it was all finished by the time she had returned to Kala. So, she could make no reply one way or the other. The diviner reiterated that the conflict was what he had seen. After a pause, he closed the impasse, by saying 'let's go' (*twende*), and continuing the divination.

This time, he asked out loud if it came from Kalwa's father. He withdrew the seed with his hand. No. He asked if it came from Kalwa's father's family. No. Did it come from Kalwa's mother's father? No. He then asked Kalwa if she had *mukalaye*.[16] No. *Kabwangozi*? No. He asked the oracle if the cause of the illness would be any of these. No.

He then returned to the original point. There had been some failure in terms of Kalwa's mother's inheritance, he said. Kaputa replied that, after Kalwa's mother had been inherited, her second husband had died. After this, there was quarrelling among Kalwa's father's kin about the inheritance.

'She was inherited then?' the diviner asked Kalwa. 'Yes.' 'But', he pursued, 'she was not absolved of responsibility.'[17] 'No', Kalwa replied, 'she was not.' Kaputa put in that, after this, she had become ill with *wazimu*.

The diviner said that he had seen a great quarrel, and this was the cause of the trouble. They should have the house cleansed, he said.[18]

Kaputa asked, if this were the cause, how they alone could be cleansed. Since the trouble applied to all Kalwa's kin, if she went back to visit them, or if they came to Mpala, the difficulty would be returned to their household.

The diviner said this would be no problem. One would simply set aside some of the medicines, and then, when Kalwa went there, she would give them some, to rub on, and thus cleanse, themselves. Or they might consider going to Kalwa's father's family and resolving the problem with them.

Kaputa replied that this would not be possible, as Kalwa's mother had had only girls, and there were no men in the family to direct the affair. Kalwa herself added that they had taken the matter to court earlier, but had lost the case; so that alternative was useless.

The diviner turned again to the oracle, saying, 'Let us look at the husband's side.' He asked it about Kaputa's father, his mother's father, his father's family, a *mukalaye* or *bulumbu* spirit. All negative.

He then asked if the illness might be due to Kaputa's adultery in town. No. The diviner repeated to Kalwa that the cause of the illness was not Kaputa's adultery.

He then said that he had seen that this was a great and fierce quarrel, and that it would finish them (that is, kill the entire family) if they did not do something to correct it. It had kept him up until dawn, and this was why he had wished to dream on the arrow two nights. He pointed at the arrow and reminded Kaputa and Kalwa that he had not invented what he said. It had all been in the arrow they had given him.

'But wait', he continued, 'let us see if it is from quarrels in the village.' He put this to the oracle, and the answer was again negative. He then said that others in Kalwa's family had died, but that this affair had previously hidden itself.

Kaputa confirmed this, saying that at the death of their first child, they had been to divine at Kala, and this had been shown to be the cause of death. Since the coming to Mpala, however, this cause had not turned up again. As everyone said that before acting upon such a divination, one must hear the same thing two or three times, Kaputa and Kalwa had done nothing further.

In any case, Kaputa followed the thought, how could they do it with no help from Kalwa's family? The diviner asked him to recall the parable he had told us at the beginning. He then looked at Kaputa for a minute before going on to say that if one waited for one's counterparts … Everyone, he concluded, must take care of his own house. They must take care of themselves and leave the others to their own devices.

After this, he said that he had nothing more to say. Kaputa asked how much it was, and the diviner told him to go and ask his wife, who was in the kitchen. She had gone to draw water while the divination was unfolding. Kaputa went to her and asked. He returned and paid the diviner 50 *makuta*.

Kaputa and Kalwa then said that they had tried to have her mother's matter arranged during the time when the elder woman's *wazimu* was not so bad, but the family refused. The diviner nodded and then repeated that he was finished. We thanked him and left; Kalwa went back to their house, and Kaputa went with me back to our house.

At the house, I asked Kaputa to repeat to me the parable told by the diviner. His version of the tale was a bit different from my own. Kaputa said that the father had told his children not to go to the pit alone, as they did not know how to remove the animal themselves. After the first child fell in, and the other sought their father, the father had gone to the bush to the single hole, and had removed only the animal, leaving the child there to die.

Kaputa went on to say that the parable meant that the affair was really one pertaining to Kalwa's seniors, not one of Kalwa herself or her siblings. It should have been settled by them among themselves, but it was not. Now, many of the principals in the case had died, so it was impossible to have the matter rightly directed. This was the point of the story: the adults had left the children without proper guidance; so now, what could the children do?

I then asked Kaputa to explain more fully the history which underlay the diviner's reference. He said that at Kalwa's father's death, her mother had been inherited. However, when the inheritor died, his family had refused to give another of their kinsmen, saying that Kalwa's mother was wasting them worthlessly. They blamed her, in effect, for the death.

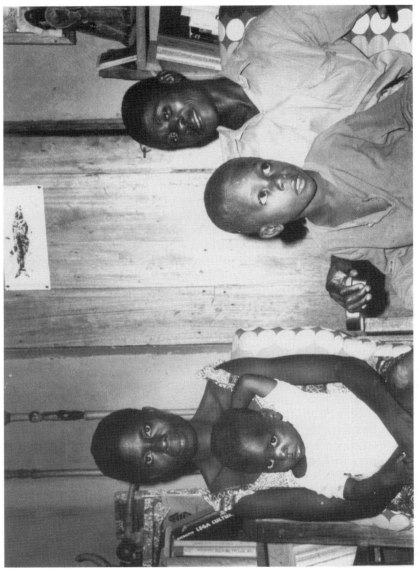

Figure 4.1 Kaputa, Kalwa and their children

The sublineage from which the inheritor was derived had not been that of Kalwa's father, because, as is the rule, the *mupyani* (inheritor) had to come from another subgroup. This second group had a *kibanda*, that is, they were pursued by the avenging ghost of a person whom they had killed through sorcery. Thus, the ghost was attached to the man who had inherited Kalwa's mother, and when the *kibanda* was found to be the cause of her grandchild's death (that is, of the death of Kaputa's and Kalwa's child), the man had admitted it to his wife, but had refused to be cleansed of it. The *kibanda* had subsequently killed him as well. However, instead of attributing his death to the ghost which had destroyed a number of them (and so admitting their guilt of sorcery), the dead man's kin had blamed Kalwa's mother.

At this, quarrelling had broken out among the subgroups of Kalwa's father's lineage. There were those who felt that Kalwa's mother was being unjustly treated; and in the end she was inherited, though not properly so. Another subgroup had taken pity on her and sent a kinsman. However, according to Kaputa, the man came 'like a thief in the night.' He slept with Kalwa's mother (thereby performing the most crucial part of the inheritance ceremony), then immediately divorced her, returning to his own village forever.

The very next week, Kalwa's mother had come down with *wazimu*, an illness brought on by the *kibanda*, who mistakenly assumed her still to be connected to the dead man. While she was still somewhat lucid, her children had tried to arrange the affair with her deceased husband's family. They, however, refused, insisting that two husbands were enough.

The children had even taken the matter to the court at Kala, but had lost the case. The judges had told them that they had the right of the matter, but could not be given it in the judgement, because they were only children. Kalwa's mother was a single child, without even a brother, mother's brother, or other kinsman to help her. She had only girl children, who did not get along well among themselves. It was said that if the case had been brought by the woman's lateral kinsmen, they would have won.

In the meantime, Kalwa's mother's illness became worse. At the time of our conversation she was not violent, but was quite incoherent. She wandered from place to place, and had even come and stayed awhile with Kalwa and Kaputa at Mpala. She behaved strangely, sleeping out of doors, not bathing, and talking nonsense. [19]

Commentary

While the above description is largely self-explanatory, two points should be underscored here. First is the great extent to which clients participate in the divination session. What the diviner provides is an index, as it were; something that indicates which among the several possible situations is the one causing the illness at hand. Since this sketch is drawn in the broadest possible outline, it is up to the clients themselves to fill in the details. They must think of how his statements apply to them, and give consideration, as well, to the consequences deriving from his hypothesis. It is on the basis of these that they will make their decision to accept or to reject his divination. It is thus the clients themselves who contribute a large part of the effort involved in the deciphering of illness. This is one of the reasons why a satisfactory divination has therapeutic effect.

Ideally, the diviner's altered or 'other' consciousness, derived from and carrying the authority of his medicines, provides a structure in which a given history can be considered and a particular sequence of future events can be imagined. In his presence the clients can 'try on', so to speak, a possibility, and see if it suits them. In other divination sessions I have attended, an important part of the diviner's role has been to prompt discussion among the assembled kin, through riddles, direct questions and similar devices. Thus, divinations are not one-answer diagnostic encounters, in which alternatives are suppressed without comment. Instead they resemble the more open-ended discussions of group therapy or seminars, when even rejected possibilities are given a hearing first. As with diagnosis, so in divinations; the proliferation of possibilities punctuated by intermittent consensus is the pattern by which knowledge develops.

The second point derives from an aspect of the first, for it is sometimes in the deciphering of a single significant illness that much of an individual's personal history is constructed and/or reconstructed. Though Kiabu's history, in Part II, provides a better illustration of this process, Kaputa's situation also shows the way in which divination functions to modify the past by selecting now one, now another factor as that which is actively operating in the present. In so far as it is partly based upon what a person knows to be true about himself, identity can thus be said to be altered by divination.

OUTCOMES

During the afternoon of the divination session, Malaika's fever went down. Though she continued to cry almost constantly, her skin felt cool for the first time that week. In subsequent days, she was much better. The *masoli* ('hives') did not return, and she began to play normally again. Tests and a check-up at the hospital in Kalemie one month later showed her to be in good health, despite the presence of intestinal worms (ascaris), for which she was successfully treated.

Kaputa consulted with Kalwa, who also agreed with the divination. He said, however, that it was customary to have a number of divinations into an affair like this. One would send another arrow to another *mfumu*, without mentioning the decision of the first. If the second diviner drew the same conclusions, one knew it to be true and then could act.

He thought that they would wait until after my departure from Mpala, at which time they would go to Kala, to attempt another divination in the company of Kalwa's siblings. Then, if the results were the same, they could all be 'thrown in the bush' at the same time. However, since Kalwa did not get along with her sisters, Kaputa doubted that anything would come of their trip. He speculated that it might be better to send a letter to the sister with whom Kalwa does get along, asking her to come to Mpala, so the matter could be investigated.

Commentary

My departure from Mpala took place nearly two months after the divination. In the intervening period, Malaika's health was not a problem, and her parents, to my knowledge, made no further efforts towards divination. Without the motivating threat of serious illness, the social and economic aspects of the task were too formidable, and the rewards for its completion too small, to warrant undertaking a second divination and the therapy which would have cleansed both Kalwa's own family and those of her siblings.

In September 1977, Kalwa was tested and examined at the hospital in Kalemie, and the unborn child was found to be normal. Kalwa herself was found to have bilharziasis and was treated for it. Kaputa became ill during the time we were in Kalemie, with *mpanga*, a chronic disorder with him. Tests showed this to be active tuberculosis, and four days before I left Zaire, I was able to get some INH (Isoniazid) for him from the regional general hospital (there was none available at any of the local pharmacies).

CONCLUSION

The divination undertaken by Kaputa and Kalwa into their daughter's illness bore all the marks of success. Reviewing these allows us to grasp both the qualities that make a particular divination satisfactory, and the contribution it makes to people's lives, beyond the immediate contribution of cure.

First, the diviner was a relative stranger to the couple, and was selected by them for this very reason. They wished to rule out a routine (hence, insignificant) repetition of hypotheses they had heard before, and the diviner's ignorance of their lives could guarantee this. The absence of surrounding gossip means the arrow can be taken to have more effectively hit its mark – even if the result should not be a new one.

The particular narrative that emerged during the divination had been latent in the crisscrossing stories of their present lives. They knew of it as it had originally happened, and they also knew that it had played a part in a previous turning point, the death of another child. In this respect it was already part of their present, but it was not active in their immediate concerns and did not figure specifically in their invocation of the arrow.

One element of the satisfaction in the divination came from precisely this moment of recognition, the shift in thought made possible by the reorganisation of a known past. The balance between the familiar and the new meant they could simultaneously see the logic of the hypothesis and yet be surprised by it.

This almost aesthetic sense of the rightness of the thing was further supported by the effective match it made between Malaika's symptoms and their probable cause. The dangerousness of her illness could not have been as satisfactorily matched to an aetiological agent less deadly than a *kibanda*, and this fit contributed to her parents' view that the diviner was correct in his representation.

Although the representation's validity could be confirmed on the spot, its final verification took the form of Malaika's recovery, which became evident that very afternoon. While Malaika continued the course of niridazole until its conclusion, the effect of the medication never intervened in Kaputa's or Kalwa's thoughts on the matter. In a way it had ceased to exist as such. This would not have been the case if the medicine had cured her on its own.

Yet, while a single narrative is enough to effect a cure, it is nevertheless not quite enough to create a turning point; and this fact is of interest in itself. When they are rewarded with recovery, people commonly fail to pursue the circumstantial therapies the diviner has suggested. This is so often the case that it is a common topic for jokes about how people, in general, behave. As such it fits into a broad set of expectations based on the presumption that frailty and folly are part and parcel of human being. Although Kaputa and Kalwa had good reasons why they could not immediately undertake the necessary therapy, everyone always has reasons good enough not to do something that will be difficult or unrewarding.

However, this common transgression of a norm is, in its way, consistent with other patterns and elements in the medical context. These include the consistent in-building, so to speak, of uncertainty as the foundation on which all gestures towards knowledge are based. People begin to know from the premise that they do not or cannot know everything, or even anything of significance to a given set of circumstances. In addition, even if they could know or come to know everything in the present, they still would not be able to know the outcome of events.

For these reasons, consultation is important and decisions are the result of collective effort, even when they are made by only a few. In this context, the repetition of a divinatory hypothesis ceases to be useless and comes to have the value of confirmation.

Finally, it is possible to see in this common deviation a generative function consistent with the functions of other gaps or 'insufficiencies' in this system. This is the proliferation of possibilities, out of which future choices can be made. By this, I mean to suggest that a hypothesis verified by recovery but not realised in therapy becomes an addition to the future's stock of possible pasts.

Problematic illness and divination reveal and heighten the respect in which the present is suspended between the past and the future. Retrospection becomes one function of a prospection that even includes a view of present events as things that will turn out to have one outcome or another, both as yet unknown.

This suspension of the present in a speculative web, this storing up of the future's pasts, is precisely the luxury of recovery. Where the illness is remorseless in its worsening, there is no time and no capacity for this. Instead, all possibilities must be exhausted in the pressing search for a cure, with narratives, like medicines, discarded as the illness does not heed them.

PART II
GENERATION OF IDENTITY,
(RE)PRODUCTION OF HISTORY

5

ILLNESS AND PERSONAL IDENTITY:
KIABU'S CASE

The description of the symptoms and circumstances of Kaputa's and Kalwa's daughter's illness provided a close view of a single instance of problematic illness and of the role divination played in making sense of and thus curing it. The history contained in this chapter shows the problems of diagnosis and the intelligibility of illness as these unfold in the life of a single individual over the course of some 18 months. Among other things, Kiabu's story demonstrates the extent to which deciphering significant, problematic illness has a profound effect on personal identity, that is, on what a person knows to be true of herself and of her life.[1]

EPISODE ONE: THE DEATH OF HER DAUGHTER

I first got to know Kiabu in September 1975, when she came to me for treatment of fever in her six-month-old daughter. This particular illness was a passing one. It responded readily to treatment with aspirin and penicillin, and I remembered Kiabu more because of her own personality than because of anything exceptional in her daughter's condition. She is a large woman, tall and big-boned. Her outgoing disposition and lively sense of humour made her the centre of attention in any group. Her way of joking with everyone on the porch at clinic hours made the time pass quickly for us all.

During this initial episode, however, she lived in another village, Mtole, to the north of Mpala and had walked to the house precisely to seek treatment for her child. Once the treatment was successful, she returned home and I did not see her again until late April of the following year.

By that time, her baby had died of another illness. In addition, Kiabu had married the local government fisheries agent, a MuHemba, and had moved to Mpala. The story of her daughter's death is as Kiabu told it to me in 1976.

In 1975, after Kiabu had returned to Mtole, and I had left Mpala for a brief trip to Kalemie, the little girl was suddenly taken quite ill with *ndege* ('infantile convulsions'). Her mother immediately packed her up and started off for Mpala, seeking treatment.[2] She had got as far as Kapanza,[3] when the child's condition became critical (*hatari*). The baby would 'start' (*stuka*) and squirm (*nyonga*) as though suffering from abdominal pain, and her mother saw that they could go no further.

At Kpanaza, the infant was treated with traditional medicines for *ndege*. These were poured over her until she urinated,[4] but, despite this positive prognostic sign, the baby's condition did not improve. She became unconscious during the night, and everyone began to grieve. Later the child briefly regained consciousness, but died at four o'clock the following morning after only two days' illness.

While this episode was unfolding, Kiabu had not neglected to seek divinatory insight. Through it, she was revealed to have a spirit which wished to 'come out' (*kutoka*) and 'be put in order' (*kutengenezwa*) by means of a *bulumbu* ceremony.

Kiabu had had a spirit when she was just a child. It had come to her through serious illness, and had remained with her until she reached childbearing age. At this time, the spirit had spoken through her to say that she would not give birth in its company, and that it was therefore leaving her, that she might have the opportunity to do so. Since then, it had not returned.

Though she was not interested in having an active spirit, Kiabu was willing to undertake the ceremony for the sake of her child. However, before arrangements could be made, the baby died, and the matter was therefore dropped.

Her child's death proved to Kiabu that the source of the illness could not have been a spirit. As everyone said, spirits do not kill, and besides, if the child is already dead, what good is having a *pepo*? Kiabu felt that if the spirits wished to kill her for refusing them, they could go right ahead and do it.

Furthermore, the illness of which the baby died could not have been *ndege*, because *ndege* does not kill. It just makes children ill and then leaves them.[5] No, the death had to be due to sorcery. What other sort of person would kill a child who had only just cut her teeth? Who would kill someone who cannot even speak and thus can have no conflict with anyone?

After the death, there were those who mocked Kiabu. They enjoyed her grief and said she deserved to lose her child because of her vanity (*kiburi* (KS) or *fiyeli* (from the French *fierte*)). Kiabu herself protested this assessment of her character. Everyone, she said, has her or his own condition. One must take people as they are. She cared for herself, dressed all right, and was clean. What sense did it make for her child to be in rags, when she, the mother, was well dressed?

With all of this in mind, then, Kiabu sought a second divination, this time into the death of the child. The seriousness of the matter[6] prompted her to select Polombwe, an itinerant practitioner new to Mpala. He had been a principal in all of the more notorious cases of 1975, was indirectly responsible for the deaths of two people whom he had publicly named as sorcerers, and was generally considered to have a very 'hot' spirit, which enabled him to get right to the heart of an affair and boldly name those who could be blamed for the illness or misfortune.[7]

Despite his reputation, Polombwe's divination for Kiabu was disappointing and, she felt, inaccurate. Prior to bearing this last child, Kiabu had given birth to two others. The first of these had died in infancy, though the second was still alive and living with his father at Rutuku, not far from Kalemie. Now, Polombwe's spirit said that it saw 'only a quarrel' (*ugomvi tu*) as the cause of the latest baby's death.

The first of Kiabu's children, the spirit said, had died 'on account of her father' (*kwa ajili ya baba yake*); that is, as a result of her father's adultery. This child had returned as a *kiswa* and killed the new baby because of the quarrelling in Kiabu's household.

Kiabu saw that this was a lie (*wongo*). If the cause of death had been the ghost (*kiswa*) of that first child, why would it return to kill the third one, while leaving the second alive? This made no sense, and Kiabu had said as much to the diviner during the session. He had had no answer for this, so they paid him 250 makuta, a white cloth, and a hoe,[8] and let the matter drop.

Prior to the last infant's illness Kiabu had planned a trip to Kalemie. Undertaking it after the death, she took advantage of the journey to seek another divination. She engaged a practitioner who lived on the north side of the Lukuga river, in a community rather distant from the nucleus of Mpalaites resident in Kalemie.

This person told her that the place where she was living, Mtole, was very dangerous. There were many bad people all around her, and the diviner had dreamt of fire every time s/he[9] had slept on the arrow. The baby had been killed by two people, both men, one of whom was near and the other far away. They had bound the child hand and foot with a magical, invisible cord. What ordinary people had seen as *ndege* had been the child's struggling against this cord, and its presence was what had caused the baby to squirm before dying.

Kiabu felt this divination to be accurate. She told me that the motives for the killing had been her refusal of the advances of one of the men, and the more general 'jealousy' (*wivu*) which is characteristic of a sorcerer's disposition. Before the child had been born, she had been living for over a year with a man whom she did not love, but who was just a friend. After a year, he had said that he was leaving her because she did not give birth. She said his departure had been a matter of indifference to her at the time. After he left, however, she discovered that she was pregnant, and told him that the child was his. He returned, but did not stay, and said he was not sure he was, in fact, the father.

Thus, at the time of the birth of the child, Kiabu was alone. She said she was careful to provide herself with clothing, soap and other necessities, because she did not have a husband to help her. As part of her earlier plan for her trip to Kalemie, Kiabu had been accumulating extra quantities of these things, so as to be self-respecting and self-sufficient. The evil (*wabaya*) people had seen this. They were jealous, and so had killed the child. This was demonstrated at the time of the infant's death, for when Kiabu brought out clothes for the burial, one of their family remarked that those things were too good for such a purpose.

After hearing the divination, Kiabu had not rested, but had gone straight to her (classificatory) sister with the news. Frightened by the danger, her sister told Kiabu that she should immediately move from Mtole. Kiabu, however, felt that flight would be to no avail. Her feeling was that no matter where you went, sorcerers could still get you if they meant to.

Shortly after this, Kiabu married the fisheries agent and moved to Mpala. The two men who killed her baby were mother's brother and sister's son to one another; and even months later, when Kiabu would go by them on the road, they would not look at her. Instead they looked at the ground, or hid their faces; and Kiabu, for her part, would pass them thinking what reprobates they were.

EPISODE TWO: SORCERY

In mid-May 1976, Kiabu came to me for treatment of an illness which she herself had diagnosed as *nkazi* ('dysmenorrhoea'). Her symptoms were lower back pain, both during her menstrual periods and between them; pain after intercourse; a menstrual flow which was dark in colour and clotted in consistency; and fever in the evening, which would remit during the day and which would be accompanied by darkened urine. She also said that her menstrual periods had been irregular since they had begun again after the birth of her child. My attempts to treat what I thought might be a urinary tract infection (with tetracycline and aspirin for the pain) were fruitless. Though she felt somewhat better, Kiabu still had pain, and still felt less than well.

Intermittent episodes of illness continued throughout June. Kiabu at one point thought she was pregnant. Then, in a dream, someone told her that her condition (*hali*) was not pregnancy. Since when had pregnancy involved such pain? No, they told her, this is illness (*ni ugonjuwa*), and they pointed out to her a tree, which she recognised as *ngenziangenzia*, and told her to dig out its roots.

Kiabu did this, and gave herself an enema with an infusion made from them. However, far from curing her, the enema caused her to have palpitations, dizziness, cold sweats, and near fainting. As she lay on her bed afterwards, she thought she was dying.[10] She couldn't understand why she had had this reaction to the medicine, as it is frequently used even on children, with no such ill effects. She thought her reaction must be due to the general condition of her body.

At another point, Kiabu's husband went to Moba, the local government seat, leaving her at home alone in Mpala. During this period, she twice dreamt that sorcerers had entered her house and 'kneaded' (*kufinyanga*) her during the night.[11] Upon his return, Kiabu told her husband of this, and he shouted veiled threats to the sorcerers for several evenings,[12] after which she slept peacefully.

Nevertheless, her sense of having been ensorcelled remained. It was increased when she noticed a swelling in the right lower quadrant of her abdomen. It would appear at some times, but not at others, and seemed to have no very fixed place, either. This, she told me, was the 'thing' (*kitu*) or the 'sorcerous medicine' (*buganga*) which had been thrown into her by the sorcerers, and it was this which was causing her illness.

Since I already had plans for a trip through Kalemie to Lumbumbashi, I told Kiabu that she could travel along with me, if she wished, and be examined free at the hospital in Kalemie. She wanted to go, but her husband refused her permission. Publicly, he said that he did not have enough money to pay for the trip. Privately, he told Kiabu that he did not want her to go because he feared she'd find another husband there, and leave him.

In addition, on the afternoon before the departure, word arrived from Kalemie to the effect that a new law had been promulgated, and without a pass, citizens of Zaire could no longer leave their zone of residence and travel to another zone. As Kalemie was in a different zone from Mpala, and it was nearly time for the local clerk's office to close, I suggested that Kiabu get a pass, giving her illness as the grounds for her travel. In so doing, she would be ready to leave at dawn the next day, should her husband finally relent, as she thought he might, and give her permission to go.

Later in the evening, Kiabu's husband came by the house, to ask us if I would purchase for him a pair of sunglasses in Lumbumbashi, and to give me money for them. He had apparently given no further thought to his wife's illness.

I became quite irritated with him because of what seemed to me to be his selfishness, and I berated him about it. I pointed out that Kiabu was ill, and that local treatment with both traditional and European medicines (*dawa ya kizungu*) had failed to cure her. If he didn't look out, he'd have another indemnity to pay.[13] That night, Kiabu's husband returned to say that this prospect had so badly frightened him that he had changed his mind, and given his wife permission to travel. The next morning, he accompanied her to the beach, to wish her a safe trip.

In Kalemie, I arranged for her to be examined by Citoyen Katumpwe, then the head nurse and administrator at the Clinique Mama Mobutu, formerly the 'Hospital Blanc' (white people's hospital).[14] I then went to Lubumbashi, expecting to return after my two-week absence to find Kiabu's illness appropriately diagnosed and treated.[15]

When I returned, on 20 July, I found that Kiabu had been diagnosed as having 'chronic appendicitis'. During the course of the two-week period, she had been receiving daily injections of a mixture of penicillin G (one million units) and streptomycin (1 gram). In addition, Dr Kabongo, of the clinic, had been scheduled to operate on her that very day. However, the other patient scheduled for surgery had not shown up, and the doctor had decided not to bother for just one person. He told Kiabu to return with us to Mpala, and to come back to Kalemie in four weeks, after he had finished his month's vacation in Europe.

The idea of putting off the operation for a month did not seem to be such a good one. There was no way I could treat an inflamed appendix at Mpala, rupture would almost certainly be fatal, and there was no assurance that Kiabu would actually get back to Kalemie at the end of four weeks. On Saturday 24 July, I approached Katumpwe about her case, and he said he would speak to the subregional doctor, Mwendy, on the following Monday (26 July), to ask that he take her on his operating schedule during that week. On Monday afternoon, Katumpwe said that Mwendy had agreed to perform the surgery, but that he thought it would be better if Kiabu were admitted to the General Hospital, rather than the Clinic.

The previous December, I had seen that the conditions at the General Hospital were unacceptable. The only food provided each day was a small bowl of beans, and sometimes even this was not to be had. Since Kiabu had no relatives in Kalemie, she would be unable to provide for herself during her convalescence. In addition, I had seen that the other patients I had brought to the General Hospital received roughly one-tenth the specified quantities of the medications prescribed on their charts. Some of the male nurses neglected their duties of administering medicines, changing bandages, and so forth. When patients complained, these people became tyrannical and intimidating.

Conditions at the Clinic, on the other hand, are much better. Meals are provided as part of the hospitalisation, and the staff are both more concerned and more conscientious. In the face of these reasonable objections, Katumpwe said he would try to arrange for Kiabu to be admitted to the Clinic at a reduced rate. She was to enter the hospital on Tuesday, for surgery on Wednesday 28 July.

The next day (Tuesday), after Kiabu had already been admitted, Citoyen Katumpwe told me that the cost of her surgery and hospitalisation at the clinic would amount to some 80 Zaires. Unaware that this was already a substantial reduction of the normal price of 150 Zaires for surgery and a five-day hospital stay, I asked my friend if he could not lower the price still further. After some hesitation, he said he could reduce it to 40 Zaires but that he would have to do so by asking Dr Mwendy to take a five-Zaire cut in his usual surgical fee, and giving Kiabu her room and board free of charge. Even at this, I paid the 40 Zaires, saying that Kiabu and her husband could repay me half this sum at a later date.

On Tuesday afternoon, Kiabu's frame of mind was quite optimistic. She told me that the night before she dreamt she had given birth to a fine baby whose father was European. They had taken the baby to the hospital for testing and had been shown three different types of medicines – all ampoules.[16] At this she had awakened. (The successsful birth, the European father, and the European medicines were all symbolic of *mukalaye*, whose proximity to Kiabu at this time was quite propitious.)

Early Wednesday morning, Kiabu was prepared for surgery, as was her room-mate. Kiabu had been given the initial dose of anaesthetic and her room-mate was in the operating room when word came from the General Hospital that some serously injured soldiers had just arrived there and were in immediate need of Dr Mwendy's attention. He had left after completing only the first operation, and Kiabu's surgery was rescheduled for Friday morning.

During the intervening two days, Kiabu's outlook became increasingly pessimistic. Having seen the post-operative condition of her room-mate, and the intense anxiety of the girl's family, Kiabu became convinced that she would die the minute her body was opened. She did not sleep a wink Wednesday night, and earlier, had been afraid to eat because a nurse had mistakenly presented her with a bill for 20 Zaires as advance payment for her room and board.

On Thursday, she told me that if for any reason she failed to have surgery on Friday, she would simply leave the hospital and we would all just go home. In addition, she expressed considerable concern about the political situation in the city of Kalemie itself.

The hub of a war zone, Kalemie during this particular period was filled with tension over the undue proximity of rebel forces. They had come down from the area to the north of the city and had taken the nearby town of Kabinda, burning the cement plant and seizing 60 captives. In addition, they burned all the fishing camps at Kasanga Mtoa, only 14 km outside of town. Bands of captured rebels were being marched by the army through the city now and then, and rumours circulated every afternoon that we would all awake the next day to find ourselves in rebel hands.

The orderly who brought her food would also bring Kiabu news of the latest events in the conflict. This included the false information that ex-Katangan soldiers had passed to the north of Kalemie on the Tanzanian side of the lake, and were crossing Tanganyika to join forces with the rebels there.

Kiabu was frightened that I would leave her in Kalemie, but accepted my reassurances that, since the other Mpala residents visiting the town (two merchants) had already left, I would await the completion of her hospitalisation before leaving. She was further consoled by the sight of those who had had surgery before her, who were up and about within two days. Even if the rebels did come, she said, if she could walk, she would still be able to make her way slowly to Kampkolobondo, where the boat was moored, and thus escape with me.

On Friday morning, Kiabu was again prepared for surgery. She was the only patient on the schedule. Her classificatory sister, who had been sleeping on the floor at the foot of her bed, was locked in Kiabu's room by Katumpwe because, overwhelmed by last-minute fears, she had forcibly tried to prevent removal of her kinswoman for the operation. At around noon, Dr Mwendy removed a 'very bad' appendix. It had been this which had been the abdominal lump she had noticed earlier.

As is the custom, the appendix was put in a little bottle with alcohol and given to Kiabu. While she was in the hospital, it sat on her night table. Compared to others it seemed quite enlarged and all the staff who saw it said that would have ruptured within three or four weeks.

During her week's convalescence, I visited Kiabu almost daily. She felt very cheerful and optimistic; and, once the pain from the stitches had subsided, her great good humour took over. She joked about her previous suspicions of sorcery, saying that one claims one has been ensorcelled, but, really, the sorcery was one's own body. They could take it out and show it to you.[17] She also ridiculed her earlier fears about both the outcome of the surgery itself and the unfolding events in the city.

The night before she left the hospital, she dreamt of a man and woman, husband and wife, who came in a car to visit her there. They told her that they had come to fetch her, and that she would come out of the hospital the next day. Husband and wife each gave her 50 *makuta*. (Husband and wife, and the car – a European thing – can also be representations of *mukalaye*. Though Kiabu did not appear to apply this meaning at the time, she later accepted this interpretation from one of the boat crew.)

We made our departure from Kalemie a few days after Kiabue left the hospital. She took her appendix with her to show her husband.

EPISODE THREE: AGAIN ENSORCELLED

During the month after our return form Kalemie, no major events occurred to disrupt the smooth flow of Kiabu's life and health. We visited or ran into one another several times in August and early September, and so I was kept up to date on her state of mind and concerns.

Though she was relieved at the successful outcome of her appendectomy, and did not attribute this illness to sorcery, Kiabu nevertheless felt that there were those who wished her harm. She cited the death of her child as proof of this, and said that had the sorcerers known she was ill and was scheduled for surgery, they would have taken advantage of these circumstances and killed her.

In addition, the death of her child seemed to have left Kiabu with mixed feelings about childbearing in general. In one breath, she would say she did not wish any more children, because they would only die, leaving her again bereft, and then go on to express concern that she might be infertile.

Kiabu said she had always had difficulty in becoming pregnant. Her son had been over three years old before the onset of her third pregnancy. In addition to a miscarriage, she had lost two infants to illness. It was for these reasons that she was nearly 30 and had only one child.

During one conversation in early September, Kiabu expressed concern that sorcerers might have made medicines to destroy her reproductive organs (*vyombo vya kuzaa*). When I assured her that the pelvic examination she had undergone in Kalemie had revealed no abnormality, she concurred, saying that Citoyen Katumpwe had told her the same thing. She went on to say that though her latest menstrual periods had been normal (unlike the ones occurring during her illness), she had been refusing to sleep with her husband for fear of becoming pregnant and having the place of the lesion rupture during pregnancy.

8 September

Kiabu's manifest ambivalence gave way to outright anxiety in response to an illness episode occurring during the night of 8 September. That night, at around eleven o'clock, she came to the house quite upset. She stopped at the window where I was working and told me she was dying; that an illness had begun not too long before, and that she did not feel at all right. Though she had been asleep, she had awakened to find her heart was pounding, she had broken into a cold sweat, and she felt dizzy, light-headed and weak. Afraid for her life, she had arisen, aroused the child staying with her (her husband was away), and then gone to the house of a neighbour – a Jehovah's Witness – to ask him to accompany them to my house by the light of the moon.

In the house, I checked her generally. Her temperature was normal and her pulse, though elevated at 102 beats per minute, was not unduly high. She felt no pain, and the area of her incision was normal.

As she talked, Kiabu expressed her conviction that she had been close to death, and that only awakening and arising had prevented her from dying. She said she thought someone was trying to *djindula* her, that is, to steal her soul for use in acquisition of wealth.[18] Since, by the limited means at my disposal, I could find nothing amiss, I gave Kiabu aspirin and suggested she come back the next day.

9 September

On the afternoon following the illness, Kiabu felt only a little better, physically; and emotionally, she felt considerably worse. She reported that she had slept the previous night after returning home and taking the medicine I had given her. While asleep, she had dreamt of sorcery. She had seen a man dancing naked around her house – in her yard. This man had had the body of one person, but the face of that person's brother-in-law.[19] In the light of her dream, an abnormal incident which had taken place the day before took on special significance for Kiabu.

She had been sitting in her yard just at dusk, sharing a small meal of *bukali* and *sombe* (boiled manioc leaves) with the little girl who stays with her, when an old man who is a neighbour passed the yard and saw them there. Kiabu called out 'good night' (*kwa heri*) to him, but, instead of calling back and continuing on his way, the man had simply stood there, looking at her. Kiabu called out 'good night' again, to prompt him to leave. After answering, he had walked on a bit, then stood rather behind the fence, and cleared his throat twice. In retrospect, Kiabu felt this to have been the act of sorcery which had resulted in her becoming ill that night. She went on to say (perhaps defensively), that she could not have offered the man any of her food because (a) there wasn't much, (b) her husband was away, and (c) her husband never ate with the man when he was home.

By this time Kiabu had become completely convinced that her illness, with its generalised feelings of weakness and other symtoms, was the result of *madjin*, and that this was the man who had done it to her. She also reported some menstrual spotting, and very slight cramping, though it was far from the date when her menstrual period was due.

10 September

The next day, 10 September, Kiabu said she felt rather better, though she still had some 'paraesthesia' (*kulewa*), and intermittent palpitations of the heart. She seemed a bit preoccupied, weak, and generally less than happy. She told me she had been to see Chief Mpala that very afternoon.

She had gone to Mpala's at one o'clock to tell him that someone had ensorcelled her and that she might die. While there, she described to him her dream, and told of how she had recognised the person in it as having the body of the old man who had behaved so strangely, but the face of the old man's brother-in-law. The chief and everyone sitting with him laughed when they heard the story.[20]

Neither Mpala nor the others had believed that the old man had been trying to ensorcell Kiabu that afternoon. Instead of sympathising, Mpala's response had been to reprimand her, telling Kiabu that in staring at her and coughing, the old fellow had been doing nothing more than begging to share some of her food. The chief pushed aside Kiabu's objections and went on to say that she had a 'bad mentality' (*akili mbaya*), that is, was mean and selfish, not to have shared her food with him, as is the custom.[21] Kiabu had retorted that Mpala nevertheless should not be surprised if he heard she had died, because she had warned him of it. After this, she said, the chief had made no further reply.

Upon arriving at the house that afternoon, Kiabu had met Mumbyoto, who was just leaving after a visit. It was not until after he had left that she told me of her visit to Mpala, and then said that she had been mistaken not to have stopped Mumbyoto to give him an 'arrow' (*mshale*) to look into the episode.

Kiabu seemed to have determined on the very spot to undertake divination and began talking about her plans for it. She said she would wait until Mumbyoto (who lived in another village) passed through Mpala again, and then give him the 'arrow'. She would then arrange with him for the divination to take place at Mtole, where her mothers were. She explained that it is better to have the divination take place where one's mothers are because the incident responsible for the illness might be something which had occurred before one was born or out of one's knowing. If one is alone and reference is made to it, one will thus deny the truth of what the diviner says. However, those who know the situation better will agree, or correct one.

Kiabu also said she wanted to have a Kalunga divine into the case, because Bulumbu diviners are 'worthless' (*bure*). When you go to them, all they ever see is *mukalaye* or other *pepo*. If you want the real truth, you must visit a *tulunga*. She concluded by saying she would invoke the 'arrow' soon, and have one of her brothers take it up to Busongo, where Mumbyoto lived.

Finally, Kiabu spoke of her physiological and social/emotional conditions. In the intervening day, the spot of blood she had seen had become menstrual flow. It was about two and a half weeks early, however, and the flow was just as it had been during her appendicitis, dark and clotted.

Her general state of mind was one of being beseiged. She spoke of the wickedness of people in Mpala, and the jealousy of her neighbours. She especially felt the jealousy of young women living near her, who were after her husband. Her symptoms of dizziness and palpitations had so corresponded to those of *djindula* that she was sure this was what had happened to her.

11 September

The following afternoon, 11 September, was the third day after the onset of her latest illness occurrence, and by that time, Kiabu was feeling rather better. When she came to visit, she said she felt no or very few palpitations, had diminished paraesthesis, and easier menstruation. She also looked better and, in her demeanor, showed that she felt better.

As she had rounded the corner to the house, she had found Kipampe, a neighbour, already sitting with me on the porch. Kiabu promptly told Kipampe that she (Kiabu) had almost got to that state where they would have sung 'that song' for her. 'That song' is the one sung at the grave site, as the dirt is being shovelled in upon the mat-enclosed body. The two women immediately began reciting its words and laughing heartily, in fact almost uproariously, between phrases.

After we had stopped laughing, Kipampe asked what had happened, and Kiabu gave her a description of the illness that combined physiology and interpretation into a neat explanatory package. She said she had been sleeping that night, when suddenly God told her to arise or risk death. Kiabu had then awakened with a start to find her heart pounding and herself in a cold sweat. She has called to the sleeping child in the next room, and then had forced herself to arise even though her body felt weak all over. She said she had been careful to arise slowly, so that she should not fall to the ground from the dizziness, because to have done so would have meant death.

She went on to describe how she had been afraid to cross the neighbourhood alone, and so had awakened the man next door, who had come with her and the child to my house. There, I had tested her but could find neither fever nor illness (further proof of the occult aetiology of the occurrence).

Throughout the telling, the story seemed to carry with it no more intensity of feeling than the average scandal; and Kipampe seemed no more shocked than she would have been over the average, entertaining bit of local gossip. That she had been a victim of *majin* was now part and parcel of Kiabu's description of her symptoms, and she concluded her story with a description of her neighbour's staring and coughing and of her subsequent dream.

After Kipampe had gone, Kiabu told me about the wickedness (*ubaya*) of her neighbours, as this had been made manifest in her latest unpleasent encounter with them. During the afternoon, Kiabu had taken her bucket and gone down to the lake to bathe and draw water. After she had washed herself and filled her bucket, a young woman arrived. This person set down her bucket, and, bending over the water, began rinsing her face and arms. While thus bent over, she picked up a rock and threw it back under her arm into Kiabu's bucket.

Kiabu reprimanded her, reminding the girl that, as one who had given birth, she was much the girl's senior. As such, she ought to be treated with respect. Why, Kiabu had gone on to ask, do you harass me thus? The other had stood arms akimbo, and, in reply to Kiabu's question, had asked 'What harassment?'

This had made Kiabu so angry her first impulse had been to give the young woman a punch. However, such behaviour was unsuitable for someone of her senior status, and so Kiabu had contented herself with telling the girl that, if they *should* get in a fight, she would completely finish her off. She would just knock her down and walk on her.

Kiabu went on to say that this bad feeling of her neighbours towards her was jealousy (*wivu*), sparked by the fact that her husband was a government employee and therefore had money. In addition, he was not adulterous, because he believed that adultery ultimately leads only to trouble and expense. All of the young women living nearby would have liked to sleep with him to get some of that money. Furthermore, they made their husbands impotent through sorcery.

17 September

Nearly ten days after the onset of her latest illness, and almost one week after I had last seen her, I ran into Kiabu on the path near her house. She was feeling much better; her strength and spirits were quite restored to normal. She remained, however, quite convinced that the episode was nothing other than an attempt to steal her soul.

She said that she had seen Mumbyoto passing her house a few days earlier and had given him her arrow. He had told her that he didn't know what his schedule would be, as he had a number of different things to attend to, including a court case. He would, however, stop at Kiabu's within a few days, and, together, they would set the date for the divination at Mtole.

18 September

The evening after our meeting on the road, Kiabu came to visit me at home. She told me that the night before she had had diarrhoea and stomach pain which had caused her to arise from sleep three or four times. During the day, she'd felt better, but the stomach pain had returned in the afternoon, and so she had given herself an enema of water. The 'filth' (*uchafu*) which had come out had been mostly water, but had contained a little blood.

Despite these symptoms, Kiabu's state of mind remained positive. Though she still spoke of being pursued, the talk of sorcery was ordinary talk, conversational in tone. Kiabu swore to me that they would not kill her without her arising as a *kibanda* to give the sorcerers trouble. In addition, her former symptoms were much diminished. She had palpitations only now and again.

Indeed, rather than illness, Kiabu's principal reason for coming was to tell me of a dream she had had the night before. In it a small wooden statue, *muzimu* as she at first called it, had come to her house. It had just walked in, then walked around the yard. In the dream, Kiabu had been astonished to see it and had asked how such a thing could move about in this way. Someone else had told her that it was not a 'tree' (*muti*, also used for statues), but was a person who had come to visit her.

Still in the dream, Kiabu had looked down at the foot of the little figure and had seen a lesion on it. Her own foot had a lesion on it too. She was afraid, but they said, 'Don't be afraid, this is medicine.' They told her to put her hand on the statue's lesion and touch it.

After a bit, Kiabu dreamt that she was in the bush, with the child who stays with her. There, they saw the large snake *ngwezie* (mamba), whose shadow, should he stand upright, is longer that that of a person. This snake tried to approach her in the bush, but she ran away. Then, as they were choosing their path home through the bush, Kiabu selected the path down which one could see other snakes of the same type. At this point, she awoke.

Kiabu said she had told others of this dream, and they had interpreted it to be of *nzunzi*.[22] The statue itself they had said was *nzunzi*, and so was the snake. After the dream, Kiabu had been afraid to go with the child to the bush to get firewood, because she was afraid she would encounter a snake there. So, she had sent the child alone.

21 September

Three days after the above conversation, Kiabu returned to tell me of yet another dream, one occurring in the intervening period. In this one, she had decided to go and buy a little meat to eat. As she described the dream, she formed with her hands a small rounded shape, indicating the size of the piece.

In her dream, Kiabu had started out to the place where the meat was being sold, but on the way she had been arrested by the police, who asked to see her national identity card (this card was meant to be carried by every citizen of Zaire). She had told them where she was going, and had asked their forgiveness, saying that her husband had taken her ID card with him to Moba. The police then took her back to her house, where Kiabu saw her mother, and began to explain to her what had happened. At this point she awoke.

Since police in a dream are representations of *mukalaye*, I suggested to Kiabu that such an interpretation was possible for her dream. She agreed that the police she had dreamt of were, indeed, indicative of spirits. I also suggested to her a thought that had occurred to me only as I was typing up my fieldnotes, the day after our earlier conversation. Couldn't the dreams of the statue and of snakes also be indicative not of *nzunzi* but of *mukalaye*?

Kiabu seemed not to have thought of this possibility before, but, hearing it, took up the idea immediately and expanded upon it. This, she said, would explain why, in the dream, they had told her not to be afraid of the little statue, but to touch it because it was medicine. It would also explain why, in the second part of the same dream, after running from the first snake she herself had chosen to go down the path where other snakes were visible.

As she pursued the thought, Kiabu began to say with greater and greater certainty that it was undoubtedly a *pepo* which was causing all her difficulties. In support of this interpretation, she went on to recount to me a series of other dreams which she had had during this same period.

For three nights running, she had dreamt of dogs.[23] She had also dreamt again of snakes.[24]

In a more lengthy description, she told me of one dream in which she, her mother and her classifactory father were walking. During the sixties, her father's arm was permanently disabled when soldiers shot him, and the dream was set after this event. As the three walked along, on their way to the lake, they saw the large snake *ngwezie*. With his sound arm, her father began to hit the snake, striking it just at the back of its head. After a few strokes, the snake turned into Kiabu herself, and she heard her mother telling her to run for her life – to run as fast as the *kwale* (button quail). Kiabu could not, and was crying out to her mother that she was bound to die, when she awoke.

Kiabu also spoke of another very recent dream in which the 'drum' (*ngoma*) of Bulumbu was being beaten for her (that is, she was having the ceremony by which such spirits are arranged (*kutengenezwa*)). She was there, sitting in the circle drawn with *pemba* on the ground; and she saw before her her husband and brothers. She heard the drum. Kiabu concluded that this dream must surely mean she was destined to have a *pepo*.

As our conversation continued, Kiabu spoke again of the spirit she had had as a child, saying it had come to her after a series of illnesses. She spoke of how she had had it until puberty, and how it had left her, that she might marry and have children. She described how her daughter's illness had been ascribed to her *pepo*. During it, the child did not defecate or urinate. Though the drum had been beaten for Kiabu, and she had fallen (a sign that the spirit has mounted to the head and taken possession of the person), the spirit would not speak. After a while, Kiabu had felt the need to urinate, and knew by this sign that the spirit had left her without naming itself. In view of this complication, they had decided to postpone a second attempt until after her baby recovered. When the baby died, however, the whole matter had been abandoned.

As she continued to consider the matter, even the characteristics of the latest illness manifested their spiritual origin. She could tell a *pepo* had been their cause, because it had nearly killed her, but had then let her return. If the cause of the illness had been sorcerers, she would have been dead long ago. No, Kiabu concluded, the cause of her difficulties was a spirit, and ultimately she would have to have a 'drum'. Her suffering was extreme, and she wished to be rid of it.

Despite her evident enthusiasm, however, Kiabu also had misgivings. No sooner would she state that, in the end, she would have a *pepo*, than she would begin to express her unwillingness to be bothered with it. *Pepo*s do nothing but bring trouble into the household with all their demands and statements.

To deal with them, one must first have a husband of strength and good character. Perhaps they will come and say they are unhappy with the way they are living, and then demand that a house be built for them that very day. What would her husband do then, Kiabu wondered aloud? Perhaps, instead of building the house himself (which she seemed unable to imagine him doing), he would pay someone else to do it. Or, perhaps, the people at

Mtole (that is, her kinsmen) would send someone to build it, to be nice to her.

In addition to these troubles, *pepo* caused other kinds of difficulty as well. You try to live well with your husband, but then 'those of conflict' (*bafujo*) come to destroy marital harmony. Everyone must listen to what they say, then sometimes they come and refuse to say anything. Then, too, Kiabu speculated as to whether she'd be able to have children, if she had spirits.

In any case, she continued, turning the matter over in her mind, Mumbyoto already had the 'arrow'. Kiabu said she would divine with him first, 'to clear out the lies' (*kutosha wongo*). She would then find another practitioner to divine with, and see what would come of it. Pursuing the thought, she went on to comment that there were many, many *wafumu* of Bulumbu at Mtole. If there was a shortage of anything, it was of clients. Further, the price of having a *pepo* arranged was much cheaper there than it was at Mpala. In the end, she summed it up, she would have to have a 'drum'.

But could you imagine her having one, Kiabu asked rhetorically? It would be a shameful thing. Everyone would see her; she would be astonishing (*ajabu*) when she fell. Then, too, there you are. As you sit there, you look about and see your husband, your brothers, and everyone gathered for the ceremony, looking at you. It would be quite something.

On the other hand, Kiabu concluded as we took leave of one another, something had to be done. Here she was falsely accusing the sorcerers of making her ill, when it was really only the spirit.

Later in the same day, I dropped in on a mutual friend of ours, Kalevela. She told me she had seen Kiabu at a funeral which had recently taken place. Kiabu, she said, had been telling her of her recent difficulties and had attributed them to sorcery, saying 'they pursue me greatly' (*wananifuata mno*). Kalevela had told Kiabu that this might be due to their jealousy, sparked by seeing how I had taken her to Kalemie to be treated, and how she had thus been cured. When she came back, she had been all well, and this had motivated the sorcerers to send other illnesses; seeing they had failed with the appendicitis, they were now trying other roads. Kalevela reported that Kiabu had replied that she'd not thought of this before, but that it (that is, continued pursuit by the same people) was definitely a possibility.

I told Kalevela that I thought it might be a *pepo* causing the current illness, and suggested that it may have been this same *pepo* which, by arranging the series of strokes of luck which got her to and through the surgery, had in fact prevented the sorcerers from killing Kiabu with appendicitis. Kalevela agreed that this was a possibility. She added that even if it was a *pepo*, it was certain that there would be a lot of trouble before it came out. They are always that way. Getting them arranged is the work of six months.

11 December

When Kiabu and I parted, in late September, she was awaiting further word from Mumbyoto confirming the date of divination, and I was setting off on a trip by boat to the southern Tabwa at the Zambian end of Lake Tanganyika. The trip had originally been planned to last three weeks, and Kiabu had agreed to wait until my return, so she and I together could go to Mtole for the divination. As things turned out, the trip actually took seven weeks, and, when I saw Kiabu on the day I got home, I was fully expecting her to say she'd already had the work done. Instead, she told me a long story, the upshot of which was that she had not been to divine at all.

It seems that at the time Kiabu had given Mumbyoto the 'arrow,' her husband had been away in Moba on government business. When he returned, kinsmen of his were staying with them. Since they were WaHemba, and eat *bukali* made exclusively of corn (rather than of manioc) flour, the woman in the party needed to pound a quantity of this, and Kiabu had been helping her. Kiabu had borrowed a sifter, that they might have two to make the work go faster, and, that evening, she had returned the borrowed item, against the other woman's wishes.

When she arrived home after completing her errand, she found her husband was very angry with her. He asked her who had given her permission to return the sifter, and went on to comment that this was precisely the sort of behaviour he disliked most in her. She was always doing things behind his back, like sending 'arrows' to Mumbyoto. He asked her why she was trying to 'go around' (*zunguka*) him in this way.

When Kiabu tried to explain that she had not meant to divine in his absence, and had only sent the arrow because she was much pursued and saw her sufferings as extreme, her husband seemed to become even angrier. Further, when she said that she was frightened and wanted to know the cause of her nightmares, her husband replied that they were because she was going crazy and would soon be like Tippu Tippu (a local lunatic who dressed in bark cords and wandered the village). His remark hurt her feelings very much, and she told him that it was a bad, bad thing to have said to her, in part because it meant he wished such a thing would happen. In response to this, Kiabu's husband began to beat her.

Relations between them continued to be strained for the next few weeks. When drunk, Kiabu's husband would beat her, and the rest of the time they were hardly speaking.

After a while, Kiabu called in a classificatory sister of hers and asked this kinswoman to approach her husband, to discover what was wrong and to effect a reconciliation. The woman approached her brother-in-law, and was told that his complaints were that Kiabu had sent an 'arrow' without permission, and that she generally refused to listen to him and follow his instructions. Finally, he confessed that he was angry, too, because she had gone to the office of the town clerk to get her travel pass, in July, without asking him first.

All of these matters were then discussed, and the conflicts resolved. Kiabu's husband admitted that he really couldn't complain about the pass, because she had been dangerously ill. For her part, Kiabu agreed to retrieve the 'arrow' from Mumbyoto without having the divination. Together with her husband, she had gone to the diviner's to do this about two and a half weeks before my return.

Mumbyoto agreed to return the 'arrow,' but said that the charge for such return was 50 *makuta*. Kiabu paid this, and agreed with Mumbyoto when he said that, do what she might, there would be no help, but that the 'arrow' would one day return to him. He went on to tell her of the contents of his dream, since he'd already dreamt, but did so without going through the other formalities of the divination.

In his dream he had seen two people, a husband and wife. They had turned to him and asked him why he had come to them. Mumbyoto had told them that he had received an 'arrow' from Kiabu, who had wished him to divine into the bad dreams she was having. The husband had at first said they had nothing to say to her (meaning, I gathered, that she was not a sorceress).

Then the wife brought out two baskets. In one of them she said was a *bulumbu* spirit. It was this, the wife indicated, that was causing the problems. But then, pointing to the other basket, she said that before the *pepo* could be arranged, they would have to do something about the *kiswa* Kiabu had acquired. Without cleansing Kiabu of the *kiswa* first, the *pepo* would never come out.

Mumbyoto had suggested to Kiabu that she had acquired the *kibanda* through the sorcery of a 'grandmother' (*nkambo*), who had killed someone with medicines. However, Kiabu said that she had had to deny this possibility because, though she hadn't been around then, and couldn't know for certain, she had never at any time during her childhood heard that anyone in her family was a sorcerer. If it had been something of which she had known, she said, she would surely have agreed.

He then suggested that the *kiswa* may have derived from Kiabu's 'prostitution' (*undumba*); that is, that she might have acquired it from one of the several different men with whom she had had fairly casual sexual relations. Kiabu said she could not say for sure if this were so, but that it was possible. After all, when one goes about with people, one knows and sees nothing. How can one tell what has gone on in the past of another person?

Taken as a whole, then, Kiabu agreed with Mumbyoto's divination. She told him that an 'arrow' would certainly come back to him for the therapy ('throwing the person in the bush') by which she would be cleansed of the *kiswa*. She would then go on to engage a Bulumbu adept to have her *pepo* arranged, because if she did not do so, 'they will kill' (*watauana*). She told Mumbyoto that she would set about obtaining the money necessary for the therapy, and, at the time I spoke to her, she was seeking a barrel with which to brew the mash for the distillation of *rutuku* (manioc liquor). By selling this (illegal) liquor, Kiabu could earn the two zaires she required.

In addition, Kiabu recently had again dreamt of Europeans, a confirmation of the hypothesis that her illness occurrence had been caused by spirits. In this dream, she had been standing with a group of people when a priest came up. He selected her from among the others of the group by pointing at her. He wanted her to come with him. Kiabu asked herself why he had chosen her. Was he crazy? She went off by another path to try to avoid him, but he went around another way, and so she found him on the same path, meeting her. They then told her that she should try to avoid him by going down along the rocks, but he met her even there. When she encountered him the last time she was startled, and awoke to find she had been dreaming.

After telling the dream, Kiabu began to laugh. The European was none other than the *pepo*, and it clearly meant that nothing would do but that the spirit must be brought out.

5 January 1977

Almost a month passed before I next spoke at length with Kiabu. From around the time of my return from Zambia, through the month of December, to the time of this meeting, her health had been somewhat better. She no longer had dizzy spells or the sensation of paraesthesia. The scar from her appendectomy hurt only occasionally. Her only problem had been a sensation of abdominal fullness or tightness (*tumbo kupanda*) after eating *sombe* (manioc leaves),[25] but this was insignificant.

Her husband had spent rather more than a month in Moba, and had just recently returned. While he'd been gone, Kiabu had been hard pressed for food and other necessities, for he'd left her no money,[26] and she had neither a field to farm in nor a hoe to weed with. During this time, as well, she suspected her husband of having taken up with someone else in Moba.

He returned to Mpala in early January, and when we spoke, Kiabu described their subsequent relations as having been quite good. They slept together frequently, which raised Kiabu's hopes of becoming pregnant. She was also flattered by his jealousy, which was so intense that he would not even permit her to get firewood alone. He insisted on accompanying her into the bush. At this time as well, her husband complained of pain in his shoulder blade, and thought he would go to Lubumbashi to have it treated. Since he had assured her that he would take her with him, Kiabu was pleased at the prospect. She had always, she said, preferred life in a big city because there is less jealousy among people and, hence, less sorcery.

When I asked Kiabu what her current plans were for her cleansing by
Mumbyoto, and the subsequent arrangement of her *pepo*, she replied by
means of a short commentary on diviners. If you go to a Bulumbu
practitioner, and he asks you 'Is your mother alive?' and you say 'no'; and
then he asks 'Do you have a *mukalaye*?' and you say 'yes'; the diviner will
become quite industrious (*atavuma sana*) (that is, he will immediately set
about rendering a decision). But if he asks you, 'Is your mother alive?'
(*mama eko?*), and you say 'yes'; 'Is your father alive?' and you say 'yes'; 'Do
you have *mukalaye*?' and you say 'no'; he will be very vexed.

She went on to say that from this I could see that she knew these people,
these diviners, very well. It was the same with Tulunga. If you go to a
Tulunga diviner, he will always say you have to be 'thrown into the bush'.

At that time, her concerns were twofold. First was her ongoing anxiety
about infertility. She had been sleeping with her husband for some time, but
was not yet pregnant. Second, though she felt no pain or discomfort, she
had noticed a lump to the left of her navel which would 'walk about'
(*kutembea*). This, she jokingly said, was probably *buganga*, (sorcerous
medicines), thrown into her by someone who had been chagrined to note
her earlier recovery.

So, now, she didn't think she'd be bothered with the cleansing process.
As for the spirit, Kiabu first said that she thought she would go ahead with
that. She would have the drum. Or, perhaps, she would 'go into religion'
(*kuingia mudini*), maybe become Catholic. It was on this note that we parted.

OUTCOMES

At various points during subsequent months, I would hear from Kiabu or
her husband, and catch up on their news. In March, her husband spoke to
me at great length about her condition, saying that her illness continued.
Some days she felt well, but on others she had abdominal pain and couldn't
work. He wondered if this might not be an internal lesion (*kidonda*) which
remained after surgery, and if it might not be better for her to go to Kalemie
for examination and treatment at the hospital. When I commented that I
doubted that it could still be appendicitis, Kiabu's husband suggested she
might try traditional medicines for a while and then go to Kalemie, if these
failed. Shortly after this, Kiabu herself stopped by to tell me she planned to
go to Kalemie, to sell ten sacks of manioc and to be seen by the doctor.

Kiabu stayed in Kalemie for two weeks and returned to find that her
husband had already departed for Moba. She told me she had sold her
manioc for 60 zaires. Of this, she had spent 20 on cloth for her surviving
child, living with his father in Rutuku. Another 23 zaires had gone to the
purchase of a bag of salt, because Kiabu had been afraid the money might
otherwise slip away from her.

During her stay, as well, she had gone to the Clinic, seeking examination.

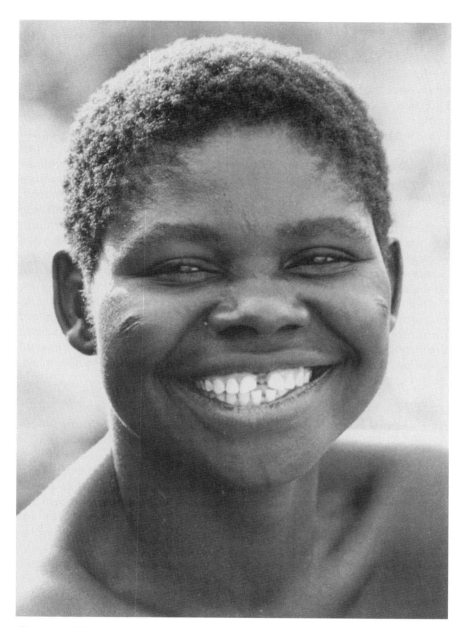

Figure 5.1 Kiabu

There, however, they had refused to examine her, saying that the clinic was for 'the wives of important people' (*babibi wa bapatron*), and that for 'us others' (*sisi wengine*), there was only the General Hospital. Kabu refused to go there, because the people were just packed in; there was no place to sit, and treatment could not be worthwhile. At the Clinic, at least, it was quiet and calm, and one could be seen by the doctor.

By May, her plan was to purchase fish from some classificatory brothers living in Mpala, using money her husband would provide as starting capital. These she would take to Kalemie to sell, and thus obtain enough money to pay for her treatment at the Clinic. When I asked her what her intentions were about being 'thrown in the bush', Kiabu indicated that she meant to go ahead with this. Her husband had consented to participate in the ceremony, too, because he had seen how she suffered from her illness. Previously, the problem had been one of coordination. When she had had the money, Mumbyoto had not been available; then, when he was available, she had already given away her money at the funerals of two close kinsmen. Now, however, everything was ready, and they were awaiting only the return of Kiabu's husband from Moba.

In September 1977, when I last heard of her, I was already in Kalemie, preparing for my departure from Zaire. She, too, had come to Kalemie, I heard, to sell fish. It was rumoured as well that she and her husband had divorced. She did not come to visit me, though I sent her word that I would welcome her company. Mutual friends said that this was due to her embarrassment at being divorced.

COMMENTARY

This description of the problematic illnesses in Kiabu's life during an 18-month period allows us to see the respects in which personal identity is reproduced through shifting constellations of symptoms, circumstances, interpretations and mood. Of significance are the attributes of the illnesses themselves, their outcomes; the openness of both symptoms and dreams to multiple narrative renderings; the subject's own state of mind and the subject's changing focus of concern as now one, now another life event necessitates speculation. Supporting the whole is a pragmatic approach to therapy and an ironic view of human frailities.

In Episode One, Kiabu's child's convulsions were classified as *ndege*. This illness, like all illnesses of the consciousness, is conventionally associated with spirits, as is the failure to defecate and urinate. These symptoms at first combined neatly with Kiabu's previous history to indicate a Bulumbu spirit as the illness's aetiologic agent. However, efforts to arrange the spirit were unsuccessful and with the death of the child a spirit had to be eliminated as the possible cause. Spirits come to aid and bless, and deadly illnesses are not characteristic of them. A second divination was discounted as false because the illness had occurred in Kiabu's third child, and not her second, as would have been the case had it derived from the *kiswa* of her firstborn. The third divination into the illness accounted for the child's symptoms by attributing them to an invisible, magical cord which had been tied around the child by sorcerers.

Similarly, Kiabu's inclination to view her second illness as deriving from sorcery was unsupported by its responsiveness to treatment. Since the symptoms of pain and swelling were readily diagnosed and were successfully treated by antibiotics and surgery, the appendicitis could not be due to the *buganga* of others.

Finally, the dizziness, cold sweat and weakness which marked the onset of the final episode were classic symptoms of soul theft (*kudjindula*). However, Kiabu's ability to arise and seek treatment despite them left her interpretation somewhat open to question. When the symptoms were both self-limiting and non-recurring, they tended to fade from the centre of Kiabu's concern.

Kiabu's approach to treatment also illustrates the freedom with which an individual may move from biomedicines to traditional medicines and treatments (called *dawa ya kizungu* and *dawa ya kinchi*, respectively), and back again. Her repeated employment of first one and then the other or of both is not unusual. Kiabu's management of her child's and her own illness, like Kaputa's and Kalwa's in Chapter 4, reflects the pragmatism governing judgement about physiological treatment. Though distinction is made between 'European' and 'traditional' medicines on a number of bases, there is a broader sense in which any sort of medication is subordinate to and will work only within the context of proper social relations – relations which neither antibiotics nor root infusions can modify themselves.

In addition, Episode Two makes clear, in a negative fashion, another critical feature of the medical environment; in rural Zaire, biomedicine's greatest stronghold, the hospital, is virtually inaccessible to ordinary people. While this alternative theoretically would be available, the high cost of transportation, lodging and food combines with the complexities of getting on in the city to form a virtually insurmountable obstacle. The social implications of hospitalisation are every bit as far-reaching as the patient's death itself. Indeed, the normal cost of treatment for appendicitis at the Clinique Mama Mobutu was three times what Kiabu's husband had been made to pay as indemnity for the death in childbirth of his other wife. In addition, since the very basis of sound diagnosis and treatment is attentiveness to the patient on the part of the practitioner, the overwhelmingly heavy case load of local doctors virtually ensures that a nondescript villager unaccustomed to city ways will not be 'seen', even if she or he is in the doctor's presence.

As with Kaputa, Kiabu's behaviour also illustrates the Tabwa truism that the willingness of the principal party to divine is directly related to her perception of danger in the illness situation. When she thought she was dying, or that she had been near death (Episode Three), Kiabu was quick to send an 'arrow' to Mumbyoto. When, however, her physical condition and social circumstances gave her no cause to worry, her credulity rapidly gave way to scepticism – only to return when she, once again, felt some discomfort. Similarly, Kiabu felt no need to divine into what, on the face of it, was a more serious illness, the appendicitis. Its responsiveness to treatment kept it from being perceived as a problematic illness.

People are quite aware of this equivocation. They regard it as one of life's major ironies and often note that scepticism emanates most strongly from a body free of suffering. People are fond of joking about how quickly they forget their disbelief in divination when they are ill; how fervently they promise to carry out the actions prescribed by the diviner; and how quick they are to forget both the practitioner and the instructions once they are well. In her response to both her personal illnesses (Episodes Two and Three), Kiabu was no exception to this rule. In Episode Two, as well, her self-awareness in this regard was one of the sources of her great post-operative good humour.

Kiabu's story also makes clear the extent to which the *experience* of an illness occurrence is comprised of both physiological symptoms and the social context in which these become apparent. In the case of Kaputa's daughter's illness, the interweaving of symptoms and history was part and parcel of the process of divination. As a consequence, it was the device by which Kaputa and Kalwa mastered the illness, stopped experiencing it and began making of it something they *had* experienced. With Kiabu's case, in contrast, the close interconnection of symptoms and social relations formed the unity of the experience itself.

Ordinarily indissoluble, components of the illness occurrence can be teased apart for inspection, and Episode Three of Kiabu's case history is especially illustrative of the way in which physiological and social situations influence one another. The actual symptoms which precipitated the crisis were neither particularly overpowering nor especially long-lasting. During the course of my stay, vertigo, accompanied by cold sweating and palpitations of the heart, happened to a number of friends and other people as well as to Kiabu. Though they also sought physical treatment, the others did not attach to their symptoms the same deadly implications that Kiabu attached to hers, the fact that such symptoms are classic characteristics of soul theft notwithstanding. It may be argued that this difference in interpretation was due in large measure to the variations in the social circumstances surrounding the occurrences. Kiabu's perception of her illness as being life-threatening may have been influenced by her awareness that there were those among her neighbours who disliked her, who envied her status as the wife of a government agent, and who would not have regretted her loss and/or her humiliation.

People recognise themselves to be jealous guardians of status equivalence. They cite such jealousy (*wivu*) as the emotion which underlies sorcery (*ulozi*). While everyone is subject to *wivu*, the intensity with which the sorcerer feels it is one of the principal characteristics by which she or he can be recognised. As Kilimamboka once put it, one never sees the sorcerer at work, but one does see his intentions (*nia yake*) as these are made manifest in his more ordinary interactions.

Kiabu's sense of threat was thus based on the social reality of others' jealousy regarding her ambitiousness and upward mobility. This reality included the possibility of sorcery and death. Numerous incidents similar to the one which took place by the lake occurred in the community during my stay, and were one of life's regular, if intermittent, irritations for all Mpala's residents. They attested to the fact that Kiabu was not unjustified in regarding her altercation with her young neighbour as but the outward and visible sign of the hidden grudges others held against her. Indeed, as some of the events in Episode One showed, this was not the first time that Kiabu had been the object of such attack.

While others' jealousy of Kiabu herself was the problematic factor of which she spoke to me, areas of difficulty about which she did not speak directly nevertheless may have contributed to a general sense of self-consciousness and anxiety. One of these was her husband's role as government fisheries agent, which caused him to be the instrument of misfortune for all of those in the community who failed to pay fishing and canoe licensing fees. Such a position carries with it the danger of ensorcellment by those whom one has 'afflicted' (*kutesa*); and the occupants of other, similar posts were always careful not to be overly conscientious in carrying out their tasks. Kiabu's husband, however, supported himself on fines and taxes during the months when his salary failed to arrive, and part of his willingness to do so may have been sustained by the fact that he was a MuHemba and thus always an outsider. The wrath which he incurred by the way he managed his job might be seen to have fallen upon his wife. She certainly could have been thinking so.

In addition, Kiabu's husband was not altogether the faithful, domesticated creature she purported him to be. He was known to have had several other liaisons around town, one of which had ended in the death in childbirth previously mentioned. He also had wives in Moba with whom he would live while there, and whom he, at one point, thought to move to Mpala. By means either of a venereally acquired *kibanda* or of sorcery deriving from a jealous lover, Kiabu could have been endangered by her husband's infidelity. Further, knowledge of his availability to others could only have heightened tension between Kiabu and her neighbours.

For her part, Kiabu was obviously anxious about her reproductive capacity. At some point after her non-divination with Mumbyoto, she revealed herself to have been in treatment for infertility with a local practitioner. She was also something of a flirt and a snappy dresser, whose low-cut bodices revealed decorative scarifications on chest and breasts. She sometimes seemed to employ traditional joking relations (*utani*) in a way which permitted more than customary familiarities in her relations with men. However, and in contrast, I occasionally had the impression that Kiabu was a bit concerned about her own past history of casual relations with men (her *undumba*, or 'prostitution', as she called it), even as she sought reassurance that she was attractive and admirably socially competent. My sense was that she would have preferred this marriage to last, and she herself to conceive successfully and bear a healthy child.

All of these ambiguities were present in the social situation in which Kiabu was living at the time she became ill. Some of them were consciously formulated problems; others were perhaps only on the periphery of her mind. It can be suggested that the sense of danger deriving from her circumstances influenced Kiabu's perception of her symptoms *and* that the occurrence of her symptoms enhanced her sense of threat.

Kiabu's dream of sorcery gave form to her anxiety and, indeed, ultimately displaced her physical symptoms as the focus of her questioning in Episode Three. It was for interpretation of her dreams, rather than for the physiological illness which precipitated them, that Kiabu sought Mumbyoto's assistance. The subsequent occurrence of diarrhoea and abdominal pain was not problematic, and had no effect on the course of action Kiabu had previously set in motion.

In rendering his decision, Mumbyoto was proposing a structure of possible meanings into which Kiabu's experience as a whole might be fitted. A *kibanda* deriving from her antecedents or from casual sexual contacts accounted for the initial physical symptoms and the other negative aspects of the illness occurrence. The *pepo* to be arranged after cleansing explained the content of Kiabu's dreams. Mumbyoto's pronouncement thus directed Kiabu's attention towards and required modification of past social circumstances. In effect, he was telling Kiabu that her bad relations with her neighbours and other aspects of her present life could not have caused this particular illness occurrence.[27] She and she alone was therefore responsible for her situation; she had control over its outcome through the therapy of 'throwing the person in the bush' (*kumutupa mutu mupori*). Finally, the subsequent arrangement of her spirit would be the *pièce de résistance*, both to the episode and to Mumbyoto's work (*kazi*), conferring upon Kiabu a blessing she could not otherwise have attained.

Episode Three thus demonstrates the complementary relation between symptoms and circumstances in the unfolding of illness occurrences. Not only does social context affect the meaning attached to symptoms even as they are experienced, but the character of the illness itself functions as something of a commentary upon the situation. Through the proper correlation of symptoms and circumstances, the diviner makes one communication out of the whole, and thus fixes with a temporary 'permanence' the otherwise fluid relations which obtain between the material and the meaningful during the unfolding of problematic illness.

PROBLEMATIC ILLNESS AND PERSONAL IDENTITY

The defining role played by divination itself leads to the other, personal aspect of illness brought before us so strikingly by Kiabu's history. This is the extent to which problematic illness which threatens life also changes it; it is not only an event which happens in the life, but is by definition something acting on the life. Though they appear to begin spontaneously, the retrospection required by problematic illnesses is the intellectual manifestation of the fact that they are not spontaneous in the least. As a consequence, much of what a person knows to be true of herself is called in question; not just a new history, but also something of a new or reproduced identity is created.

Substantial parts of personal identity consist of what an individual knows to be true of herself, what others take or know to be true of her, and basic assumptions of the continuity of capability and motivation over time. Personal identity is thus as circumstantial in its constitution as it is substantial, even though its 'substance' is identified with ourselves. It is also more labile than most of us would like to think, vulnerable to the identifications of others and so to their misrecognitions and to their perhaps malicious misidentifications as well.

What Kiabu's illnesses demonstrate is that a person has numerous experiences during the course of her life, and that she organises these in such a way that some function to support or confirm her identity, others are 'noise', and still others undermine her sense of herself. Identity is thus not only a thing inherited and a history which happens, but also a thing worked on. Careful consideration of a diviner's interpretation involves the reorganisation and reinterpretation of all elements, especially how one is seen. This is the work itself, and the change in what one knows is its result.

Such was the case in Episode One, when the third divination into Kiabu's daughter's illness revealed it to have been caused by sorcery. At the time of the first divination, the illness had been attributed to a *bulumbu* spirit. Kiabu had had one of these in her childhood, but it had left her. The attribution of the child's illness to the spirit made this past, inactive aspect of Kiabu's history into something of salience for the present.

When, however, the child died and a subsequent divination defined the death as the result of the evil acts of two men, 'one near and one far away',

Kiabu could not help but rethink her personal history. Part of what became salient as a consequence was a remark made during the child's funeral. Someone had said that the clothes Kiabu presented for the burial were too grand for such a purpose. In accepting and pondering the divination, Kiabu connected this with other interactions to determine the exact identities of those responsible. Aspects of her personal history which had perhaps been of minor significance thus became major contributors to Kiabu's knowledge of her life and herself living it.

Similar, though more elaborate, transformations took place during Episode Three. After experiencing the first of her symptoms, Kiabu dreamt of sorcery. This dream performed something of an ideological function. It confirmed her impression that she had been ensorcelled, it coalesced Kiabu's anxiety around the person appearing within it, and by these means it constituted the grounds on which she reconstructed the events of the previous day.

The throat-clearing incident of that day had been an insignificant, though incongruous, moment. When she came to me for help that night, Kiabu made no mention of it. In the light of her subsequent dreams, however, the moment took on a different meaning. The next day, Kiabu saw it as the very act of ensorcellment, and reported it as such to the chief.

In addition to these, there were many other aspects of Kiabu's life during this period that seemed to require renewed definition. During lengthy conversations, she would indicate her ambivalence towards pregnancy and childbirth; towards her neighbours; towards her past history of sexual relations; towards the acquisition of a *pepo*; and, to a lesser extent, towards her husband. Early on, she spoke of how there was no longer God in the world, 'only *shetani*' ('devils', a term applied to *bulumbu* spirits as well as to *vibanda* and, metaphorically, to sorcerers). She said one could know which was the right path to follow, but the *shetani* would grab you by the neck and force you down the wrong road, anyway.

That Kiabu's identity was at a crossroads, so to speak, was also manifest in the content of her dreams. Many of them were ambiguous and were susceptible of two different interpretations. In the earlier dream, the statue and snakes which she saw could have been signs of sorcery and of *nzunzi*, the sorcerer's agents; or, as Kiabu later reinterpreted them, they could be signs of the proximity of a *pepo*.

In a second dream, Kiabu first was witness to the sighting of a snake, then became that snake herself, chased by her father and virtually killed with stones. Though she readily interpreted this to indicate the presence of a *pepo*, her father's response to it – typical of the way non-spiritual snakes are treated – may have reflected her ambivalence towards the idea of having a spirit herself.

In a third dream, the 'little piece of meat' Kiabu set out to purchase might be seen as a reference to pregnancy. A number of *viabiko* (fertility medi-cines) make use of a small piece of meat to represent the developing foetus. That Kiabu was stopped in her progress by policemen (representative of *mukalaye*), who demanded her identity card of her, and that her husband, away in Moba, had this card, can be seen as a model of the situation in which she then found herself. Kiabu had yet to conceive, and might properly have expected a *pepo* to help her do so. However, a large measure of her ambivalence about acquiring a *pepo* had to do with her husband's reaction to such an eventuality. To the extent that she felt herself to be torn between her husband and her *pepo*, Kiabu's identity was held by the former in opposition to the latter, with Kiabu herself as passive victim in the conflict. Finally, in this dream, she was returned by the police to her mother's house, where she explained to her mother her circumstances in a turn of events clearly comparable to the divorce Kiabu may have felt to be imminent, and of which acquisition of spirits might have been the preci-pitating factor.

Perhaps to a greater extent than would be true for other people, then, Kiabu was uncertain about crucial aspects of her life and identity. The presence of problematic illness is sufficient, of itself, to cause intense questioning on the part and/or behalf of the afflicted; and a problematic situation makes the experience of any symptoms more intense. In this case, each of the two competing aetiological hypotheses – that Kiabu's illness was due to sorcery or to a *pepo* – implied a particular structure of experience. Each structure would bring certain events to positions of prominence, while others would be relegated to less significant spots in the memory.

Had Mumbyoto's divination confirmed Kiabu's initial suspicions, the incident with the old man and the subsequent altercation with her neigh-bour would have become meaningful events in Kiabu's life. Had Mumbyoto found Kiabu's illness to be due to the sorcery of one of her husband's lovers, his prolonged stays in Moba and his lack of concern for her would have become significant determinants in the overall value attached to their marriage. In either case, Kiabu would have become someone who was 'much pursued' (*kufuatwa sana*) by envious others. She might have consi-dered moving to another section of Mpala or divorcing her husband; and her previous history would have had no relevance to her present situation.

What Mumbyoto found, however, was that Kiabu's own past behaviour had caused her suffering. In accepting his conclusion, Kiabu was, in effect, disengaging the symptoms and dreams of Episode Three from the apparent complexities of her current social life. She was saying through this acceptance that the cough of the old man was nothing other than a cough, and the altercation signified nothing more threatening than the hostility of a young adult.

Simultaneously, however, Kiabu was bringing into prominence her previous identity as a *kapondo*, or human vehicle of a *bulumbu* spirit. The acquisition of such a spirit could be expected to cause some changes in Kiabu's lifestyle and marital relations, most particularly if the spirit were one which had come to divine. Indeed, it was on these very grounds that Kiabu was quite hesitant to go ahead with the arranged ceremony, and, in fact, had not done so at the time of my departure from the field some eight months later.

Taken as a whole, then, Kiabu's case history, covering a period of almost two years, allows us to see how the impact of illness on identity is experienced by people themselves. In her selections among alternate diagnostic theories and methods of treatment, Kiabu showed the extent to which the form of the illness occurrence and the recurrence or remission of symptoms both play crucial roles not only in the interpretation of disease but also in the reproduction of identity.

Kiabu's case history also shows the extent to which the illness occurrence is a phenomenal totality comprised of both physical symptoms and features of the social situation in which the patient finds himself. Perception of one affects perception of the other, and diagnosis of problematic illness must take both into account. The solutions offered, when substantiated by cure, can result in modifications of personal identity, changes in what a person knows to be true of herself, and therefore alterations in who she takes herself to be.

Visible, though perhaps understressed in this analysis, is the respect in which this reproduction is, at least in part, a collective process. The interpretation of identity-transforming events is a project worked on by many, as many as the person wishes to include in the circumference of her conversation. Talk about what might have been and assessments of what might be are all governed by rules which condition probabilities and codes which condition the iconography of dreams. As elsewhere, talk functions to proliferate possibilities out of which a choice can then be made.

6

ILLNESS AND LOCAL HISTORY: MWANGA VILLAGE

Expanding on the points explored in Chapter 5, the case history presented here will allow us to explore the processes by which the changes to personal identity caused by problematic illness in individual lives become part of lineage group history or instead are in some sense excluded from it.

The episodes covered here comprise the major illnesses occurring within a single lineage group over the course of two years. Through their unfolding we shall be able to consider the complex interrelations between social dramas and illness occurrences.

The complexity of this interrelation derives from several characteristics. Primary among these is the resemblance between the processual form of the illness occurrence (whether problematic or not), and that of social drama.[1] The 'breach' phase of social drama, in which a disruption of social relations is signalled by a public breach or non-fulfillment of a social norm, has its correspondent in the onset of illness, in which the presence of symptoms indicates that normal circumstances no longer prevail in the body.

The 'crisis' phase of social drama is characterised by the spread of the conflict throughout the group as factions are formed. A similar phase in illness occurs when symptoms persist or worsen in the absence of adequate medical treatment.

In the third, 'redressive' phase of the social drama, measures are taken by leading members of the social group to resolve crisis, and to restore balance. In an illness occurrence, this is the curative phase in which differing treatments are undertaken.

In the final phase of the social drama, reintegration of the conflicting parties is achieved or schism between them is recognised. In illness, the corresponding phase consists of either a remission of symptoms or their exacerbation and possible progress to a subsequent developmental stage.

This similarity between the processual forms of the two types of episode has perhaps resulted in a confounding of the two in anthropological literature. Indeed, early interpretation of African 'traditional' thought posited a direct relation between the two. The reasoning was that since natural death was impossible from an African perspective, in theory any death or serious illness could result in accusations of sorcery or other political crisis. Illness occurrences became analytic invariables, extensions of social situations which were the true subjects of anthropological contemplation, the true agents in ethnographic texts.

That such confusion should occur is not surprising in view of the fact that a problematic illness may precipitate or form a significant part of a social drama. What is made clear by peoples' approaches to illness and treatment in Mpala, however, is that the relation between the two is not direct, but is quite delicately articulated. Conflict and illness occurrence affect one another in oblique, not straightforward ways.

This case history demonstrates the point in some detail. It consists of eight problematic illness occurrences, and the dramatic episodes (including divination) to which they gave rise. The history also includes the episodic social dramas which were the form taken by the long-standing conflict then functioning to split the lineage group. Observing the relations between the two types of interruption we come to understand how the re-production of social order through the management of illness is parallelled by the production of local history.

SETTING AND CONFLICT

During the time of my stay, the village of Mwanga, in which most of this history unfolded, consisted of no more than four of five inhabited houses, and about an equal number of abandoned buildings or their ruins (*matongo*). Situated on a point about one kilometre south of Mpala and, like it, overlooking Lake Tanganyika, Mwanga had once been both more popular and more important than its somewhat deserted air led one to believe.

The village had originally been established nearly a century earlier, long before the present village of Mpala had come into existence. It was founded by Mumbwe Kiembo and was the birthplace of many of the older members and antecedents of the Bakwa Mumbwe lineage, whose role in contention for the chiefship of Mpala is recorded elsewhere.

At one time, Mumbwe fled to Nkonda, because he had several wives, and the mission's priests would not allow polygamists near their post. When he returned, he brought with him Kaponda, a renowned Tulunga diviner and healer, who had come up the lake from Zongwe and had lived for a time at Marasini village before moving to Mpala. It is said that Kaponda was called to Mpala to practise his curative arts for the priests as well as for the local people.

Some time after Kaponda's arrival, Kimpinde[2] moved to Mwanga from Nzawa. As many people did in those days, Kimpinde had moved first to Marasini, making the migration in two steps.

Kaponda, now influential because of his medicines, saw that Kimpinde's character was good, and so suggested that the latter become headman of the village. The diviner/curer worked to protect the village from sorcerers and was perhaps the 'power behind the throne' while Kimpinde was 'he who stood before' Kaponda (*musimamizi mbele yake*), and dealt with ordinary affairs.

At its peak, the, limits of Mwanga extended almost to Mpala's present borders but, local people say, internal disputes and accusations of sorcery caused residents to move away. At the time of my stay, Mwanga was inhabited almost exclusively by the members of one lineage, all of whom were Kimpinde's children. The long-standing conflict of which this history is a partial account was a significant (indeed, at times, defining) aspect of the relations between two of them, Muvimbo (C4 on Figure 6.1) and her younger sister, Kibambo (C11), though they were rarely the primary actors in its unfolding.

The actual origins of the conflict are somewhat obscure. People living outside the village trace its beginning to a conflict over headmanship beginning after Kimpinde's death in 1972. Those closely involved say that this only crystallised an opposition which had begun years before.

Kisile (D3), second son of Muvimbo and a man in his forties, says that the tension between his mother and her sister Kibambo was already in existence as he and his siblings were growing up. Though the two had been friends as children, relations began to change during their adulthood, and by the time members of Kisile's generation 'became conscious' (*kukalamuka*), the lines were already set.

More specific, however, were a number of grievances to which Muvimbo's children could point. Among these were disagreement over the operation of an outboard motor and a dragnet sent to the local lineage group by one of its members, Kafindo (C10), who was an officer at a bank in Lubumbashi. Each of these items represented a substantial investment as well as the possibility for the accumulation of considerable wealth. Instead, conflicts over the use of both items and the management of their proceeds resulted in the near splitting of the group and the cessation of all collective commercial activities.

Kisile and Kakonge (Muvimbo's youngest child (D9)) say that, of their sibling group, it was really this which began their 'disagreements' (*mizongano*). At the time the motor was in operation, Kibambo's husband, Matipa (C12), was stricken by what would be considered biomedically as a psychiatric illness, and was permanently disabled. Though he regained coherence, Matipa was thereafter unable to leave the house and so could no longer earn money by fishing or hunting.

During and after the acute stage of Matipa's illness, Kalandu (B2), Kimpinde's wife, and mother of Muvimbo, Kafindo and Kibambo, began helping her youngest daughter in quite specific ways. Kalandu thought that, since all Muvimbo's children were grown and all her daughters were married, Kibambo should receive the better part of the proceeds deriving

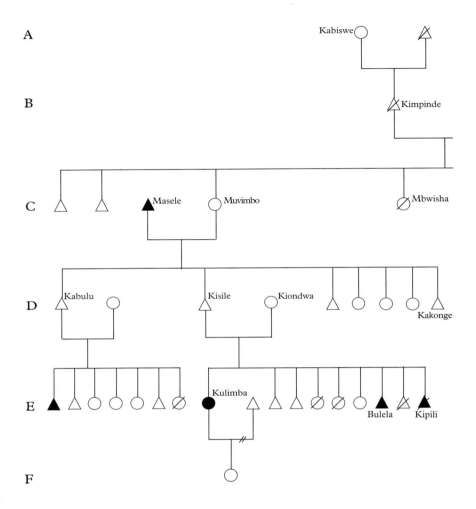

Figure 6.1 Genealogy of residents of Mwanga village

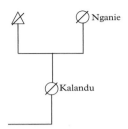

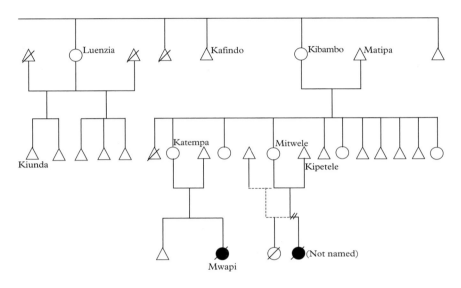

Key

△ = Man

○ = Woman

△—○ = Marriage

△—○ = Divorce

△—○ = Siblings

△ = Deceased

● = Illness figures in case history

from operating the outboard motor. Kalandu reasoned that Kibambo had small children and no husband to help her raise them, and Kalandu would therefore give her daughter money from the motor's cash box, and even gave her the lengths of cloth Kafindo sent to her from Lubumbashi. Once, when Kalandu lay dangerously ill, she even told Muvimbo that if she died, she would have nothing to leave her elder daughter but the very blouse she wore. Everything else she had given to Kibambo.

In addition, instead of keeping the key to the cash box herself, Kalandu turned it over to another daughter, Luenzia (C7), who gave it to Kibambo when she later moved with her husband to another village. After this, Kibambo would regularly help herself to money to buy such things as salt, soap and kerosene

Such differential treatment violated a basic principle of kin relations, viz., status equivalence among all occupants of a given kinship category. Balancing this principle of equivalence of all against individual differences in life circumstances, principles of individual ownership, and, of course, the very real personal preferences and distinctions that characterise kin relations is a delicate social process not always successfully achieved. Muvimbo and her children interpreted Kalandu's generosity to Kibambo as favouritism.

Their sense of alienation from Kibambo was increased by quarrels between them and the children of Luenzia, who operated the motor and, with their mother, tended to side with Kibambo in conflicts. The pre-existing tension caused Muvimbo's children to confine their commercial effort to the operation of the dragnet. When their kinsmen refused to transport their children to school free of charge, Muvimbo's children responded with an equivalent refusal to share freely fish caught in their nets. This, too, violated a basic principle of kin relations; that is, the obligation of mutual assistance and nurturance among relatives. Finally, the group decided that both motor and net should be in storage, because the quarrels they generated were too destructive, and that is pretty much how it was during my stay.

While Muvimbo and her children envied Kibambo her access to money, for her part Kibambo began to complain bitterly of the differences between her situation and her sister's. Muvimbo had a sound husband and healthy children. These had given birth to many grandchildren, and Muvimbo's descendants were growing great in number.

Kibambo's children, by contrast, had difficulty in conceiving and in giving birth. Her husband was unsound. Her grandchildren were sickly, and many died. Especially when drunk, Kibambo would lament her misfortune and would ask herself why she was so 'wretched' (*masikini*).

Kisile and Kakonge felt that the polarisation of the group was enhanced by the death by drowning of Mbwisha (C5) shortly after the purchase of the motor.[3] A sister whose order of birth placed her between Muvimbo and

Kibambo, she had also been an effective arbiter of their disputes. When Kimpinde or Kalandu settled the sisters' conflicts in a way that favoured Kibambo unduly, Mbwisha would speak privately with their father and obtain a more equitable judgement. Without Mbwisha to act as go-between and to maintain harmony among these family members, bad feelings and petty slights grew into genuine factionalism.

The next major episode in the lineage group's underlying conflict occurred after Kimpinde's death in 1972, when the terms of the conflict and the personnel shifted somewhat. At this time his sister's son, Ngandwe, inherited the headmanship of the village, much to the chagrin of Kimpinde's children, who thought it should have been theirs. They made this clear to Ngandwe, by saying that they felt the village was of members of the Bena Mumba[4] clan – their own in contradistinction to their father's clan, the Bazimba.

Such conflict between the rights and privileges of a man's maternal kin and those of his children is a constant in social life. Kibambo felt that she should have succeeded to her father's position; and eventually Ngandwe began to suspect that she was ensorcelling him. He accused her of rubbing magical medicines into incisions made on certain of his domestic animals. Finally, his own senior maternal kinsmen concluded that Ngandwe did not have sufficient support within the village, and that continued residence there placed him in jeopardy. At their prompting, Ngandwe left Mwanga and moved to Mpala.

After the departure of Ngandwe, conflict over the headmanship flared up between Kibambo and Muvimbo's elder son, Kabulu (D1). Each claimed the right to arbitrate disputes in the village, to shout public warnings to sorcerers (*kupiga mbila*), and to transmit local news to Chief Mpala.

During the course of this episode, Kabulu's eldest son (E1) was taken ill with a strange sickness that no one could recognise and which caused his skin to become 'very black'. His parents went to several different diviners for diagnosis of the illness, and all of them found it to derive from Kibambo. One of the practitioners, a man who lived beyond Kala (some two days' walk away), they brought back with them to the village. There, he undertook treatment of Kabulu's son and such other patients as came to him.

The presence of this *mfumu* gave Kibambo reason to believe that Kabulu meant to kill her with sorcery. One day, while drunk, she went to the house of Muvimbo's husband's younger brother and stood before it, telling him in a loud voice that his children were sorcerers. She said they 'drank *tufwabubela*' (large black weevils with red dots, *Brachycerus apterus*, which are filled with medicines, either protective or aggressive), that they buried medicine-filled horns in their houses, and that they made medicines to kill her and her children.

Ultimately, the conflict over headmanship of Mwanga was settled by Mpala. He determined that the village should no longer be regarded as an independent entity, because it had so few inhabitants. Instead, it was placed under the headmanship of Kafwanka, who was completely unrelated to anyone there, and Mwanga thus became a part of his section of Mpala. Kabulu was made responsible for the internal affairs of the village, but was to work closely with Kafwanka and to keep him informed of current events.

Though I arrived several years after the conclusion of this particular set of incidents, considerable bad feeling remained in Mwanga, and the conflict's ideological form appeared to have been determined more by the last episode than by any other. Principal foci of the factions were Kibambo and Kabulu, each of whom felt the other to be a sorcerer. Kibambo believed Kabulu was determined to destroy her descendants, while Kabulu believed Kibambo to be jealous of the fecundity of his mother and her children. When quarrels would erupt, it was these suspicions, rather than complaints or grievances deriving from earlier episodes, which would be cited by the parties concerned.

It is upon this set of circumstances, then, that our case history opens. During this two-year period, the lineage group resident in Mwanga suffered approximately eight significant illness occurrences.[5] The management of these, their effects upon the long-standing central conflict, and their relations to the social dramas by which other conflicts unfolded form the topics to be outlined and discussed below.

PROBLEMATIC ILLNESS EPISODES
Episode One: Kulimba's difficult labour

On 23 August 1975, Kisile's daughter, Kulimba (E8), gave birth to a baby girl after a prolonged labour lasting some sixteen hours. During it she was assisted by her mother's mother, her father's mother (Muvimbo), and one of her father's sisters. Her mother, Kiondwa, had also been present, but had played only a passive role, praying for a successful delivery while the other women actually worked. (To have been more actively involved would have implied that she did not think the others capable.)

Contractions had begun at around 4:00 a.m., but were intermittent, sometimes subsiding altogether. By late afternoon, Kulimba was exhausted and said she simply could not push anymore.

At 5:30 p.m., the baby's head was seen. However, instead of coming down and being born, the baby had mounted; returning inside her mother's body. It was at this moment that those present decided to seek outside medical assistance.

Kisile came first to the house, but I was not home. He then sought the help of the local nurse, who came to the house and administered two injections, one to aid the delivery and another of vitamins to give Kulimba strength (*kumuletea ngu'vu*).

When there was no substantial improvement in Kulimba's condition, traditional medicines were tried. The formula was one known to the women assisting her, and even while they were administering it, they dispatched the young woman's father and uncle to make inquiries in Mpala regarding other effective formulas. Kabulu even sought advice from a practitioner living one and one half hours' walk away from Mwanga.

During this same, especially difficult, period, Kisile also went to a nearby village (a twenty-minute walk from Mwanga) to seek divination into the cause of his daughter's difficult labour. He went alone, and carried with him the 'arrow', so that divination was immediate. The diviner, Kisimba, was a *bulumbu* practitioner whose spirit was quite new, and was said to be very accurate. This spirit attributed the difficulty to the anger Kulimba felt over harsh words of her husband's, uttered during a quarrel. At that time her husband had said that he didn't care if she lived or died. It was all the same to him, because if Kulimba died, he would just pay the indemnity and be given another wife. The spirit indicated that these words had made Kulimba feel great anger, and that, when the time came to give birth, this anger made her say to herself, 'let me just die!' (*nifwe tu*), just to be done with the matter.

The spirit concluded by recommending that Kulimba confess her anger and its causes to the *wangomba* (midwives) attending her, and then ask for the assistance of her *mizimu* in safely giving birth to a healthy child. Kisile paid 20 k for the divination and took back the spirit's insights and recommendations.

Kulimba confessed her anger and asked for assistance, as she had been instructed, and the baby girl was born shortly thereafter. The afterbirth was not delivered for an hour, however. The dispensary nurse gave Kulimba another injection to facilitate this process.

During the unfolding of this episode, Leya, classificatory sister of both Muvimbo and Kibambo, heard of her grandchild's situation, and immediately started off to see her. When she arrived at Mwanga, she stopped first at Kibambo's house, and there was told that she should go no further. Kibambo said that she herself had not been called to assist during the delivery, and she lived right there in the same village. Furthermore, it was she to whom Kalandu had told all her medicinal formulae for facilitating birth.

She could only conclude from this that Muvimbo and her children wanted no one to help, and that Leya would do best to return home. Since Matipa, Kibambo's husband, also concurred in this interpretation, Leya thought it best to refrain from offering assistance and so returned to Mpala.

The next day, Leya went to visit her grandchild, and to see the new baby. At that time she explained why she had been absent during the time of difficulty and outlined the sequence of events described above. Though reproached, Leya was ultimately excused for her omission, and blame for it was placed on Kibambo.

Despite their resentment, however, Muvimbo's children said nothing to Kibambo herself about either her own absence, or her deflection of Leya's intended course. Instead, they simply tolerated (*kuvumilia*) it.

Later, when I asked Kisile why they had not called Kibambo (which was itself a breach), he cited a number of different reasons. First, she had not been home at the time they went to inform her. Then, in any case, a grandmother should not have to be called for such a thing, but should just come. Further, in notifying Leya, were they not informing and calling her senior, and was that not the same as calling Kibambo herself?

In addition, Kisile said that they had not called his mother's sister because, when Kulimba had been ill earlier, Kibambo had never come to look in on her. Since she lived in the same village, but had never visited Kulimba even once, they felt they could not call her to attend the young woman during her labour.

Finally, they did not call her because they felt uneasy about Kibambo's constantly voiced envy of her sister Muvimbo, whose children were so much more fertile than her own. How could they call her to assist in the labour of one of Muvimbo's grandchildren, when Kibambo's own children had so much difficulty?

Commentary

Several important points are to be noted regarding this initial illness occurrence. First, the results of the divination into Kulimba's difficult labour focused upon the young woman's relation to her husband, rather than upon the strained relations among members of her own lineage. By thus disengaging the difficulty from the ongoing, intralineage conflict and by relating it to Kulimba's own anger deriving from a quarrel, the diviner took a conservative course. He both refrained from making outright accusations of serious wrongdoing, and placed the means of redressing the situation entirely within Kulimba's power. His divination took Kulimba's point of view, and made her the subject to whose will her body was subjected. Her successful delivery of a healthy baby after complying with his recommendations was proof of their accuracy, and, in effect, made this definition into the truth of the situation.

Despite the fact that it was in no direct way related to the conflict, the illness nevertheless contributed to the conflict's unfolding. In outlining the above events, Kisile used the term *mizongano*, a word that described the collective circumstances of his maternal kinsmen and him. In KiSwahili, *kuzongana* means 'to wind, bend about, or coil around'. People in Mpala use the noun form to give an acute image of the process by which everyone in such a situation misunderstands everyone else's motives. They oppose this to the term *kusikilizana*, which literally means 'to heed one another', and is used more generally to mean 'to come to an agreement'.

The term *mizongano* gives the impression of people talking past one another, or circling round one another, always failing to arrive at a consensus, a single domain of understanding. In this way, Kibambo could feel herself insulted because she had not been called to aid her classificatory granddaughter, while everyone else could feel that Kibambo should not need to be called. Each side made the incident into a test the other had failed. At one level, such *mizongano* are a failure to agree upon the applicability of social norms and obligations to a given situation.

There are, however, other levels as well. These were illustrated in the series of reasons given by Kisile for not calling Kibambo during the crisis. The first set can be described as legalistic technicalities: Kibambo had not been home; she should not have required special invitation; she should have assumed herself to be called because Leya, her senior, was sent for; etc. These are the kinds of statement one would expect to hear during the arbitration of a dispute. They refer only to norms, and not to underlying motives.

A slightly different level of misunderstanding was revealed in Kisile's mention of Kibambo's failure to show concern during her grandchild's previous illness. Though he conceded the impropriety of his failure to inform Kibambo, Kisile justified this lapse by placing it in the wider context of his suspicions regarding her motives. These suspicions in turn appeared to be founded on Kibambo's expressed envy of her sister's fecundity and numerous descendants.

Kisile in his final statements described his basic comprehension of Kibambo's ultimate motives, and much of his perception of her proximate behaviour was based upon this interpretation. Kibambo's failure to visit the ill Kulimba therefore was seen in the worst light, and this breach, in turn, led to another.

Finally, and equally important to our understanding, is the observation that *nothing was said* to Kibambo about either her failure to attend Kulimba or her prevention of Leya's intended visit. The day after the baby's birth, I visited Kulimba and found *everyone* present, including Kibambo herself. Relations appeared cordial at this time, and it was only later, in the telling of the story, that Kisile mentioned the breach.

Situations of significant illness occurrence are frequently those in which there also exist hidden tensions or grudges, which the divination may bring to light. The unspoken alienation existing among lineage members at the time of Kulimba's difficult labour is clearly an example of this circumstance.

Leya, whose motives were never doubted and against whom little bad feeling existed, was openly reproached regarding her breach of obligation. Similarly, she openly explained what had prevented her attendance, and awaited reciprocal explanation from her junior kinswoman and descendants. Through such discussion based on trust, misapprehension of intent is

obviated, and relations are restored to normal, with but one reality including all social interactions.

Since Kibambo's motives were suspect, however, no attempt was made
to discuss the breach with her. By simply 'tolerating' one another's breaches
of obligation, the group was in fact furthering misunderstanding. Each
social interaction thus might have attached to it numerous different, even
mutually exclusive, meanings; people's perceptions of and thoughts about
the situation could 'coil around' (*kuzongana*) one another, never meeting or
coming to agreement.

This is the sort of smaller misunderstanding which precedes the more
significant breach that opens social dramas. In addition, it might also be said
that social situations in which numbers of hidden *mizongano* exist become
those in which it is increasingly difficult for people to make sound judgements as to appropriate social behaviour. Under ordinary circumstances,
the fundamental ambiguity of social relations is contained by actions whose
meanings make clear that the abiding intention of another is precisely that
those ambiguities should be contained. In contrast, with *mizongano* that
other is seen to be taking advantage of those same ambiguities to conceal a
malicious motive; it is their intention that ambiguity should *not* be contained. Under these circumstances, one can know but with great difficulty
to which of an action's aspects or agent's intentions to respond.

Episode Two: Kulimba's *mushindo*

About six weeks after the birth of her child, Kulimba again became ill. The
illness began while I was away from home, and had been going on for a week
when I returned. Kisile described its onset and its progress to me.

He said Kulimba had these 'things' (*vitu*) which appeared on her arm and
itched. When she scratched, they ruptured and water came out. When I
asked Kisile if the illness was not *upele* ('skin eruptions'), the diagnostic
category whose description matched the one he gave, he said that it was not
upele but 'a thing, an event of the land' (*ni kitu, tukio ya nchi*). By this he
meant that it was sorcery.

Kisile went on to say that at the time Kulimba had given birth, she had
only a few little papules or pimples (*chunuku*) on one arm near the elbow.
Since then, however, it had spread to all parts of her body, from the neck
right down to her feet.

The arm on which the *chunuku* had originated was quite swollen, and
very painful. Kulimba could not stand even to move and had to be forced to
nurse her new baby. While itching was tolerable during the day, at night
Kulimba's suffering was so great that it made tears come to one's eyes just to
watch her. The baby cried, the young mother cried, and nobody in the
house got any sleep.

Two days after the illness first appeared to be spreading, Kulimba's family had taken her to the dispensary, where she received two injections of penicillin. When these proved to be of no avail, they thought the illness might respond to treatment with traditional medicines, and so had sought out a *mfumu*.[6]

Though the family had first diagnosed the illness as *lunanu*, Kisile himself had been of another opinion. The lesions of *lunanu* begin with very small *chunuku*. These itch and emit water, but do not hurt when they are scratched. With Kulimba's illness, however, the lesions had been large (*unene*), and although they also released water, when scratched, they hurt. The spread of the lesions from one place to the entire surface of the body was also not characteristic of *lunanu*, and made Kisile suspicious.

When he looked into the matter five days after its onset, the *mfumu* engaged by the family ultimately found the illness to be nothing other than medicines thrown on Kulimba by 'adulterous partners of her husband' (*wapuzi wa bwana yake*), who wished to eliminate her, that 'they might live with him'.[7] 'They' had originally thrown medicines upon her that were meant to descend to her abdomen and cause her either to deliver a stillborn infant or to die herself in childbirth. Luckily, however, Kulimba had left the village where she lived with her husband and come home to be delivered. She had thus escaped the greater part of the medicine, but the remainder of it appeared as this illness. Her sickness was thus *mushindo*, for such is the name applied to any illness coming from 'the path of people' (*njia ya watu*).

Since the diviner had so effectively recognised (*kutambua*) the illness, and believed it could be cured, the family decided that it should also be he who undertook treatment. So, they sent him another 'arrow' for the preparations of medicines, and he brought several different kinds.

Primary among them were the roots of the *mululuzia* tree (*Veronia colorata (Willd.) Drake*). These were to be dug, pounded in a mortar, and the pulp heated (with a little water) in a metal pot. The resulting mash was to be rubbed over Kulimba's body, and the water poured over her as a rinse.[8] The *mfumu* also provided a black, powered medicine (made by burning its ingredients and grinding their ashes), the contents of which were unknown, but which was to be sprinkled on the worst lesions, those on Kulimba's arm.[9]

In addition to his physiological therapy, the diviner also provided for the treatment of the aetiologic agents responsible for the illness. This took the form of a *kafwabubela* beetle whose abdomen had been filled with protective substances. Kulimba wore this around her neck during the day, to be protected from sorcerers. At night, she put the insect at the head of her bed, so that it could tell her through dreams the identities of those who had made her ill.

Jural action was also taken. The divination had been made in the presence of Kulimba's classificatory mother-in-law, who agreed with its results. Kulimba's husband was sent for, and arrived at Mwanga a few days after my own return. He was expected to confess his wrongdoing, name the female person(s) responsible for his wife's illness, and pay an indemnity to his wife's family for the injury he had caused their daughter.

At the time of his arrival, local rumour had it that the culprit was a woman with whom the young man had been sleeping even before his marriage to Kulimba. After he married, he had continued to see her, and, when this woman's husband divorced her, Kulimba's husband had established the woman in a house near Kulimba's own quite as if she were his second wife. It was said that the woman had grown tired of sharing her 'spouse' with Kulimba, and so had made medicines against the girl, so that she could have the young man all to herself.

Local opinion notwithstanding, however, Kulimba's husband consistently refused to name his adulterous partner. In subsequent weeks, as her illness began to remit, it was the refusal of her husband to cooperate that became the outstanding feature of this episode in Kulimba's life.

By 26 October 1977, Kulimba was physically completely recovered from her illness. Not only were the lesions themselves healed, but the behavioural milestone of resumption of work had also been passed. Kulimba had again begun to go to her parents' fields, to pound manioc, to cook, and to gather firewood.

The young woman's social situation, however, was not as well or as quickly resolved. Kulimba's parents and other members of her family were both definite and vocal in their opinion that she should not return to her husband. Kisile told me that the matter would not be considered completely closed until the divorce was settled and the diviner had again examined the case, to be sure no evil remained within Kulimba's body.

Though her family were strongly opposed, Kulimba herself seemed to be unsure about her course regarding her marriage. In the weeks that followed, she wavered among several different points of view. At some times, she would say that she had no intention of returning to her husband. At others, she said she would return to him, but only if he agreed to move elsewhere (a compromise that satisfied her parents). At still other points, Kulimba would insist that 'a husband is a husband' (*bwana ni bwana tu*), and that she would return to him no matter what.

On 2 December 1977, nearly two months after the onset of her illness, Kulimba's parents met with the diviner, to inform him of their daughter's recovery and to ask him to name his fee. I attended the session, which lasted little more than ten minutes. The *mfumu* named a fee of five zaires and a chicken, and agreed to look into the matter once more before Kulimba returned to her husband. When asked by him, her parents said that they didn't know quite what the girl would do; and her mother added that she wanted the diviner to tell Kulimba that if she went back to her husband she'd be sorry.

Ultimately, Kulimba remained in Mpala for some weeks, staying on to care for her younger siblings while her parents were away.[10] During this time, and for months afterward, she continued to wear the *kafwabubela* that the diviner prepared for her. Though the girl had resolved to return to her husband by this time, her mother later told me that Kulimba's *bulumbu* spirits possessed her several times to say that they saw evil awaiting her, should she go back to him.

Finally, her husband sent for her. He underwent a ceremony in preparation for her return in which he foreswore future adultery in the presence of a *mwendo* (pl. *baendo*; clan joking partners and therapeutic intermediaries). Manioc flour was placed in water, and both men then drank from the infusion. The remaining liquid was spilled out on the ground, and the pot inverted over it. On 21 January 1976, Kulimba returned to her spouse after a meeting in which the *mfumu* refused to indicate future danger, despite pressure from her parents that he do so.

One or two months later, another illness occurrence prompted her to leave him for good. During its course, she was completely incapacitated; and neither her husband nor his mother and sisters did anything to help her. Instead, she had to rely upon her father's mother's sister, Luenzia (who then resided in the same village), for help with such basics as drawing water, finding firewood, making food, and caring for her daughter. Kulimba said she saw from this that to stay with her husband would be to die; and so she came home to her own parents.

When she requested divorce (*kukata tumbako*, 'to cut tobacco'), her husband refused, saying 'a wife is a wife' (*bibi ni bibi*). His sister, however, agreed to play his part in the divorce ceremony; and so it went forward. At the time of my departure from Zaire, Kulimba had only recently stopped wearing her protective amulet, which she had continued to wear after the divorce on the grounds that when one becomes ill and does not have such a thing, it is easy for sorcerers to 'know your name' (*kujua jina lako*).

Commentary

As with Episode One, this significant illness occurrence is noteworthy for the way in which its interpretation and management remained unrelated to the principal social conflict unfolding within the lineage group. That Kulimba's husband's adultery was known was probably no more responsible for this separation than was the girl's structural position as one on the edge (so to speak) of her own matrilineage.

Kulimba's status, as recently married and a new mother, placed her on the adult side of the border dividing that state from childhood. Her situation was reflected in her return to her natal home to deliver the very child whose birth marked her transition to the status of 'big person' (*mukubwa*).

The birth of the first child marks accession to adulthood; yet it is customary for a woman to return to the place where she was a child to have the protection of her mother at the time of the birth and right after. This relative marginality lent the diagnosis plausibility. As she was no longer completely her parents' child, her illnesses could not necessarily reflect her parents' social conflicts.

Of significance as well is the way in which the social aspects of the episode outlasted the specific symptoms of the illness occurrence which gave rise to them. Kulimba recovered from her itching lesions[11] fully one month before her parents felt it safe to consider her cured and to ask the *mfumu* his fee. She had resumed work, and she was able to return to her husband, several months before the diviner made his final pronouncement.

This discrepancy between social and physiological aspects of an illness episode is in part due to the fundamentally negative nature of the 'cured' state. In it one is *not* sick; one does *not* have symptoms.

One of the characteristics of sorcery is precisely the way in which the patient can have appeared well, displaying no symptoms, even as her body has been penetrated by illness. Problematic illness emphasises this mystery and raises profound questions regarding the difference between 'ill' and 'well', showing them to be states more easily opposed in thought than in fact. It is precisely this uncertainty which makes it necessary that a substantial period of time should have elapsed without recurrence of symptoms before an individual may be considered to be completely recovered. Such a period permits her transition from a state wherein her symptomlessness is, in fact, a marked (though featureless) condition to one wherein symptomlessness is normal (or unmarked).

In Kulimba's case as well, problematic social factors came to displace physiological ones, for as her symptoms remitted, her husband's uncooperative attitude came to the fore. His earlier transgression was compounded by the fact that he was unwilling to demonstrate repentance by naming his partner, even though his wife's life was at stake.

In such a situation, the specific truth of the matter is less important to people than is the willingness of the culprit to confess. With a matter of such relative unimportance as adultery, one who quibbles over particulars and insists that he never committed such or such an act is to be faulted more because he fails to show concern for his counterpart than because he has committed a wrong that 'everybody does' (*wote wanafanya*) in any case. Kulimba's husband's initial unwillingness even to go through the formalities of severing himself from his adulterous partner was taken as a strong indication of the extent to which he would not properly protect his wife in the future. This, in turn, increased her parents' unwillingness to have Kulimba pronounced well and to permit her to return to him. Long after the illness was ended, the question of Kulimba's relation to her husband remained.

This very question, in fact, leads to yet another significant feature of this illness episode: viz., the role played by Kulimba's own *bulumbu* spirits. In her childhood, spirits had come to her, though then, as at the time of my stay, they did not 'mount' (*kumupanda*) her often, but came only in time of crisis. This is characteristic of all *bulumbu* which do not come specifically to divine.

Noteworthy here, however, is the way in which the spirits sided with Kulimba's parents and family, rather than with Kulimba herself. From the analyst's perspective it is evident that, through them, Kulimba could respond simultaneously to both of the divergent impulses pulling her. In other situations, as well, *bulumbu* spirits take postures quite distinct from those of their human vehicles (*kapondo*). In speaking of their *kapondo* with other family members, *bulumbu* thus permit a discussion in the third person, as it were, by those who might otherwise be too closely involved in a situation to do so directly. It also makes things hypothetical; and, thus, as in other areas of life, knowledge or decision begins or proceeds by a device which promotes the proliferation of possibilities and points of view, out of which consensus intermittently emerges.

Finally, it is to be noted here that, despite her parents' very definite and definitely expressed wishes, the *mfumu* would not forbid Kulimba to return to her husband. The relative neutrality of diviners is a significant part of the divination situation. Indeed, it is precisely this which, in practical respects, underlies the credibility of divination as an interpretative procedure, enabling individuals to see into a situation in ways that are not otherwise available and yielding results that are in some sense unexpected.

Episode Three: Premature birth of Kibambo's grandchild

On 7 November 1975, slightly more than one month after Kulimba's *mushindo* had begun, Mitwele (D20), a daughter of Kibambo, gave premature birth to a baby girl. Born after a pregnancy of only eight months' duration, the child was not given a name while the family waited 'to see her condition' (*kuona hali yake*). On the day she was born, the baby's father, Kipetele, came to me to ask for vitamins 'so that she might gain strength' (*apate ngu'vu*) and begin to nurse normally.

Two days later, on 9 November 1975, Kipetele returned to say that the infant's condition was still not good. She had not yet nursed effectively. Since birth, all she had consumed was a little sugar water given her from a spoon.

At my suggestion Mitwele and Kibambo brought the child to the house the next day. She was tiny and red and moved slowly and feebly. She seemed able to suck and swallow, however, and, though she was very weak,

I nevertheless had hopes that she might survive. By this time, her mother's milk had come in, and she was being put to the breast regularly, but could not nurse effectively. I supplied powdered milk, and an eye dropper (all I had), and suggested that she be given a little something at frequent intervals during the coming days, so that her strength could gradually be built up. I suggested that the infant be brought back to me on 14 November , four days later.

When Mitwele did not return with the baby on that day, I knew it meant that the infant was considered to be either out of danger or beyond saving. I had observed during the earlier visit that, though her navel cord was dried and almost ready to drop off, the family had not tied a little piece of cloth over her genitals, as is usually done.[12] These things, in conjunction with their unwillingness to name her, told me that the family had not invested much hope in the baby.

Then, on the morning of 17 November, ten days after her birth, the baby died. Kabulu stopped by the house to get smoking paper for the funeral, and told me that this was the second child Mitwele and Kipetele had lost. Though the baby had never been named, because of her poor condition, they were having a funeral because the umbilical cord had dropped prior to her death. However, rather than relatives sleeping there the three days customary for the funerals of adults and those of children after the first, they were only going to sleep one day. By this, my sense that the death was not unexpected was confirmed.

Slightly more than two weeks after the baby's death, on 2 December 1975, Mumbyoto divined into the situation surrounding it.[13] I did not know him well at this time, and was present as a guest of the family.[14] Also present were Mitwele herself and Kibambo, who paid for the session (one small white chicken and 150 *makuta*), as well as a father's sister of Kibambo (*shangazi*). Representing his side were Kipetele himself, his brother's wife, and a close friend. Mumbyoto had with him a young man who served as assistant

The divination took place in much the same way as Kaputa's (Chapter 4). Water was boiled in a clay pot, and Mumbyoto used it as an oracle. He asked questions of it, then plunged his hands into it to retrieve (or fail to retrieve) a seed dropped there.

The situation was a difficult one, perhaps made more complicated by my presence. Mumbyoto began his discussion with a parable spoken in KiTabwa which I did not fully understand. It was a story about a rabbit attempting a journey who found one road blocked by a lion and the other by a hippopotamus. I did not know if Mumbyoto was referring to his clients' or to his own situation. For her part, Mitwele was uncooperative, speaking KiTabwa at first, then, when her husband insisted that they all speak KiSwahili, refusing to speak at all. Kibambo similarly did not have much to say. Their very unwillingness to talk was later interpreted by Kipetele's sister-in-law as evidence of Mitwele's culpability in the case.

In any event, after examining his *nsuko* gourd and asking questions of his oracle a number of times, Mumbyoto focused upon marital discord as the source of Mitwele's and Kipetele's difficulty. At first neither of the young couple would respond to his questions about their marriage. When asked, they would just shrug their shoulders and say nothing. The medicated *lukusu* seed stuck again and again to the bottom of the pot, however. Finally, Kipetele began to open up.

Saying, 'Let us open it, sister' (*tufungue dada*), Kipetele first asked Mitwele to begin describing things with him; then, when she refused, went on himself to say that there was, indeed, conflict in their household. He said that the problem in a nutshell was that he and Mitwele simply did not get along. Their strained relationship had been further weakened the previous July, when (undoubtedly during an argument) he had told his wife that he was not sure this pregnancy was his.[15] That, Kipetele concluded, was more or less the end of their marriage. He thought they ought to divorce and leave it at that.

Once the situation had been 'opened' (*kufunguwa*), the discussion continued, pursued largely by Kipetele and Mumbyoto, with the oracle validating Mumbyoto's pronouncements. The concluding hypothesis was that the death of this child had been caused by the spirit of the first.

The first child had had 'two fathers' (*bababa bawili*), said the diviner. So saying, Mumbyoto held up three fingers, one of which he said was the husband, the middle one the wife, and the third one the lover. Since the child had had two fathers, it had been, when it died, 'like an animal' (*kama vile nyama*). It had not known whether to go to the 'side' (*ng'ambo*) of the husband or of the lover, and so had just stayed hovering there.

Then, with the pregnancy that had just ended, the dead child had seen that his mother had forgotten him. She was treating him as though he and his problem did not exist. So he had come to kill this child. Now, Mumbyoto concluded, addressing Kipetele, it was up to the young couple to cleanse the marriage of 'your [plural] adultery' (*upuzi wenu*).

'My adultery?!'; Kipetele pulled himself up. Mumbyoto promptly replied that it was *both* of theirs because it was in *their* house. He pointed to me as an example, asking if something of the sort were to happen in my house, would my husband and I not both be involved? Kipetele stopped protesting, though he did not go on to agree with the diviner's assessment.

Mumbyoto went on to say that he had also dreamt of a snake which was sitting up in one of the corners of the room, along the top of the wall, looking into the room itself. He also had seen the same snake standing near Mitwele's and Kipetele's bed, looking into that.

Under the line of questioning indicated by this dream, Kibambo revealed that there had been a dead kinsman of theirs who had brought a *bulumbu* spirit to Kibambo herself. The spirit had fled, however. Now, Mumbyoto said, the dead antecedent wished to return to be born to Mitwele and her husband. It was frightened of their marital discord, though, and this was why it could only hover on the periphery of their lives, unable to enter. Like the dead child, this spirit, too, had no place. It was up to Kipetele and the family members to resolve their conflicts, be cleansed of their adultery, and arrange matters so that the spirit could be born to them.

Even Kibambo herself was not exempt from his commentary. Mumbyoto told her that she just 'threw her cash up' (*kutupa makuta juu*). She wasted it on beer and similar things, and then was reluctant to come up with the necessary money for the arrangement of spiritual matters. In the face of his remarks, she, like her daughter, just sat, silently unwilling to respond.

Mumbyoto's final remarks were directed to Mitwele herself. Throughout the divination she had been unresponsive and had seemed to me to under-estimate the extent to which Mumbyoto sympathised with her. At this point he spoke to her, reiterating his assessment of the situation, and telling her that if she did not believe him, she should make beer dedicated to the spirit itself. She was to buy millet and corn and, as she prepared the mash, she was to say 'we are two' (*tupo wawili*, meaning she and the spirit were alone). If what Mumbyoto said was true, the spirit was to leave the beer so that it 'ripened' (*kuivia*). If, however, what he said was not true, the spirit was to make the beer sour (*kuchacha*). By this means she could herself test the validity of his statements.

With this, Mumbyoto concluded his divination. He was paid by Kibambo, packed up his things, and departed – telling us that it was not his policy to stay around after he divined. The next day, Kipetele's sister-in-law came to the house to visit and to hash things over. She said that despite Mumbyoto's conclusions to the contrary, Kipetele was determined to divorce his wife. Kipetele's friend, who accompanied her, was even more adamant, and clearly blamed Mitwele for everything. He said she had said little during the divination, because she had nothing to say. She was simply a bad person; they had already lost three children to her adultery; and they had decided to divorce long before the occurrence of this particular death. While Kipetele definitely wanted the divorce, Mitwele and her mother did not; probably because under these circumstances – with everyone knowing of Mitwele's adultery – such a course would mean that she would never get a good husband again. Though he didn't know just what the couple would do, the friend concluded, he thought they might just leave one another (*kuachana*).

Several weeks after this, the pair were separated. Mitwele returned to her natal home, and Kipetele moved to Moba, where he took another wife. Their situation remained at an impasse for the following two years. Then, in the spring of 1977, Kipetele began seeing Mitwele again during his visits to

Mpala to visit relatives and to purchase dried fish. After consultation with a *mwendo*, the two again took up residence together. For awhile, Kipetele continued his second marriage, though, at the time of my departure from Mpala, he went only rarely to Moba. At this time, as well, he suffered intermittently from *mpanga*, a male illness affecting the lower back and testicles.

Commentary

In this, as in the previous two episodes (the second of which overlapped in time with this one), the significant illness was attributed by the diviner to the poor marital relations of the patient and her husband, rather than to the major intralineage conflict simultaneously in progress. At the time the divination took place, in 1975, I was unaware that such conflict existed;[16] and it was not until much later that I came to ask myself if this had not played a role in Kibambo's and Mitwele's unwillingness to cooperate freely in the divination session.

It was Kibambo who had sent the 'arrow' and, as noted above, it was she who paid for the divination, even though it took place at her daughter's husband's house and not her own. The knowledge of hindsight makes this appear to have been a strategic move on Kibambo's part, notwithstanding the fact that divination into an untimely death is always considered an appropriate course of action. Given the state of the marital relations obtaining between Kipetele and Mitwele at the time, and given the past history of infant deaths, it was important for Kibambo, on her daughter's behalf as well as on her own, to appear to have nothing to hide. Such openness would perhaps enable the marriage to continue or, failing this, would clear Mitwele's name, and thus improve her prospects of finding another husband. In addition, there was also the possibility, not to be overlooked, that the premature birth and death were due to the sorcery of Kabulu, Kibambo's sister's (Muvimbo's) son. Such a diagnosis by Mumbyoto would have served both to exonerate Mitwele before her husband and to precipitate a breach in relations between Kibambo and her sister.

As we have seen, however, Mumbyoto did not come to this conclusion. He also did not give the diagnosis most desired by Kipetele and his kin; viz., that the fault for the death lay with Mitwele, and that Kipetele should divorce her at once. Instead, Mumbyoto steered an adjudicative course between the two, completely satisfying neither side, while upholding higher principles of social order.

Two days after the session, I was told by my friend Mumba, a Bulumbu diviner and protégé of Mumbyoto's, that the latter had stopped by to see her after his divination. He had told her of the session; and she went on to tell me of Kipetele's and Mitwele's early marital history.

It seems that before they were married, Mitwele had had an extended affair with another man (who lived at a large fishing village down the lake). Though it was never clear whether or not the affair had continued after the marriage, it certainly went on through the engagement. After the marriage, Mitwele found herself to be pregnant, but it became apparent (*kujulikana*) that the child was not Kipetele's, and he publicly repudiated it prior to its birth.

Both Mitwele and her lover were jailed, and each was required to pay 20 zaires as a fine to the court, and 20 zaires indemnity to Kipetele. At the end of her term, Mitwele gave birth, but the child died shortly thereafter. A second pregnancy resulted in miscarriage, and now the third had resulted in premature birth and death.

This background history provides a context in which the meaning of the specific diagnosis made by Mumbyoto and his handling of the divinatory session can be seen better.[17] Though she was in no mood or position to appreciate it fully at the time, Mitwele was not, in fact, being blamed by Mumbyoto for the death of her child.

In stating that it was a *kibanda* deriving from her past adultery, the diviner was both declaring the young woman's innocence in the present, and describing the way in which the past continually arose, so to speak, between her and her husband. The ghost of the repudiated first child, like the shadow of the early adultery of which it was the product, acted to destroy current fertility. In a similar manner, Kipetele's inability to forgive his wife tainted their ongoing relations. It was clear even at the time that the two things fed upon one another. The more they failed to get along, the more Kipetele nursed his grudge. The more bitterness he felt, the less they got along. The misfortunes of repeated miscarriage only exacerbated the problem by giving it concrete embodiment.

In suggesting the diagnosis of a *kibanda*, Mumbyoto was providing an opportunity for all to put an end to that particular phase of their relationship. Treatment of such a ghost would be the ceremony of 'throwing the person in the bush' (*kumutupa mutu mupori*). In it, both partners would confess their grudges and bad feeling and then, conflicts resolved and with clear hearts, be therapeutically cleansed by Mumbyoto or another *tulunga* diviner.

The acceptance of this approach would have presupposed a willingness on the part of Kipetele to make Mitwele's wrong his own, and thus to forgive her in a sense more profound than the jural one previously employed. It was this attitude that Mumbyoto was in fact suggesting when he used the phrase 'your [plural] adultery' (*upuzi wenu*) in speaking with Kipetele during the session. That Kipetele reacted so quickly and vehemently to this shows the importance of Mumbyoto's move, as well as Kipetele's own intense feeling about and his sensitivity to any suggestion of compromise.

Kipetele and those on his side were determined that the two should divorce. In fact, Mumbyoto's own assistant (who was something of an upstart, and whom I never saw in the diviner's company again) dipped in during the discussion to say that he agreed with Kipetele, and thought that Mumbyoto should tell or permit the two to divorce. Mumbyoto sharply disagreed with this, and insisted that it was better for the couple to try to resolve matters between them.

To the 'stick' of the *kibanda* Mumbyoto had seen in his dream, he added the 'carrot' of the *muzimu* who wished to be born to the pair. The presence of such a being virtually insured that Kipetele's and Mitwele's resolution of marital discord would result in successful conception and delivery of a healthy child. Such a birth would constitute something of a benediction on the marriage, returning to Mitwele and her matrilineal kin by rebirth one of their number who had been lost to them through death.

Ultimately, however, all these dream visions and Mumbyoto's best persuasiveness were to no avail. That Kipetele had already determined to leave his wife was evident even as the session was unfolding. It was his belief in her continued adultery, I think, that had combined with the baby's condition to convince him of the futility of giving the child a name.

Indeed, as mentioned above, this was not the only indicator of the extent to which people felt the baby's case to be hopeless.[18] There was thus a sense, well conveyed by everyone's passivity during the session, that the whole thing was just a matter of going through formalities. Separation seemed inevitable, an impression confirmed by my conversations the following day with Kipetele's sister-in-law and his friend, and it was on this note that Episode Three was closed.

Episode Four: Death of Kalandu

Some six months after the above episode, in early June 1976, Kalandu (B2), widow of Kimpinde, and mother of both Kibambo and Muvimbo, died of old age. The old soul had been socially ineffective for some years before her death, and I had never known her to be competent. Early in my stay, the wedding of Muvimbo's youngest child, Kakonge, had taken place in Mwanga village, but Kalandu had not actively participated in the festivities. Instead, she continued to sit on her mat at the end of town, oblivious to events around her. Despite her decrepitude and senility, however, and despite its state of advanced disrepair, Kalandu had continued to live in her own house, triangulated between her two daughters. Her children provided her with food and kept her clean, and her grandchildren saw to it that she was taken outside to sit or snooze in the sun every day and then taken back into her house in the evening.

Kalandu's death was not the occasion for conflict among her children themselves. She was old and feeble, and though distressing, her death was accepted as inevitable. Her burial and the funeral surrounding it passed almost without incident. There was, to my knowledge, no divination.

Episode Five: Bulela's critical illness

At 10:31 p.m. on the night of 19 August 1976, some two months after Kalandu's death, we were interrupted in our preparations for bed by Kisile's voice calling outside. When we opened the door, he entered, carrying Bulela (E15), his three-year-old son, on his back, and his bow and arrows in his hands. With him was his wife, Kiondwa, who carried the baby Kipili (E17). They had come to seek help for Bulela.

At about nine o'clock that morning, Kiondwa had taken the child to Kisimba, the *mfumu* who had divined into Kulimba's difficult labour, and who lived not far from Mwanga. Kisimba had given the child a cup of an emetic/purgative meant to cleanse his system. Kiondwa did not know what medicine this had been because, as is the custom, Kisimba had kept it secret. She had, however, noted that the liquid in the cup was milky white.

At the time he drank the medicine, Bulela had complained of stomach pain. This was expected and caused no alarm. Kiondwa carried him home, where the diarrhoea and vomiting induced by the medicine began. This continued until around one o'clock in the afternoon, when the little boy began to show signs of being 'extremely tired' (*kuchoka mno*). At this point, he was given an antidote (*mutompololo*) of cooked sweet potato leaves (*matembele*).

The *mutompololo* slowed the diarrhoea somewhat, but Kiondwa was still alarmed by Bulela's weak condition, and so took him to where Kisile was working at making bricks of sun-dried clay. After seeing his son, Kisile had stopped work and gone over to Kisimba's to tell him of the child's condition and ask if there was not another antidote that could be used. Kisimba said they might gather the leaves of the *kibwabwa* of the bush (*Curcurbita moschara (Lam.) Poir.*), then cook and administer these to the boy. Kisile did this, and Bulela's diarrhoea completely stopped.

In the afternoon, Bulela had eaten a little food, but as time wore on, his parents could see that he continued to 'weaken' (*kuregea*). That night, observing the ongoing deterioration of his condition, they decided to bring him to me.

What I saw was a child in shock. Bulela was conscious but indifferent to his surroundings. His skin was cold; his pulse, though strong, was 150 per minute.[19] He would not lie still, but constantly tossed about, agitated.

I was totally without the means to treat such a case, and had only the mild medication given by the doctor in Kalemie for use in such situations. I explained the situation to Kisile and Kiondwa, and asked their decision. They wished to go ahead, and so I administered the appropriate dose, then waited for it to take effect. While we waited, we had tea, and discussed what medicine Kisimba might have employed. By its milky colour and Bulela's symptoms, we concluded that the plant had been *kanoka* (*Euphorbia grantii Oliv.*), a medicine whose dangerousness is well known.[20]

At the end of an hour and a half, Bulela seemed a little, though not much, quieter. At 12:30 a.m., Kisile and Kiondwa gathered him up to start home. I told them they should call me if his condition became worse during the night. After walking them partway along their road, I returned to the house and went to bed.

At 2:30 a.m., we were awakened by Kabulu calling outside the window to tell me that Bulela's condition was 'no good any more' (*hakuna nzuri tena*). While he went on to call the boy's maternal grandfather (for whom the child was named), we gathered up our things and started off for Mwanga.

We arrived at Kisile's to find the room full of people, all residents of Mwanga itself. The area had been cleared of tables and chairs, and mats had been spread on the floor. The men sat to the north of the room, the women to the south, on the side with the child. Everyone was quiet and tense, eyes fixed on Bulela, who was being held and cared for by Kibambo. It would have been clear, even had I not already known it, that a crisis was unfolding in that room; Bulela's condition was critical (*hatari*, 'dangerous'), and the group of people gathered there could become his first mourners if their treatment of and intense concern for him were not to be enough.

As I made my way over to the women's side, Kibambo changed her position and held the child out to me, so I could examine him. By this time, Bulela's pulse was so weak I could not feel it. He tossed and turned constantly, and I could measure its beat only by putting my hand directly over his heart. I calculated its rate at 171 beats per minute. His rectal temperature was elevated (38.5°C/101.3°F), while his skin still felt quite cool. The only positive sign was the continued ability of his dilated pupils to contract in the presence of light. Regretfully, I informed everyone that they had been correct, that Bulela's condition was much worse, and worst of all, that there was nothing we could do about it.

During the time I was looking at the boy, Bulela's maternal grandfather and namesake had arrived in response to Kabulu's call. Now, the old man sat next to the child and began calling his name and speaking to him first in KiSwahili, then KiTabwa. The elder spoke using the intonations employed when addressing the deceased at funerals, saying 'Bulela! Bulela! Is it truly the voyage? Then let us go together. No. It is better for me to precede and you to remain behind' (*Bulela! Bulela! Ndiyo safari? Kumbe, twende pamoja. Hapana. Afazali nitangulie na weye ubakie*). As he spoke, others in the room began to cry silently.

Kisile had sequestered himself in the bedroom, but could be heard sniffing and sobbing. After a few minutes, he left the house, and then could be heard sobbing loudly outside and speaking unintelligible words in a high-pitched voice. His father followed him, and after a few minutes more, Kisile fell silent.

Shortly after this, Kisile re-entered the house and the bedroom. From there, he called out to Kulimba, asking her to call her brother so that he could hear him answer (*umuite aitike*). She called Bulela several times, but he did not reply. Finally, Kabulu suggested to his mother that she call him, from there, where she held him on her lap. Muvimbo did this, and Bulela at first answered feebly, then did not respond at all.

Upset at his son's silence, Kisile came out of the bedroom and squatted on the floor near Bulela, holding out his hands though not touching the child – and speaking lamentations to him. 'My son, let us go together. My son, poor one. What has happened to you? Bulela, don't die worthlessly' (*Mwanangu, twende pamoja. Mwanangu, masikini. Ilikufikilia nini? Bulela usikufa bure*). Seconds later, Kisile arose and returned to seclusion. There, he began to grieve openly.

Speaking in a high, strained voice, he described the events of the night. He told of how they had seen Bulela's condition to be worsening; of how they had come to our house in the dark to seek help; of how I had examined the boy and given him medication; of how we had had tea together while we waited for his condition to improve; of how the medicine had failed; and of how they had returned home, where Bulela had become worse.

Kisile repeated his description of the night's events several times. With it, he alternated lamentations about their grief-stricken future. What, he asked Bulela, would the baby Kipili do? Whom would he have to play with now? At eating time, Bulela would not be there. Who would take him places?

Kisile's open expressions of grief made everyone more upset. Kiondwa, in her turn, approached her son, and squatted before him. Like her husband, she too spoke of the events of the night. She also spoke of how Bulela would have grown big in time and would have gone to the lake to fish; she spoke of the 'last tea' (*chai ya mwisho*) we had had with him that evening and of how the blanket we had lent them would turn out to be the last he was to lie upon.

By the time the two parents finished speaking, all of us were in tears. No one else grieved quite so openly, but tears, sniffing, and stifled sobs were perceptible around the room. As his weeping began to trail off, Muvimbo reprimanded her son, asking him if crying was good. Between sobs, Kisile replied that there was nothing to crying but what one thought about it (*hakuna kitu isio mawazo*). Nevertheless, he stopped and a few minutes later stepped outside to wash his face in water that had been drawn there for him. When he returned, we all sat in silence.

At 3:55 a.m., we heard the first cock's-crow. Outside it was still dark. Kisile, hearing it, began to lament again, commenting that now was the hour at which many people die. Warm water was brought, and by means of a cloth, Bulela was massaged with it. His body was completely slack; his eyes were partly opened, but only the whites showed. He seemed dead, and the method his grandmother used to massage him was identical to that used to close the mouths, arrange the faces, and loosen the joints of the dead.

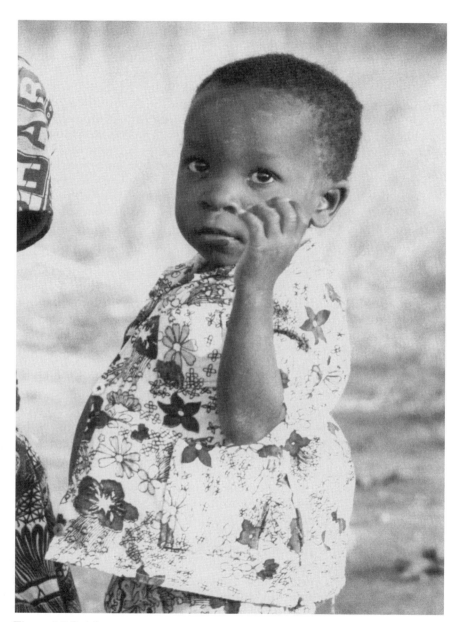

Figure 6.3 Bulela

to assist at Kulimba's difficult labour, and, Kisile went on, had wished to ensorcell his children because she was jealous of their large number. This mention was the first I had heard of the long-standing, bitter quarrel between Kibambo and her sister Muvimbo, described above.

During the next few days, Bulela's condition first stabilised, then gradually began to improve. By 24 August, some five days after the incident, the child was walking around the house, and, though he still tired easily, had complained of hunger for the first time in days. The household itself had returned to normal. The table and chairs had been returned to their places, and only members of the household and casual visitors were present at any given time. At the end of two weeks, the boy had completely recovered.

Such, however, was not the case with the social relations of his lineage group. On the contrary, two days after Bulela's crisis, these had taken a decisive, and seemingly irreversible, turn.

That day, 21 August 1976, was a Sunday, and, as was their wont, many residents of Mpala and neighbouring villages, including Mwanga, were spending the day drinking. During one of the earlier parts of the day, Kibambo was seen at a local bar, drunk, dancing and singing. Someone present had reproached her, asking her if she did not feel a bitterness over the death of her mother which would prevent her from dancing thus. Kibambo had replied by asking if her mother was not already dead. Was she not already buried? And she herself, Kibambo had concluded, would follow her mother.

Later in the day, she had gone to drink at one of the households where beer had been brewed for that day. There, she had quarrelled with someone and, leaving the house, had begun reviling Muvimbo and her children, insulting them loudly and publicly, as she made her unsteady way home. She began with the people of her own generation, and went all the way down until she had insulted Muvimbo's grandchildren, who had only just attained adulthood. She said that they were all sorcerers and that they put medicines in the beer of her children so that, after drinking, they would wander all over town instead of coming home. Perhaps they might be stricken with insanity (*wazimu*) and end up wandering off into the bush. She claimed that if it were not for her strength, Muvimbo and all her children would have died long ago. It was by her strength that they all ate, wore clothes, and had possessions.

At Mwanga village, meanwhile, Kabulu, Kiondwa's brother, and Kabulu's father, Masele (C3), were sitting in Masele's house drinking *rutuku* (distilled manioc liquor). They were shocked and upset when Kibambo burst into the room to ask them how they could be sitting there drinking when Bulela had just died up the street. There was nothing to do but to bathe the corpse, she said. Kibambo then departed as abruptly as she came, leaving everyone sitting in stunned silence.

Kabulu and his brother-in-law decided to investigate. They went to

Kisile's house, approaching from different directions and meeting again beside Bulela's mat. There they squatted down to examine the boy as he lay peacefully sleeping.

From Kisile's the two men went directly to Kibambo's, and asked her what she had meant by her statement. Her reply, that she had only been joking with her *mwendo* (Kiondwa's brother), was not accepted, and the discussion quickly deteriorated into hot argument. Kibambo told Kabulu that his siblings and their mother were bad people. Because of them, the village had been filled with sorcery, and they were sorcerers themselves.

For their part, Kabulu and his brother-in-law had replied that Kibambo had made her 'joke' because she was jealous of the way her sister had given birth. She was chagrined to see how her sister's children had given birth and become numerous, while her own children were few and not fertile. For this reason, she had 'joked' that Bulela was dead. She had said that because she wished it were true.

By the end of the discussion, it was obvious that a complete impasse had been reached. Since it was a family affair, the court was considered an inappropriate forum for its settlement. Kabulu offered to go with his mother's sister to the BaLuba to divine, to have the *mfumu* state which of the two of them was the sorcerer, but Kibambo refused. Muvimbo's children then decided to call in senior lineage elders and *baendo* to hear the matter and adjudicate (*kuamua*) it. Things were allowed to rest a day, Monday, and were scheduled for discussion on Tuesday.

Monday went by uneventfully, with nothing said of Sunday on either side. On Tuesday, three elders (including Leya, classificatory elder sister of Kibambo and Muvimbo) were called to preside at the discussion among lineage group members. The matter, however, was not well settled.

First, Kibambo refused to attend. Then, when she did arrive, after someone had been sent for her, she had proceeded to insult everyone present, including the arbitrators. She repeated that Muvimbo and her children were all *walozi*, and had spoiled Mwanga village with their sorcery. She said that the arbitrators selected were unacceptable to her, because they came from too close by. However, she again refused to go to BuLuba (Lubaland) with Kabulu to divine. She also spoke of her unhappiness at living among so many sorcerers and evil people. Hearing her statement, someone in the group commented that, if she felt so strongly about it, she ought to just move.

In response to *this* remark, Kibambo became even wilder and more abusive than before. She concluded by removing her *kikwembe* (cloth, worn like a sarong) and, insulting them with her nakedness, swept it back and forth in the dirt while telling her kin she would not spend even one more night in their company. By that very evening, she and her husband Matipa had moved down onto the beach below the village. There, they cut saplings and erected a rude shelter for themselves by spreading mats over these.

In subsequent days, Kibambo and Matipa confirmed their resolution by cutting grasses and building themselves a more stable temporary dwelling of straw. They took the long path into Mpala, to avoid using the one which passed behind Mwanga village. Their children continued to reside in Mwanga, however, and other residents showed some concern over the breach.

Everyone said the move had been precipitate. With Matipa unwell, it was better for them to remain in the village, where others could look after them. If something happened to Matipa, his kin would say that, in moving thus, Kibambo had failed to take proper care of her husband. An elder *mwendo* even went so far as to approach her, in an attempt to prevail upon her to return. He pointed out to her that she had no way of knowing 'who would precede her' (*ni nani atakutangulia*, that is, who would die before her). Perhaps she would find herself in old age with none but Muvimbo's children to care for her. If she did not repair this breach, what would she do then?

For their part, despite their anxiety about the breach *per se*, those of Muvimbo's children whom I knew remained resolute in their opinions of their mother's sister. Kisile commented that, ever since he could remember, Kibambo had been one who preferred her own children to those of her sister. She had kept the two groups quite separate. Now, she saw how fecund Muvimbo's were, and she was not happy. These had given birth, and now *their* children were starting to give birth, while Kibambo's children were few and had reproductive difficulties. Kabulu's wife said that Kibambo was starting to kill her sister's children with sorcery, so that she and her sibling could be equivalent as they had previously been and united in their misfortune.

When I commented on the irony of it all, noting that Kibambo had been the best and tenderest nurse of Bulela during his crisis and observing how quickly she had responded to his needs, everyone nodded in agreement. But, Kiondwa commented, all the same, in her heart, Kibambo had not wished him to recover.

Commentary

Of eight episodes surrounding the occurrence of problematic illness, this one, for reasons both obvious and subtle, was probably the most socially decisive for the residents of Mwanga village. During it, the conflict which they had earlier recognised as existing among them became a definite breach between some members of the lineage group. Though Kalandu's death itself had passed without open display of disunity among her children, one might speculate that its effect was felt indirectly in this, the first social drama to unfold after it.

Prior to the period of my stay, Kalandu had ceased to be fully coherent and to have any clear social impact upon the relations among her children. At the time of her death, no one seemed particularly embittered; everyone expects that an old and feeble person will eventually die. She was never mentioned by anyone as a unifying figure in lineage affairs.

Nevertheless, Kalandu may have served in some unstated way as a reminder of lineage group unity. Despite her own decrepitude and her home's equivalent disrepair, she continued to live in the house she had shared with Kimpinde. Her situation could not help but recall to everyone the days when their father had been headman and the residents of Mwanga village had been numerous.

In addition, with Kibambo living opposite, and Muvimbo to the south, Kalandu seemed to be mediating between the two at least in some structural sense. After her death, the house remained empty, and eventually fell into ruins. The person in whom both sisters shared was gone.[21] It is not impossible that their mother's death left Kibambo with no reason even to attempt to maintain co-residence with her sister.

In a manner reminiscent of Episode One, the social drama began with a breach which was related to but not embodied in a specific illness. The inappropriateness of Kibambo's joke about Bulela was taken to be directly indicative of the inappropriateness of her attitude toward him. Everyone assumed that she would not have made such a remark if she had not wished it were true.

Kibambo's justification of her statement on the grounds that she had only been joking with her *mwendo* (Kiondwa's brother) could have been regarded as acceptable had there been no previous history of ill will. *Baendo* are not only clan joking partners, but also those upon whom a lineage group calls for ritual and social mediation, as well as for funerary services.

The special relation that obtains between joking partners is given particular form in the content of the jokes said to pass customarily between them. These are usually mock accusations of sorcery, and false tales of the death of distant kin.[22]

During my stay, such jokes were the common substance of passing remarks between *baendo* meeting on the road, and on at least one occasion two people were sent rushing to the deathbed of a kinswoman (six hours' walk north of Mpala) only to find her returning, hale and hearty, from her fields. However, the ill will existing between Kibambo and Muvimbo's children, particularly Kabulu, excluded the possibility of such a joke being taken lightly.

In addition, the bad feeling had been heightened by a divination of which I did not learn until two weeks after the incident. It had taken place some-time before, had crystallised Kisile's and Kiondwa's suspicions of Kibambo, and had defined the situation to which Kisile had referred on the morning after Bulela's crisis.

Apparently, the onset of Bulela's original illness had been insidious. He had been born healthy, but subsequently had grown sickly so imperceptibly that at first neither parent had noticed it. Then, one day they had suddenly observed that the child was thin and that his stomach was swollen. He did not eat well, and, after eating only a little had noticeable abdominal distension (a condition known as 'rising of the stomach' (*tumbo kupanda*)).

The concern of Kisile and Kiondwa had become genuine alarm several weeks earlier, when Bulela's stomach had 'risen' (*kupanda*) so abruptly and acutely during the night that the child seemed unable to breathe. Kisile was away at a fishing camp at the time. Kiondwa, seeing her son's state, began to fear for his life, and so, during the night, had aroused Masele's younger brother, and had gone with him to Kisimba's to divine. It was there that she had learned that the illness was due to 'poisons' (*sumu*) Bulela had been given when eating at Kibambo's house.

The diviner had given Kiondwa some medicines to use during the night and told her to supplicate (*kutambikia*) her *mizimu*. They had agreed there and then that emesis/purging would be attempted as soon as Bulela had recovered from that particular episode and regained his strength. The child had recovered from the acute illness in a few days, and it was the attempt at definitive treatment which had nearly killed him on 19 August.

It was this definition of her prior acts and motives which formed the context in which Kibambo's joke was interpreted. Under its influence, what might, in other circumstances, have been viewed as a lack of good judgement came to be seen as a definite breach of the norms governing behaviour in time of misfortune.

Kibambo was generally known to behave in an unseemly fashion when drunk. Indeed, public opinion at Mpala held that everyone at Mwanga village drank too much and was therefore too quarrelsome. It was because of drunkenness that settlement of the bitter exchange was held over a day, and drunkenness might have been used as an excuse for Kibambo's remark. However, her sister's children were disinclined to excuse her, and Kibambo herself failed to repudiate her behaviour voluntarily

She might have done this by using a social tactic well known to local beer drinkers, that is, by approaching Kabulu or Masele the next day and asking them if she had by chance done anything offensive the day before. They could then have recounted to her what she had said and done, and she might have responded by disclaiming any memory of her behaviour and asking their forgiveness. Such an approach, though by no means stated as a rule, is nevertheless standard practice on Monday mornings around Mpala. That Kibambo did not do so was indicative of the extent to which she, for her part, remained as resolute in her judgement of Kabulu and his siblings as they did in theirs of her.

Ironically, none of the powerful tensions extant in the situation was evident the night of Bulela's illness. As noted above, the whole time I was present, Kibambo and Muvimbo worked together to nurse the child. In fact, Kibambo was the more sensitive of the two, and responded more readily to the child's stated wishes. Though Kisile and Kiondwa had previously determined that it was Kibambo who originated their son's illness, this could in no way be detected in their behaviour. When Kibambo took the boy, they made no protest.

Interesting as well is the fact that no open accusations of active sorcery were ever made. Quarrels were in the same terms as always, with Kibambo accusing Kabulu of having ruined the village, and Kabulu saying that Kibambo was jealous of Muvimbo's children's fertility. Though a breach was made, and, for a time, no one was speaking, no open action was taken to blame Kibambo for Bulela's illness. This restriction of discussion meant that relations could resume at a later date, and confined the conflict to the two sublineages then resident at Mwanga village. An open accusation of sorcery would have meant the forswearing of interaction once and for all, and possibly the widening of the breach to include factions comprising all of Kalandu's children.

Despite the almost accidental nature of the breach, and the limitations quickly imposed upon it, the interlude was nevertheless decisive, and, in some ways, it seems, irreversible. As subsequent discussion will show, unofficial interpretations of significant illnesses following this one all had a much more stridently accusatory note. After Bulela's illness, periods of cooperation were interrupted by quarrels and slights of a much more serious nature than had previously been the case.

Though highly revealing of the complex interrelation between illness occurrence and a social drama, Episode Five is also of significance because it displays many characteristics worthy of more general note. Most obvious of these is the transitional nature of the critical phase of illness. People describe this condition as 'dangerously ill' (ugonjuwa hatari), and its social aspects include features which characterise funerary practices.

When, like Bulela, a person becomes dangerously ill, the attention of the entire household and extended kin group becomes wholly centred upon him and his condition. Other work is stopped, and it is customary for a large number of people to visit the sick person and sit for some time with him. At night as well, family members gather to keep watch; they relieve one another of nursing cares; and lamps remain lit through the hours of darkness, giving one day the value of two, as people say.

The number of people gathered in this way seems directly proportional to the intensity of threat of death. Older people arriving may examine the patient for coldness of limbs and irregularity of heartbeat, both signs that he is dying. The people who are gathered are not only those who wish most fervently that the patient should not die, they are also the group that will form the core of his mourners, should their wishes be denied.

As in the situation described above, the phase ugonjuwa hatari is structurally marked as well. The furniture ordinarily kept inside the house is removed and the floor spread with mats on which the guests, who leave their shoes outside, sit in silence.

Lamentations such as the ones spoken by Kisile and Kiondwa to Bulela may also characterise this phase, though they are considered somewhat in bad form until after the death has actually taken place. (It was for this reason that Kisile's mother reprimanded him.) The crying out of lamentations such as these is one of the roles of formal mourning as well as one of the ways in which grief is more personally expressed. To grieve in advance of the formal mourning is thus almost to wish death upon the patient, but people cannot help themselves at such a time and may lament nevertheless.

Like Kisile's statement to his son, lamentations are addressed to the patient or to the deceased and delineate the events of the illness, leading up to the death. They also always outline the bleakness of the future that awaits those of the person's kin who must remain behind and learn to live in a world where he no longer exists. Like certain kinds of invocation, lament- ation thus serves to make of the moment a fact of consciousness, suspended in the web of words linking past to present and making of the present the future's past. Each of the points of the illness, of the life, of the events surrounding the death, and of the future is described and delineated. In this way, the whole that was the life and is the transition is marked in all its particulars and held quite distinctly in mind.

In many respects, such a speech is the verbalised, rhetorical form of the processes of public historisation described in previous chapters. Like the death to which it may lead, problematic illness marks an era in the life of a patient and of the group to which that life belongs.

Besides the transitional character of the phase *ugonjuwa hatari,* Bulela's critical illness demonstrates still other features of problematic illness occurrences. These are the almost continuous holding of the patient, especially if a child, in the arms of his kin, and the equally constant, active care, given primarily in the form of manioc gruel (*uji*) and hot water massages. These massages are given to keep the patient's body loose and relaxed, so that the blood may move about freely in the veins, for cessation of such movement will result in death. *Uji* is the only appropriate food for a patient, and small amounts of it are given at frequent intervals.[23] Holding the patient has no explicit medical rationale, though it very clearly expresses the anxious concern described by the term people use for nursing, *kutunza* ('to care for', 'to protect').

Briefly observable in this episode as well was the extent to which the moment-to-moment management of the patient is determined by the patient himself. It was Bulela who decided when he would lie down and he who determined that he would be taken outside to urinate. In all matters, and to an extent that increases with the maturity of the patient, care of the ill is organised by and around the will of the sick person. People feel that such things as lack of appetite and crankiness *are the illness itself* being manifested and not mere recalcitrance. They make no effort to have the patient eat more than he desires or remain in a position or situation that he dislikes.[24] Unpleasant remarks made by a person when suffering are not held against him. In this sense therapy management de-emphasises the removal of an individual's agency as the prerequisite of nursing care.

Finally, note should be made here of the role played in all of this by Kisimba, and the relations he subsequently had with Kisile and Kiondwa. At the time of the incident, Kisimba had not been long in practice. His was a *bulumbu* divining spirit which had been 'put in order' (*kutengenezwa*) by the divining spirit of my friend Mumba. Kisimba's spirits, however, had not remained on good terms with their 'mother', and, according to Mumba, had refused to await proper instruction before beginning pharmacological practice.

Other practitioners, such as Kalwele, took the incident in their stride, shrugging and commenting that the fault had to lie elsewhere, because a remedy given to many without mishap could not kill the few unless something else (that is, sorcery or avenging ghosts) were also present. Mumba, however, was quite distressed, and felt that Kisimba's behaviour would result in all diviners being driven from the area. She blamed Kisimba totally for what happened, saying it was due to his ignorance of posology. She herself got most of her medicines from Mumbyoto, who, she said, was very experienced, with well-tested formulae.

For their part, Kisile and Kiondwa also felt that the accident had been due to Kisimba's poor judgement. As is considered proper, the *mfumu* had been to visit the boy twice during his illness, thus showing he had nothing to hide in the matter.

Though relations between them remained formally open, Kisimba never came to bring other medicines or to discuss at length what had happened. Had he done so, Kisile and Kiondwa had decided to terminate the relationship by returning to him his medicines and asking him how much they owed. They both felt that further use of traditional medicines might kill Bulela and that people would say they had done it deliberately.

For a time after his crisis, Bulela was treated with European medicines, in the form of anti-thelmenthics, chloroquine and the like, but without success. At one point, Kabulu considered taking the boy to Kalemie for examination and, perhaps, surgery, to remove the thing inside that made his stomach swell. Ongoing military operations in the area, however, made this impossible, and, finally, a lay herbalist came forward who said he recognised (*kutambua*) the illness as *mpanga*. Bulela was being treated for this with traditional medicines at the time of my departure from Zaire. At that time, Kisimba, despite a year's lapse, still had something of a special relationship with Kisile, who felt obliged to give him fish occasionally because it was he who had initiated the connection (*nimekwisha kumuchokoza*).

Episode Six: Kipili's death

After the decisive turn of events in the month of August, life at Mwanga went on uneventfully for a time. In October, I began a trip to Zambia by boat, and was away from Mpala for seven weeks. During the time I was south of Moba, I was completely out of contact with Mpala and heard no news whatsoever of it. When I returned to Moba, in early December, I found that Kipili, Kisile's infant son, had died suddenly several weeks before, and that his death had been closely followed by that of Mwapi, a granddaughter of Kibambo.[25]

As soon as I arrived in Mpala, I went out to Mwanga village to visit Kisile and Kiondwa, to pay my respects, and to find out how such a robust and healthy child, who had never been seriously ill since I had known him, could have died so suddenly. As it turned out, Kisile and Kiondwa were asking themselves the same question.

Apparently, Kipili had been a bit sick for a while before the acute stage of his illness. His parents had been treating him with the aspirin and chloroquine tablets I had left them, and then with similar medicines I had left at the house for emergencies. This course of treatment had been successful for a time.

Then, the Monday before his death, Kipili came down with a high fever. On Tuesday and Wednesday he seemed a bit better. Then on Thursday, the fever returned and was quite intense (*kali kabisa*). At that time, too, the child was stricken by 'infantile convulsion' (*ndege*). The emergency medicines I left were used and exhausted, but the illness did not respond. Traditional medicines were employed for the convulsions, but they didn't work, either. People began to ask themselves what sort of illness this was, that failed to heed medicines (*ni ugonjuwa ya namna gani isiosika dawa?*).

Kipili remained feverish and somewhat stiffened with convulsions all day Thursday, Friday and Saturday. That he had severe *kimbeleka* had been demonstrated by the fact that his *safura* ('spleen') was clearly visible in his abdomen, sticking out below his ribs. During this whole time, however, he would drink *uji* when given it, and would ask for water. He never tossed about (*kujitupa*) the way people often do when they are dying.

Early Saturday morning, it was decided that they should seek divination into the cause of this intractable illness. At 5:00 a.m., Kisile set off with an 'arrow' for the house of a diviner who was from Mpweto and who had come to Mpala to visit distant kin. On his way, Kisile stubbed first his right toe, then his left; events which he took to be a bad omen. When he got to the diviner's house, he found others just leaving.

Kisile put the coin on the ground, from whence it was taken up by the diviner's classificatory sister. As soon as he looked at it the *mfumu* refused to take the case, saying it was useless because the person 'had already passed' (*amekwisha kupita*). After some discussion, however, Kisile prevailed upon him to at least come and look at the child, before deciding once and for all.

So, shortly after 5:00 a.m., Kisile and the diviner together went out to Mwanga village. Arriving there, the *mfumu* examined Kipili, noted the manner in which he was breathing, and then said that though he was not sure the child would recover, they might nevertheless attempt treatment if they had a medicine called *kitupa*.[26]

Kitupa did not grow in the area around Mpala and Mwanga, though it was known by Kisile to grow elsewhere, much further off. Finally, someone remembered having seen it growing in the hills to the southwest of the village. Kisile, Kabulu and their father, Masele, set off to search for it.

They went to the place where it had been seen, but it no longer grew there. They returned to Mwanga, and Kisile had just started off for the diviner's when Kipili's 'soul split' (*roho inapasuka*), and the baby died. He had never grown thin, never seemed comatose. He just closed his eyes and died 'just like that' (*hivi-hivi tu*).

The first divination into the child's death was made before my return from Zambia. At it, the *mfumu* said that the death had derived from a deceased mother's mother's brother of Kiondwa. This man had been accused of sorcery during his lifetime, and had been driven from the village and cut off from his relatives. He had not, however, been a sorcerer, and so had died with great bitterness, unremembered by his kin. He was never called upon by them, nor were children named for him. So, he had killed Kipili.

The diviner had said that they were to fabricate a *musambwa* for the antecedent. However, they themselves had also asked him if he could not make medicines for them to put into their house, so that their children would be born and grow up without trouble. He had agreed that this also could be done.

When I asked her opinion of the divination, Kiondwa replied that her own mother, who had been present, had been unable to respond positively to this hypothesis. If it were true, the events had taken place at a time when she herself was only a child, and she could not confirm them. Later, Kiondwa added that it didn't make sense for a thing such as that to have caused a death such as this one. Similarly, Kisile said that the elders had decided that it would be better to seek another divination before following through on the first. If the second diviner came up with the same thing, they would go ahead.

In the weeks that followed, a grief-stricken Kiondwa could be seen around Mpala. Without Kipili on her back, she seemed strangely incomplete. She never smiled, and, for a long time, could hardly converse at length

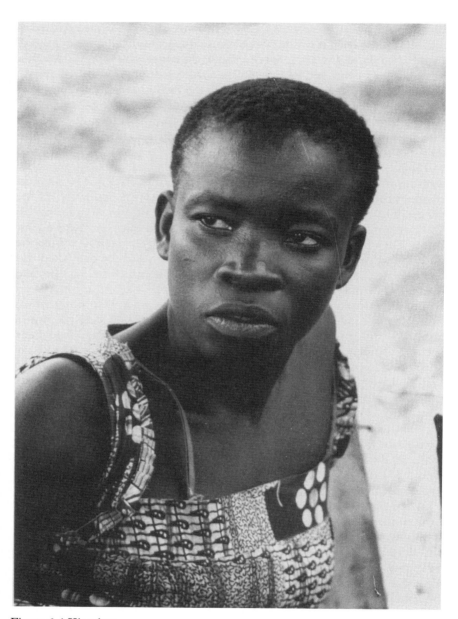

Figure 6.4 Kiondwa

without breaking into tears. She was sorely distressed that the healthier of her two smallest children had died, leaving only the 'weakling' (*musaifu*), the chronically ill Bulela, on whom they had tried medicines until they 'were tired' (*mpaka tunachoka*), but whose condition failed to improve. During this period, as well, Kiondwa was subject to fits of weeping that alarmed everyone. Especially after drinking beer, she would sit and lament her lost baby boy, crying and talking far into the night until she fell asleep, exhausted. At this same time, Kiondwa was twice stricken with strange, excruciating abdominal pain which kept her up until almost dawn.

Kisile and Kulimba were quite upset at the intensity of Kiondwa's grief and bitterness. They tried to forbid her mourning in this way, but to no avail. Kisile told her that the intense grief she felt might well make her ill, or, if ill from some other cause, might serve to kill her.

Finally, early in 1977, Kiondwa found she was pregnant again. This made a substantial improvement in her spirits, and at the time I left the Mpala she was in a much better frame of mind.

A second divination into Kipili's death yielded a more plausible aetiologic hypothesis. For this one, they had gone to the same diviner who had been called on the day of the death. Present at the divination were Kisile and Kabulu, Kiondwa, her brother, and her parents.

The diviner found that the cause of Kipili's death was a sorceress then living within Mwanga village itself. He could not, he said, name names, but he gave a description of her as a big, heavy-set woman who had been a sorceress for a very long time. He said she made medicines so that the children of Mwanga village would be sick all the time. These she kept in a pot, down by the small stream between Mwanga and the next village to the south. At night, she would go down there to get them, and bring them to Mwanga village to cook. This brought a bad wind (*pepo*) to the village, and it was this that was responsible for the death of Kipili and of Mwapi, as well as the death by drowning of the woman's own grandson in late 1975.

The woman referred to in this case was a classificatory kinswoman who had been taken into Mwanga village the previous dry season. At that time, she had been accused of giving a young girl human blood to drink, and, after a celebrated court case, was driven out of Marasini village along with her grown children. Several days after their settlement at Mwanga, a grandchild of hers had accidentally drowned in the lake while playing with friends.

A few months into the new year, and after the above divination, this entire lineage group moved from Mwanga village to Moba. They made their move 'like thieves' under cover of night, carrying their belongings down to the beach after dark, and leaving without even saying goodbye. They had not been terribly agreeable in any case, and their manner of taking leave of those who had given them sanctuary confirmed everyone's impressions/ suspicions of them.

Episode Seven: Mwapi's death

The day after Kipili's death, Mwapi (E19), daughter of Katempa (D16) and granddaughter of Kibambo, fell seriously ill with diarrhoea. She was a baby who was just beginning to sit when she fell ill, and she died about three days later. Prior to the beginning of this particular occurrence, the ongoing intralineage conflict had surfaced in the form of two minor incidents.

Kabulu and other men of the group had been preparing to go to their dry-season fishing camp when they observed that a plank in their boat had rotted. They hired someone to repair it, but the replacement board and tools had to be provided by the family. These things were stored in Katempa's house, and when Kabulu went to get them, Mwapi fell ill with diarrhoea and fever, from which she recovered. Then, when Kabulu went to return the tools to their place, the infant fell ill once more. Her mother blamed Kabulu for it, saying he had done something to the child each time he'd entered the house.

In view of the suspicions, when Mwapi came down with severe diarrhoea, her parents immediately set off to divine, seeking the insight of the same diviner to whom Kisile had gone during Kipili's illness. In a response similar to that for Kipili's case, the *mfumu* told Katempa, her husband and her mother that it was too late to save the child.

He gave as the cause of Mwapi's illness the tremendous conflict taking place in Mwanga and said that, at the very least, such conflict created a bad atmosphere in the village. The very injuries (*asara*) to which it gave rise were enough to cause sickness. At worst, continual fighting provided sorcerers with a perfect cover under which to operate.

Though the case seemed to him to be nearly hopeless, the diviner told them that they might nevertheless try to clear up the grudges that divided them. He said that all were to sit together and state their mutual grievances. After this, they were all to make an offering (*kutambikia*) to their *mizimu*. In this way, if there was a chance of the infant's recovering, she would; and if not, at least she would 'go well' (*kuenda vizuri*).

In response to the diviner's instructions, an attempt was made to clear up the long-standing grudges dividing the residents of Mwanga. Everyone came together in a group, but no one seemed willing to air his or her grievances. When asked why she had moved, Kibambo at first could give no reason and denied that anything had been said or done to drive her out. For his part, Kabulu refused to admit that any ill will existed between him and his mother's sister. He said that to see one another was to exchange greetings as they passed, and nothing more.

Katempa was the only person willing to speak openly and honestly about what disturbed her. She said that her grievance was that no one would make any overt statements about the matter, but when she made food and called all the children, those of Kisile and Kabulu would refuse to come, saying

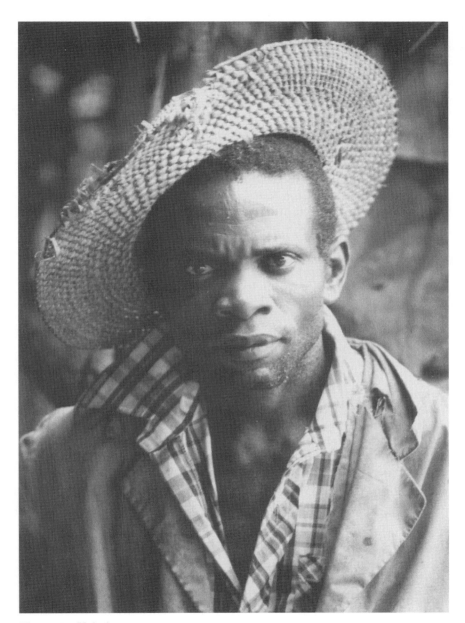

Figure 6.5 Kabulu

they had been forbidden by their fathers to eat at her house. She resented this, and felt it was an unjust, unspoken accusation of sorcery.

In the end, Kabulu and Kibambo sat together to make an offering to their *mizimu*. But, as Kisile put it, 'they were already too late' (*wamekwisha kuchelewa*), and the child died anyway. After this, there was no further motivation to get to the bottom of the matter, and/or to have the grudge-removing *mutimbe* ceremony.[27] Though Kabulu went to Kibambo's with another offer to divine among the Luba, she again refused.

Following her death, Mwapi's parents and grandmother went to yet another *mfumu* to gain insight into their loss. Like the first, this practitioner was also a young man from out of town. Despite the fact that Kibambo and Katempa strongly suspected Kabulu of having killed their descendant, and might have liked to have their suspicion confirmed, the *mfumu* said it derived from the husband's 'grandmothers', and not from Katempa's side at all.

The young parents denied the validity of this divination and set off for Maseba, in the interior, to seek another one. It was rumoured that while there, they had attempted to purchase a thunderbolt (*radi*), to strike Kabulu at Mwanga and so to kill him. The *mfumu* had told them he could sell them such medicines, but that the thunderbolts it made would only follow them, as they were accusing Kabulu unjustly. Hearing this, they let drop the matter, but they moved from Mwanga village, and went to live at Kirungu, the district seat just outside Moba.

Commentary

Taken together, Episodes Six and Seven illuminate several important aspects of illness occurrences and the relations these have to social dramas. One of their most obvious features is the way in which these post-Episode Five incidents were immediately assumed by the parties involved to be directly reflective of the ongoing intralineage conflict. Though neither faction ever said so explicitly or was ever successful in its attempts to have its suspicions confirmed, members of both groups leapt immediately to the conclusion that the sorcery of the other group was probably at the bottom of the illness. This unofficial attribution of the occurrence to sorcery highlights the extent to which the terms of the continuing conflict had been escalated by the incident following Bulela's illness. It also demonstrates the extent to which divination is not entirely in the control of those seeking it, and does not always provide them with the answers they want.

The events of Episodes Six and Seven also illustrate the more subtle point that there is a certain amount of latitude to be derived from leaving hidden grudges as they are. As long as the true depth of the hostility is unmeasured, there is always the possibility of smoothing over by equally indirect means the many little slights to which it may give rise.

Once the terms are clearly set, however, little slights become breaches in social relations, gaps which cannot be overlooked. Thus, Kibambo had been central to the drama of Bulela's critical illness, even though she was suspected of having been its ultimate cause. Mutual assistance in time of common misfortune might be said to have diminished somewhat the bad feeling.

However, so extreme a violation of kin relations as undressing oneself so that one's relatives might be insulted made manifest the intensity of Kibambo's hostility towards Muvimbo and her children. When they subsequently attempted to air their grievances, Kibambo's insistence that she bore no ill will was patently belied by her previous behaviour. How could she not hate them, people such as Kabulu and Kisile asked, when she had treated them thus? Their awareness of this contradiction justified their own unwillingness to confess. In the end, it was only Katempa whose concern for her child was sufficient to prompt true revelation.[28]

This way in which hostility can distort priorities, making the maintenance of the grudge as important as the saving of a life, was commented upon by those diviners who told both factions that it was their quarrelling which was indirectly responsible for their children's deaths. Such divinatory conclusions also direct our attention to the related point that the conflicts surrounding problematic illness have more to do with social norms than with the illness itself. In both cases, diviners attempted to minimise the social structural significance of the deaths, by separating them from a currently unresolved breach of norms. Something similar was said by Kalwele to have occurred in times of epidemic in pre-Europeanised days.

In those days, in response to widespread disease, the chief would make a large pot of medicines to 'close' (*kufunga*) the village to the epidemic. After confessing and resolving their grievances and grudges, villagers would wash in the medicine. Husbands and wives would then refrain from sexual intercourse until the epidemic had passed. In this way, Kalwele said, people would know that those deaths which might happen anyway were insignificant (*bure*), that is, that they were unconnected to social conflict.

Had the diviners' opinions been accepted by the residents of Mwanga village, the deaths of Kipili and Mwapi would have been no less tragic. They would not, however, have been the cause of further fragmentation. That they were such is indicative of another important point, viz., that once a spontaneously occurring problematic illness is tied, even by suspicion, to a given social relation, its outcome becomes as much a significant variable in the situation as any social fact.

In such a case the body itself becomes like an oracle, demonstrating the truth of diagnostic hypotheses through remission or recurrence of symptoms. When Katempa's child died instead of showing improvement, the rival factions of Mwanga village saw that further efforts to remedy their situation were useless.

In addition to the above demonstrations of the complexity of relations as between illness occurrence and social drama, Episodes Six and Seven also bring to our attention other features which generally characterise instances of being sick. Among these are the question of availability of requisite medicines.

For all its wealth of plant life, a given area of woodland, with its small riverine forests and specialised termitary ecology, may nevertheless be lacking in a particular medicinal plant. Under ordinary circumstances, people make use primarily of plants and trees that grow in their vicinity. However, they also make note of places where individual specimens of unusual plants are located, so that they can find them in time of special need. Among practitioners, this knowledge is part and parcel of the esoterica that includes knowing the right combination of medicines to effect cures. When they went to look for *kitupa*, Kisile, Kabulu and Masele were doing so on the basis of this sort of observation.

Another feature of significance here is the refusal of the diviner to undertake divination into and treatment of the cases of the two children. This refusal is part of the social form governing the relations of practitioner and patient. A diviner or herbalist who will not take a case is said to be telling the patient's family that their efforts will be to no avail, for the person cannot recover.

Finally, Kisile's and Kiondwa's refusal to accept the initial divination into Kipili's death (like the similar refusal of Mwapi's parents) in some sense reflected the inability of the proffered hypothesis to absorb the intensity of their grief fully. As they spoke of it, I had the distinct impression that the plausibility of the diagnosis was questioned not only because the kinsman concerned was beyond memory, but also because a wrong done in so distant a past seemed small by comparison to the magnitude of the pain felt in the present. That someone should actually wish them ill, no matter how indirect the connection, made more sense to Kisile and Kiondwa than did the idea that Kipili died for no immediate reason at all. In contrast, the second hypothesis (that is, that the death was due to the sorcery of the classificatory kinswoman) managed effectively to accommodate the extremely negative aspects of the case and so was satisfactory even though it did not implicate Kibambo.

However, despite the fact that Kibambo had been exonerated, Kiondwa continued to suspect her. Even after her grief had subsided, and Kiondwa had found herself pregnant again, she continued to make oblique references to her husband's mother's sister's envy of her fecundity. In many a conversation she would comment about how 'they' would see one had had many children and lost only a few; of how 'they' would see that one's children, in their turn, had begun to bear; of how 'they' would see that one was still oneself fertile; of how 'they' would be unable to contain their jealousy at how one's children were growing numerous while one was still young; and of how 'they' would decide to reduce their number (*tuwapunguze*) to accord with the modest size of the group of 'their' own offspring. In the same vein, Kiondwa would then go on to comment on the falseness of diviners and the difficulty one invariably had in getting them to cite sorcery and to name names when diagnosing illness.

Episode Eight: Masele's accident

For a period of slightly more than two months, life unfolded quietly at Mwanga village. During this time, relations gradually became somewhat normalised between Kibambo and her sister. Most of the former's children had continued to reside in Mwanga village in any case, and during this period those who did not had begun to take the short path to Mpala again. Kibambo and Muvimbo had an apparent improvement in mutual relations during the month of December when the two of them had worked together to nurse Leya, their classificatory elder sister, who had nearly died of acute, explosive diarrhoea. It was in this climate of tentative calm and restored relations that the final significant illness of the lineage group occurred.

On Sunday 13 February, there was beer at Kisile's house, and Kisile and Kabulu had been drinking it along with one of Kibambo's sons. After everyone was appropriately drunk, Masele decided to go home to bed, but was unable to do so without help.

They had begun the short trip (of a few hundred yards) in the proper fashion, with Kabulu helping his father by holding him under the armpits. Then, partway along, Kibambo's son decided he had a better idea. He picked up the old man and began carrying him over his shoulder, with his head hanging down behind and his feet sticking out before.

A bit further on, the younger man stumbled and fell forward. As he did so, he threw the old man over to one side, where he fell on his head and almost broke his neck. That night, everyone sat up watching over him, certain he would die, but he survived.

Everyone brought medicines to treat him. Each person tried his or her own, but it was to no avail. The old man remained weak, and his right arm seemed paralysed. Finally, they went back to Kisimba for a divination.

Kisimba divined that Masele had been made ill because of his continued skill and energy in farming. Though in his seventies he remained a vigorous man. Seeing this, a jealous person had left medicines in his field that made Masele fall ill and thus fail at farming.

After thinking over this divination, Masele rejected its results. He couldn't think of who such a person might be or how this could be the cause of his accident. Another 'arrow' was sent to a local *kashekesheke* diviner.

This man conducted his session at Mwanga itself. Looking into his apparatus, he determined that the accident was caused by Masele's mother's brothers. These had seen the way in which the old man had quarrelled violently with Kiunda (D10), one of his wife's sister's (Luenzia's) sons who tended to side with Kibambo's faction. Kiunda was a hopeless drunk and marijuana smoker whose condition had deteriorated considerably since the beginning of my stay.

Not too long before, Kiunda had quarrelled with Masele, calling him names, and insulting him to a point where the old man had got quite beside himself and had begun responding to the young one in kind. Masele's mother's brothers, the diviner said, had found this behaviour between a father and son to be highly inappropriate. They had decided that he should die on the spot of the fall. At the last second, however, they had taken pity on him, and so had spared him, leaving him in his sickly state.

The diviner said that Masele should take out the *misambwa* of his mother's brothers and of his mother and speak to them, asking that they should help him recover, and disavowing his previous quarrel. Masele did this, but did not recover with any rapidity.

After a few more days, Kisile began to wonder whether or not they ought to seek yet another divination, as the old man did not seem to be improving at a great rate. He consulted with another kinsman, who suggested that he first ask his father exactly what he had done when speaking to his *misambwa*.

It turned out that old Masele had been so weak at the time the diagnosis was made that he had not risen from his bed to speak to his *misambwa*. Instead of speaking to them at the threshold of the house, he had therefore spoken to them there, where he lay. Everyone felt that this was inappropriate and might account for their failure to help him. So, Masele spoke to them again in the correct fashion, sitting at the door to his house (back door, for privacy) just at dusk. Shortly thereafter, he began to recover, and about twelve days after the accident he had got back a good part of the use of his arm.

About a month after the incident, I commented to Kisile and Kiondwa that I doubted the correctness of the divination, saying that I didn't see how someone's *mizimu* could kill them for quarrelling with such a worthless person as Kiunda. They agreed that it was not too probable but with Masele's recovery the question was no longer pressing.

Commentary

This final instance of significant illness forms something of a denouement to the high melodrama of the episodes which preceded it. Though centred on an affine (Masele), it is nevertheless included here because all other principals in the case were members of Mwanga lineage. That the most intense phase of the social drama's crisis period had passed is indicated by the fact that accusations of sorcery or of ill will did not figure in the case at all, even though the very person who was responsible for Masele's injury was one of

Kibambo's sons. The old man's survival and recovery kept tensions to a minimum, and also worked to minimise the number of divinations sought.

As before, the diviner's diagnosis carefully wove together a cause comparable to the degree of danger or intensity of feeling involved, and a secondary responsibility which was under the patient's control and without which the illness might not have happened. In this way, Masele was as much to blame for his illness as anyone else. Conflict was not only kept to a minimum, but Masele's symbolic control was maximised.

CONCLUDING INCIDENTS

Our case history of significant illnesses of Mwanga village is now complete. However, there remain a few more general incidents to describe and some final remarks to make.

Beginning just after old Masele's accident, and continuing for some weeks beyond this, relations between Kabulu and Kiunda took a sudden very violent turn. When they would meet on the beach, Kiunda would try to fight his mother's sister's son, or would cut up the dragnet the lineage members held in common. On one occasion, failing to arouse Kabulu with insults, Kiunda began to cut up the former's clothes. The next time they met, Kabulu returned the favour, slitting the inseam of Kiunda's pants, so they would flap about 'like a woman's skirt' (*kama vile kikwembe*). He also attempted to drown Kiunda by holding his head underwater, but was stopped by passers-by. Indeed, the hatred between the two men was such that for a certain period, not a Sunday would pass without Kiunda staggering out to Mwanga to stand before Kabulu's house and hurl insults at him until far into the night.

Residents of Mwanga took this to be an indicator of the fact that Kiunda was not quite right in the head. They said that all his years of drinking and dope smoking had 'spoiled his intelligence' (*kuharibu akili*). As proof of this they pointed to the fact that the sort of exquisite hatred for one person that Kiunda felt for Kabulu is also characteristic of *wazimu* ('insanity'). A person with this illness usually has a 'friend' (*rafiki*) about whom he can drive himself into a frenzy of destructiveness.

They also noted that Kiunda had effectively managed to alienate his own brothers by his insults and inappropriate behaviour. The two lived near Kiunda, but never called him to eat with them any more, despite the fact that he had no wife to cook for him, because he repaid their kindness with harassment.

Finally, the group took the matter to Chief Mpala. The Chief concluded that since Kiunda acted like a crazy person, he had, in some sense, to be treated like one. He suggested to the residents of Mwanga that they simply grab Kiunda and beat him soundly the next time he came to insult and harass them. They were to be careful not to kill or seriously injure him, but were to beat him sufficiently soundly that he would remember not to go back there again. (This was similar to the method of treating the local crazy person when his incursions into others' kitchens became too much for a neighbourhood to bear.)

In August 1977, word came from a lakeside village near Moba that a grandchild of Kibambo's had been born prematurely and had died. When word of the death arrived, Kibambo immediately dispatched a messenger to inform her classificatory sister Leya of the event. No one, however, was sent to inform the nearer Muvimbo, who took this omission as a serious breach of relations, amounting to an accusation of sorcery.

The funeral itself was subdued and less than formal in character. It was decided that no one would sleep over, due to the small size of the house. Instead everyone would mourn and sing during the day, and then go home at night. Many people did not even know a funeral was in progress, and Muvimbo heard of it only by accident.

After learning of the funeral, Muvimbo went over to her sister's. Eventually, she called Kibambo to one side, asking her bluntly what she had meant by not sending a messenger. She noted that it could be taken to mean that Kibambo was accusing her of sorcery in the case, and wanted to know if this was so.

Leya was present at the time of the conversation, and intervened with Muvimbo on behalf of Kibambo. She smoothed the matter over by saying that Kibambo had been so overwrought at the news that she had simply forgotten to inform her sister. On this note, the matter was outwardly dropped.

In private, however, Muvimbo's children sneered at the excuse, saying that it could not undo the wrong their mother had suffered. They also noted that her intervention only confirmed the preference Leya had for Kibambo, to whom she had always been close.

Several days after the funeral, I arrived at Mpala's to find Kibambo just leaving. When I went in and chatted with him, the Chief said Kibambo had just come to tell him that it was Muvimbo and Masele who had employed sorcery to kill the infant at the other village.

Mpala attributed the sisters' accusations and counter-accusations to the conflict over headmanship of Mwanga village. Mpala described the affair as a struggle between the lion and the bushbuck over who would rule. In the end the bushbuck had moved down to the beach, and left the village to the lion and her children.

Mpala went on to speak of how destructive such a conflict is to the life of a village. In permitting themselves to quarrel this way, Kimpinde's children had destroyed the village of which their father had been headman. Where there had been many people, there were now only a few, all the rest having fled the conflict which brought illness and misfortune to the village as a whole.

A village, Mpala continued, was meant to grow. People would come there and settle down. Those who were 'carried by the wind' (*kubebwa na pepo*) would arrive there and stop their wanderings. Those who had been born there would themselves grow up and continue to live there. In this way a village grows large, as a village was meant to be.

But the people at Mwanga just spoiled everything with their quarrelling (*ugomvi*). Eventually everyone had begun to move away, and now the whole village was shrunk down to nothing. It was just a few houses and nothing more.

At the time of my departure, lineage members were awaiting the imminent arrival of Kafindo, scheduled to spend his vacation among them. Both factions were making careful note of the twists and turns their conflict had taken of late, and they were assiduously collecting documentary evidence pertaining to the mismanagement of both motor and dragnet. Everyone anticipated Kafindo's just arbitration or adjudication of the affair(s).

Commentary

Though the case history of the Mwanga village lineage group was in some respects different from those of other lineage groups in Mpala, its exceptional aspects differed only in degree of explicitness and intensity, not in kind. Their internal conflict was both well known and of long standing. However, as the cases of Kaputa and Kiabu have demonstrated, the indirect, contrapuntal relation between illness occurrences and social drama was by no means unique.

Many residents of Mpala looked to this lineage group as prime examples of how not to live. Like Chief Mpala, people felt that it was the group's conflict which had ruined the village and forced others to move away. Indeed, in describing the pair of sisters as the lion and the bushbuck, Mpala was doing Kibambo no real service. People say the bushbuck is an inappropriately truculent, pugnacious animal which has the audacity to bark at *you*, the owner, should you encounter it in your fields. In referring to Kibambo in this way, Mpala was pointing out that she, too, was at fault for the conflict and the way in which it was unfolding.

Other outside opinion held that the members of this lineage group drank far too much, and that it was, in fact, their drinking which really lay at the heart of their difficulties. When drunk all could be most aggressive, and, it was thought, the drinking they had been wont to do together had, little by little, led to a build-up in hostilities.

Still others said that it was inappropriate for members of Mwanga village to live as exclusively with other kin as they did. Such was the pattern of living in rural, rather backward, places, and this kind of living could only lead to sorcery. It was much better to live in larger villages or even cities. Where many people were gathered together, jealousy could not become so intensely focused, and the sorcerers had much more space for their nocturnal dancing.

On the whole, public opinion tended to side with Kibambo in the affair. It was unfortunately true that, much as I liked Kisile and his siblings, their mother tended to be abrasive and greedy in her behaviour. During the time her children were away attending to their court case, Muvimbo would come to ask for salt, kerosene and soap, and then refuse to share these things with her own grandchildren. It is greed of this sort more than any other personal characteristic which causes people to be suspected of sorcery.

Finally, from the analyst's perspective, the lineage group of Mwanga village showed structural signs of splitting as well. These consisted not only of the cleavage of the residential unit, and of the intensity of the conflict's accusations and counter-accusations, so characteristic of schism, but also of the exchange of *bapyani* (sing. *mupyani*) among two of the sublineage groups.

A *mupyani* is one who inherits the name and certain aspects of the identity of a kinsperson after that person's death. Such an heir, however, may not derive from the same sublineage as the deceased. Instead she or he must be chosen from among comparable members of a sublineage related to that of the deceased at the level of the grandparental generation or above. As genealogies are not very deep, this is the precise level at which the memory of the connection begins to fade. Frequently, only one or two of the very oldest members of the subgroup remember the connection exactly. Mature adults define the connection ambiguously, saying the two subgroups are both one 'abdomen' (*tumbo*) and two; *both* the same lineage *and* different ones.

Early in the history described here, a son of Kibambo's (D15) who was teaching at a lakeside village to the south of Mwanga was killed by the sorcery of a neighbour there. His wife was pregnant at the time, and was brought to Mpala to live. The *mupyani* produced to inherit the woman was another of Kalandu's descendants. He was one of Luenzia's sons (D11–D14).

Such a choice at that particular stage in the history of the group seemed a bit precipitate. Ordinarily, subgroups of this type might not begin exchanging *bapyani* until the mature women (that is, Muvimbo, Kibambo and Luenzia) were in their dotage. That the lineage group of Mwanga village had already done so was indicative of the way in which they were on the cusp, so to speak, of major structural change. While speculation as to primacy of one aspect of the situation over the other could be questionable, that the two parts, cleavage and conflict, exacerbated one another is clear.

Equally clear is the indirect relationship revealed by this history to exist between illness occurrences and the social dramas with which they may coexist. This very indirection in some sense justifies an analysis of social drama apart from the illness which may precipitate it. Should such be the case, however, it must be remembered and made clear that the picture of society so presented is in some sense inadequate. In it, problematic illness is seen as inevitably causing and/or as being attributed to only the most salient social conflict.

This development of a case history which uses instances of illness themselves as the constants demonstrates the bias of such a view. Instead, the connection of illness to conflict is seen to resemble rather the inter-relations among melodic lines in a musical piece. Now and again, the lines of illness and of salient conflict almost come together. Frequently, the two resonate in their repetition of comparable themes and relations. More often, however, the one affects the other obliquely. The illness begins, measures are taken to control or diminish it. Suspicions may be aroused, but remain unconfirmed. Divination forms a switch-point at which physiological, historical and aetiologic elements converge, to be recombined and contained in a usable narrative of local, interpersonal history and of personal identity. The illness remits, but the conflict is driven forward by breaches in social norms which have taken place during the occurrence's unfolding.

PART III
INTERVENING IN THE
SUBSTANTIAL REAL

7

BODILY THERAPIES

Like their west Zairian contemporaries, the BaKongo (Janzen 1978), the people of Mpala have long resided in and become accustomed to a situation of medical diversity. In it, not only may they choose from among several different varieties of divination, but when considering bodily therapies, they may also select between two more broadly defined categories of medical technology: European medicines (*dawa ya kizungu*) and traditional medicines (*dawa ya asili*). Although both are part of a single medical culture (Last 1981), clear distinction between the two is made and used by people themselves. Distinguishing features include the form taken by each, the sources from which it may be obtained, its capabilities and benefits, and its limitations relative to its counterpart. A description of the therapeutic alternatives available to people must therefore include discussions of both and of the articulations between them as these existed in the area around Mpala during the time of my stay.

DAWA YA KIZUNGU

Though defined or labelled in terms of its origin, these days *dawa ya kizungu* can no longer be said to be associated with Europeans as a population. Though the impact upon it of the White Fathers' missionary effort was immense, the area never knew dense European settlement. After independence, much of the small foreign community withdrew from the larger towns in the vicinity, making the situation one wherein there is virtually no contact at all between the two racial/status groups. In the medical as in many other domains, then, the term *ya kizungu* is now used more generally to denote things of or pertaining to industrial manufacture,[1] the environment in which they are found, and the market economy in which they are exchanged.

Physically, *dawa ya kizungu* is distinguishable from *dawa ya asili* by its form and method of administration. European medicines consist of 'pills' (*vinini*, sing. *ki-*), liquid medicine (*kinini likid*), and various injectable medicines (*dawa ya shindano*) which come in single-use ampoules. The term *kinini*, used for pills, would seem to derive from the French *quinine*, while the modifier *likid* is also a Bantuisation of the French *liquid*.

In Mpala and vicinity, during the time of my stay, there were several sources, local and non-local, of European medicines. Among the local sources were the village dispensary, people skilled in intramuscular and intravenous injection, circuit priests, itinerant merchants of medicines, and the ethnographer.

Mpala had the only village dispensary in operation along the 300-km stretch of lakefront extending from Kalemie to the Zambian border. The dispensary was run by a male nurse, a grandson of a previous chief, Kansabala. He had begun his career as a *fundi wa shindano*, one skilled at giving injections, and was given nine months' instruction at the hospital at Moba after a shocked government doctor discovered how little formal instruction he had had.

At the outset of my stay, the nurse had not been paid his salary for approximately one and a half years. He lived by fishing and farming, and selling the medications intermittently issued to him by the administrative head of the hospital at Moba. He also purchased quantities of medicines from the circuit priests who came to Mpala at three- to four-month intervals, and from the pharmacy in Kalemie. These he sold to residents of Mpala at a profit.

The economic crisis precipitated by the crash in the copper market of the early seventies (and exacerbated by the government's nationalisation pro- gramme) made a shambles of the hospital's provision to dispensaries of free medicines as well as of the nurse's profit-making plan. As time wore on, he had medicines less and less often. Quantities became more and more limited, arrivals more and more irregular, and supplies more and more rapidly exhausted. For long periods the nurse simply would cease practising altogether, although he would continue for a time between shipments of medications to conduct the simple faeces, urine and blood tests of which the dispensary was capable.

Slightly more than halfway through my stay, even this was stopped. The nurse felt that his time was wasted in this practice. Despite the fact that testing was done for a fee, as were injections of medicines purchased by others, the income provided was not enough to live on, or to justify his neglect of his fields. Toward the end of my stay, he applied for transfer to another village, and was given it. He was replaced by another nurse whose practice was as intermittent as his predecessor's had been.

Fundi wa shindano, persons skilled in administration of injectable medi- cines, were another source of *dawa ya kizungu* in Mpala. Resident in the village were several individuals who owned hypodermic needles and syringes and who charged for their services on a per-injection basis. Prices varied according to whether the medicine provided belonged to the patient or to the *fundi*. As is often the case in rural circumstances, the conditions under which hypodermic needles and syringes were kept were less than sterile. A number of those receiving injections would subsequently suffer subcutaneous infections.

In addition to practising their art, *fundi wa shindano* tended also to occupy other skilled Europeanised roles, such as primary school teacher and merchant. Foremost among them was the town photographer, who took, developed and printed the pictures required to complete the identity cards of Zairian citizens. It was frequently this man, and not the nurse, who was called in the middle of the night for emergency treatment.

A third source of European medicines, in existence at the outset of my stay, was the circuit priests who came to Mpala every third or fourth month. In addition to their evangelical duties, they would also sell medicines at cost to those who needed them. Their supplies were derived from the Catholic charitable organisation CARITAS, and the prices they charged covered transportation fees. Not long after my arrival, however, the Zairian government forbade the importation of medicines by private companies and agencies, and this source dried up.

Another, less regular source of *dawa ya kizungu* was itinerant merchants who came to Mpala seeking the dried fish to be bought relatively cheaply there. Quantities of medicines might be bought in Kalemie and then sold at a profit in Mpala. Even those who were not merchants, but were simply travellers visiting relatives, or students returning from school for the holidays, might engage in this sort of petty commerce. Medicines sold off gradually during the course of their visit helped defray the cost of the trip.

Another source of European medicines in Mpala was the ethnographer.[2] Though my initial idea had been to refrain from this practice, social demand (in the form of increasing numbers of people coming and asking for help) backed me into it. On Monday, Wednesday and Friday mornings we operated a dispensary out of our house, using medicines we purchased in Kalemie and sold at cost (and often less) or traded in kind. During the course of our time there we came to treat and have records of over 600 individuals. The dispensary became the forum in which I first learned of the diagnostic categories outlined in Chapter 1.

Though our clinic primarily handled simple problems, as time wore on, the illnesses brought to us and those we became capable of handling became more complex. Occasionally, we would be supplied with free medicines and with advice by hospital administrators/doctors in Kalemie and Moba. People with difficult illnesses could come along on our bi- or tri-monthly trips to purchase supplies, and be treated free of charge through the generosity of the same administrators and doctors. Finally, when we ran out of medicines, and the petrol shortage prevented our making trips to Kalemie, we continued to treat people when they could obtain the necessary medicines themselves.

The economic situation prevailing in Zaire during the time of our field stay was little short of disastrous. As mentioned above, the copper market collapsed shortly after the government's programme of Zairianisation of private businesses had got under way. Prices soared with an inflation rate well over 100 per cent per annum. Lack of foreign exchange meant that necessary items such as medicines could not be imported, and for a time smuggling from neighbouring countries was the principal means by which the eastern border areas of Zaire were supplied with manufactured goods. Though there was always a trickle of medicines coming into the area, then, over the years we watched the quantity and variety diminish, prices rise unbelievably, and thus the possibility of obtaining the correct quantity of the appropriate medicine become almost nil.

In addition to local sources of *dawa ya kizungu*, residents of Mpala also had several non-local sources available to them, at least in theory. Nearest was the hospital at Moba. Built and equipped before Zairian political independence (1960), this small hospital was capable of performing more complex diagnostic tests (including blood sedimentation rate, X-ray, culturing, etc.) than was the local dispensary. It had a small number of beds, and a maternity ward with a nurse capable of performing Caesarean sections.

Staffed by Zairian nurses and orderlies, and by European nursing nuns, this hospital had been without a physician for two years at the time of my departure from the area. In addition, much of its equipment was in such poor condition as to be virtually worthless (the X-rays, for example, were often so blurred as to be practically unintelligible). The task of the nursing staff was made still more difficult by the fact that crates of 'medicines' sent from Kinshasa (the capital) would arrive empty or filled with rocks, the contents stolen along the way, or never shipped. Patients were expected to supply their own bedding, their own food and, in time of hardship, their own medicine.

At Kalemie, the number of hospital facilities and of physicians was much greater, although most of these would be inaccessible to a resident of Mpala travelling there. Both the railroad company and the textile mill headquarters in Kalemie had clinics and doctors of their own, reserved for their own staff.[3]

In addition to these were two government doctors, and two public or semi-public hospital facilities, the Hopital General and the Clinique Mama Mobutu. Located near what was the outskirts of the city, and literally on the 'other side of the tracks', the General Hospital was formerly operated by the colonial government for the African population of the Belgian Congo.

During my residence at Mpala, a stay at this hospital necessitated payment of a daily room fee. In addition, the patient was required to provide his own bedding, and to have food brought in. One rough blanket and a daily bowl of beans were all that was provided by the hospital. Further, as was the case in Moba, patients or their relatives were often required to provide their own medication as well.

At the General Hospital, the case load was so heavy and medicine so scarce that doctors saw only the most exceptional cases, and these were seen only upon admission. The course of treatment prescribed by the doctor often was not followed without payment of a bribe to one of the ward nurses.

Located on a hill, with terraced rooms overlooking Lake Tanganyika, the Clinique Mama Mobutu was formerly the hospital for white residents of the Congo. At the time of my stay. it was the medical facility for the Europeanised and wealthier residents of Kalemie. Among its clientele were families of local government officials, clerks for the local fisheries, school teachers, and well-to-do Omani and Zairian merchants. In 1976, hospitalisation at the Clinic cost a minimum of four zaires a day. Though this included meals and bedding, the price was well beyond what most residents of Mpala could afford to pay.

In both Moba and Kalemie, treatment with *dawa ya kizungu* could also be had privately. Medical assistants and nurses in both cities had private practices to which they attended at their homes in the hours before and after work. For many people local to these cities, this was the most satisfactory alternative. In it, the treatment came to the patient and spared him the social complexities and long wait of the hospital itself.

The final source of European medicine in Kalemie was the local pharmacy. At the outset of my stay, there was only one in operation. A year or two after my arrival, however, the subregional doctor opened a second pharmacy, which was run by his wife. At either place, medication could be had by prescription or by diagnostic consultation with the pharmacist. Pharmacists also freely substituted one medication for another prescribed substance they might be lacking. Moba was without a pharmacy as such. Medicines might be purchased from nurses and government health agents, who might buy medicines in Lubumbashi for resale at a profit.

These, then, are the forms and the sources of *dawa ya kizungu* as it existed in the environment surrounding residents of Mpala. European medicines are distinguished from traditional ones on other bases as well. Each type is thought to have its benefits and its limitations. The distinction drawn between the two becomes the basis for opposition only in certain specific social circumstances, to be discussed below.

People say that foremost among the strengths of European medicine is the precision of measurement (*kipimo*, literally 'measure') it offers through diagnostic tests and a specific posology. People say that by means of microscope, test tube and X-ray, the doctor of European medicine is able to see inside the body, and thus to determine the cause of the illness. He can then study his medical text, find the therapy most appropriate to the illness in question, and apply it immediately.

With traditional medicines, people say, one has no idea of what the illness might actually be. The therapist simply brings one medicine after another until he hits upon the one that works.

Similarly, European medicine is more effective because of its refined posology. The quantity of medication administered is geared to the body size, age and physical condition of the patient. People contrast this to traditional medicines, in which, they say, there is no posology (*kipimo*) as such. Medicine is simply mixed and administered without regard to the specifics of the patient's physiology.[4]

Finally, *dawa ya kizungu* has as a benefit the possibilities of surgical repair, bone setting and Caesarean section. Also by means of it, the health of an unborn child can be determined, and the exact stage of parturition ascertained.

Despite these many obvious benefits, European medicine does have its limits. It is ineffective against certain prevalent illnesses. Such illnesses as *mpanga* ('lower back pain leading to swelling of the testicles'), *kimbeleka* ('infantile malaria'), *ndege* ('infantile convulsions') and *mkola* ('tuberculosis') cannot be treated by *dawa ya kizungu* with any lasting success. Indeed, some people go so far as to insist that treatment with European medicines of a chronic illness such as *mpanga* does nothing but exacerbate it. The symptoms diminish, but the illness is really simply hiding in the body, to return, fully 'mature' (*yenye kukomaa*), at a later date.

Dawa ya kizungu is equally ineffective against illnesses caused by sorcery. Sickness derived from 'the path of man' (*njia ya mutu*) will only hide itself (*kufichama*) during testing and surgery. European doctors will find nothing, and the sickness will return as soon as the patient is away from the hospital.

This capacity of *ulozi* to hide itself in the body is what accounts for those cases of chronic, debilitating illness in which faeces and blood tests reveal no parasites (*wadudu*). In such a case, a negative test of this sort is said to have revealed that the person had 'no sickness' (*hakuna ugonjuwa*), and this absence becomes an important feature of problematic illness. Though I have never heard it mentioned in court or at divination, when news of a patient's condition circulates as gossip, this fact becomes grounds for the suspicion of sorcery.

Just as its means of testing cannot reveal *ulozi*, so European medicine's methods of treatment cannot affect it. If any medicine is to work against sorcery, it must be *dawa ya asili*. In fact, European medicines are considered so ineffective as almost to be declined out of hand. However, pragmatism is the salient value governing people's approach to treatment, and more often than not both sorts of medicine are employed, even while it is being observed that only the traditional ones are likely to work.

Further, like the *miti* traditionally employed in treatment of physiological disease, *dawa ya kizungu* can work against problematic illness only if divination is also sought. Once the full social and spiritual situation of the illness occurrence is known, recovery is possible. Prior to this time, all attempts at effective treatment will be futile.

People know that foreigners are inclined to be suspicious of divination as a therapeutic device. The indirect relation between physiological condition and aetiologic agent is such that one can be spoken of without reference to the other, and this was usually the practice when seeking treatment at hospitals or mission dispensaries which were run by Europeans. In these post-independence days, however, the subject of divination can be broached to Zairian doctors of European medicine, though the work itself must be conducted outside the hospital, and run parallel to medical treatment. I would frequently ask patients suffering with complicated illness if they had been to divine, and would inevitably get 'no' for an initial answer. When I would then (honestly) comment that I thought divination might improve the patient's rate of recovery, people would almost inevitably tell me that they had, in fact, already been, and they would then go on to tell me the hypothesis the diviner had given.

Another, great, limitation of European medicine is its relative inaccessibility. The centre of *dawa ya kizungu* is the hospital, while that of *dawa ya asili* is the *mjini* (village). Though the distances of Moba and Kalemie from Mpala are not insurmountable, the social and political distances dividing the hospital from the village are such that to consider entering the hospital for any length of time is tantamount to considering a complete change in social identity; a change in every way comparable to that attendant upon the death itself of the patient. A brief outline of what would be required in such a case will suffice to illustrate the difficulty.[5]

A person whose 'therapy management group' (that is, spouse, siblings, parents and matrilineal kin, as in Janzen 1978) have determined that he or she should be admitted to the hospital must first ascertain that the patient is well enough to withstand the trip by canoe or small boat from Mpala to Kalemie. This comprises some 27 hours of virtually non-stop rowing on Lake Tanganyika (a trip to Moba takes some 12 hours). For this, three or four people must be found who are willing to transport the patient and the person(s) who will accompany him to care for him in the hospital. A canoe or small boat must also be secured, and, like the rowers themselves, its owner must be compensated with money for the use of his boat if he is not a close kinsman of the sick person. Prior to departure for Kalemie, a travel pass must be obtained from the town clerk for each of the persons making the trip. Required of all Zairian citizens travelling outside their zone of residence, this pass must state the reason for the journey and show its day of issuance. A fee is charged for this document; it must be renewed within four days of arrival at Kalemie, and revalidated at the office of a local chief every two weeks for the duration of the stay. (If the patient is taken to Moba, no such pass is required.)

Arriving in Kalemie, passes and identity cards must be shown to the
soldiers who patrol the beach, or these agents must be effectively evaded.
One must live with relatives and must have money to buy food. Though it is
customary for a guest to bring along a sack of manioc, fish that might have
been caught at Mpala must be purchased at Kalemie by those who do not
have licences or boats, or who, like most women, simply do not fish. Urban
dwellers usually eat only once a day, in contrast to the two meals taken by
Mpala residents; and the quantity of food cannot be significantly increased
to accommodate visitors. Guests are thus caught in the double bind of being
both hungry and unwelcome if they stay for more than a short time.

Once patient and guardian have overcome the obstacles of trip and
lodging, they can turn their attention to obtaining the knowledge necessary
to manoeuvre the intricacies of hospital access routes. One can either go and
wait all day at the hospital clinic, or one can begin to approach kin who are
residents of Kalemie and who might know ways by which corners can be
cut. Such people might have contacts at the hospital itself, or know someone
who does. It might also be through them that one might arrange to borrow
a bicycle to transport the patient from Kamkolobondo, on the south of
town, to the hospital, on the far northern end, several miles away.

Admission to the hospital means payment of a daily room and board fee,
unless one is declared indigent. If the latter alternative is the case the fees for
hospitalisation must be paid out of the budget of the village chief, Chief
Mpala, and the forms and permission for this must be obtained prior to
departure. As noted above, hospitalisation also requires that the patient
provide his own bedding, and that his relatives bring him his food.

In the wards, life for a rural dweller unaccustomed to city ways can be
quite complex. One may be bullied by the nurses or mistreated by them.
One can also be simply overlooked and not treated until one pays a little
something extra for the privilege. The prescriptions written on patients'
charts are for the most part incomprehensible to them, and, though
adequate in theory, it is certain that most patients do not receive what has
been prescribed. Daily rounds by the doctors are not made, and there is no
possibility of complaint or redress of grievance.

I wish to make very clear in this text that the above description by no
means applies to all Zairian nurses, or even to all nurses at the General
Hospital. Indeed, some of the most dedicated individuals I met during my
stay in Zaire were the nurses who continually struggled to bring what health
care they could to an overwhelmingly large patient population. They often
practised seven days a week, and worked despite deficiencies in supplies and
facilities that would stagger the average urban American physician. The
number of lives saved by these men and women and the good they do
cannot be overestimated; nor can it be adequately described here.

Despite these exemplary people, there are a number of nurses who take advantage of the almost continual critical shortage of medication and supplies to further their own personal interests. It is the contact, however limited, with them that makes the hospital into an environment of trauma instead of one of cure. As everyone knows, the threat of a single rank humiliation can obliterate in the mind the potential of a hundred small kindnesses.

From the above description, then, it can be seen that the hospital, for most residents of Mpala, is only a theoretical alternative. Gaining admission to and pursuing treatment in it requires monumental effort on the part of the patient and members of his therapy management group.

Indeed, from their point of view, such effort would amount to little less than a complete, profound transformation of their lives. In the wet season, especially, the patient's kin would be giving themselves over totally to his illness, neglecting their fields and the next year's subsistence. *Bouleversement*, or overturning, of this sort is no less intense than that which people would suffer if the patient should die, and is probably more so. Indeed, during my stay, no one of whose illness I knew asked that his kin take such trouble for him. Though mothers would sometimes take their children to Moba for treatment, going on their own and on foot, there were rarely any instances in which a sick person himself sought treatment in Kalemie, and definitely none in which a disabled person was taken that far by concerned kin.

Treatment at Moba was sought somewhat more often,[6] but the patient was frequently moribund or had been very nearly so when the decision was made, often dying before he or she arrived at the hospital. I found that my offers of assistance with hospital visits were accepted precisely because I provided transport, certainty of a fixed date of return, and easy access to medical treatment. Kiabu's case illustrates the response an Mpala resident could expect when unprotected by the privilege of foreignness. After I had seen the realities of hospital life, I stopped my (at times somewhat strident) insistence that more complicated illnesses be taken there.

The point, in short, is that seeking treatment in the hospital is, in many instances, equivalent in stress and difficulty to permitting the patient to remain at home and there await the working out of his fate. Like Hamlet's, people's attitudes about their ends are that these remain, in some ultimate sense, unchanged, 'rough-hew them how we will' (*Hamlet* V, ii, 10–11).

For the most part, then, the *dawa ya kizungu* extant in people's social setting and under their control has a somewhat different aspect from that brought to mind by the phrase 'European medicines'. It is a smaller, more domesticable form of medical technology, and the use of this form of *dawa ya kizungu* is governed by a body of local knowledge.

Though they do not always adhere to this in practice, people know that their first step in seeking treatment of illness should be the completion of blood, faeces and urine tests at the dispensary. As noted above, the idea that

parasites cause illness is now quite clearly a feature of lay medical knowledge, and it is expected that abdominal pain, backache (unrelated to
heavy work), fever and malaise may occur as a consequence of *wadudu* of
various kinds. Tests made at Mpala's dispensary can detect such parasites
as ascaris, hookworm, whipworm, schistosomes, trichomonas vaginalis and
malarial gametocytes. The presence of albumin can also be detected, as can
anaemia.

While people know that each sort of parasite has its own medicine, knowledge of exact correspondence is differential. Often, those without much
experience in these matters will simply purchase a treatment of the correct
medicine from the nurse, or show their test results to someone who can
advise them what to buy.

The *dawa ya kizungu* most commonly in circulation at the time of our
residence at Mpala were as follows.

Antibiotics

Penicillin was the most common and widely used of the antibiotics. It was
given by injection for fevers (*homa*) and used for generalised illnesses, where
the patient 'feels his whole body' (*kusikia maongo tu yote*). Some considered
its use was inappropriate during the early stages of measles, because,
according to them, it inhibited high fever and prevented the papules from
'coming out' (*kutoka*), as they ought. It might safely be employed only after
these had shown themselves. Penicillin was also known to be the cure for
gonorrhoea (*sofisi*). In powdered form it was sprinkled on wounds, to
prevent or treat infection. Streptomycin was almost always used in
combination with penicillin by the doctors in Kalemie. In the village it was
considered a less effective medicine than penicillin, though one which could
be employed in the same circumstances.

Other antibiotics were in circulation in the area from time to time. There
were occasional quantities of chloramphenicol, used in the same fashion as
penicillin, and there was sometimes tetracycline. Tetracycline was the only
antibiotic to be offered in capsule form, and, as with ambilhar (niridazole),
there was a general belief that a single capsule constituted complete treatment, in the case of urethritis and/or venereal disease.

Aspirin and cafenol

These were taken in treatment of fever, headache and malaise. Cafenol
tablets, manufactured in Tanzania, contained caffeine as well as aspirin,
and came packaged individually.

Ambilhar

This was the common treatment of schistosomiasis once it had been discovered through diagnostic tests. Ambilhar (niridazole) would not auto-

matically be employed to treat symptoms (vague and non-specific as these are) of bilharziasis without such confirmation. As noted above, the value of this medication was exaggerated by biomedical standards, perhaps because the orange tint it gave the urine and the side effects it could cause provided perceptual proof of its strength. People often believed that a single 500-mg. tablet was effective against bilharziasis, and individual tablets sold for as much as 250 k by the end of my stay.[7]

Mintezol
This brand of thiabendazole was the commonest anti-thelmenthic available. Its effectiveness against the parasites ascaris, hookworm (*Necator americanus*) and whipworm (*Trichoceohalus trichiurus*) was well known. For children, it would be employed after fever, malaise or ochre-coloured faeces had prompted diagnostic tests which revealed one or more of these parasites to be present. In adults, treatment would follow diagnosis similarly sought in response primarily to abdominal illness.

Nivaquine
This was the commonest brand of chloroquine in circulation in the area, though as the economic crisis wore on, even this became, for the most part, unavailable. In Mpala, it was never used prophylactically. Instead, nivaquine would be given children suffering from high fever, or adults stricken with either fever itself or general aches and pains (often the only clinical manifestation of chronic malaria). It might also be sought and administered in response to positive test results.

Kali-sumu
This was the Swahili-ised name applied to injectable calcium–vitamin C mixtures. A near homonym to the French pronunciation, the term *kali-sumu* means 'fierce-poison', and refers to what people described as its capacity to produce fever after intramuscular injection. Though it was never readily available during my residence in Mpala, *kali-sumu* was highly regarded as a medicine capable of curing serious illnesses, and of correcting the generalised itching (urticaria) attendant upon bilharziasis.

Vitamins
Injections of B vitamins were sought to correct anaemia (*kuleta damu*) and to 'strengthen' (*kuleta nguvu*). An example of the latter use was in the case of Kulimba's difficult labour, described in Chapter 6. In that instance, the nurse gave her such an injection to strengthen her during and immediately after parturition. Vitamins (*vitamini*) are known to be necessary for the healthy development of children and for robustness (*afia*) in adults. It is *vitamini* as well which bring milk to the breasts of new mother. They are to

be found in certain foods, such as beans, meat, corn, and leafy foods like the
manioc, squash and sweet potato leaves people often eat.

Vitamini are also found in the *kibuku* corn and millet beer people are fond
of drinking, but not, say, in the illegally distilled *rutuku* which is 'just smoke'
(*moshi tu*). Vitamins likewise are not found in *bukali* (manioc flour polenta),
only in that made from corn meal.

These, then, were the principal European medicines in general use among
residents of Mpala. Other, less significant medications employed were
merchurochome (*tenturi*), which was painted on wounds; petroleum jelly
(*manteka*), spread on skin eruptions; talcum powder, used in treatment of
'heat rash' (*piakusu*); and potassium permanganate, used in infusion as
enemas and sitzbaths for treatment of *kidonda tumbo*. Permanganate might
also be rubbed into *machanjo* incisions (see below), as might the filling from
torch batteries and also petrol, in a treatment of pain which combined a
traditional method with an industrially manufactured substance.

In addition to the above, other medications seemed to be in circulation,
though limited to those who were *fundi wa shindano*. Among these were
small, single-injection ampoules of vitamin K, phenobarbital and oxytocin.
As a rule, the *fundi* owning them would know something of the physiological
circumstances in which they were used. However, exact dosage frequently
was unknown, as were contra-indications and possible complications.

Finally, knowledge of *dawa ya kizungu* included awareness of the fact
that many medicines 'rot' (*kuoza*) and must be disposed of after the
expiration date stamped on the bottle. Often, this date was scandalously
close to the date of purchase, frequently being less than one year. In
addition, medicines whose use had been forgotten or whose labels obliter-
ated by time were considered inappropriate to administer and were thrown
away.

This is the sum of *dawa ya kizungu* as it forms a part of the medical
culture in which people live. Opting for or against it is a matter of specific
judgement as well as individual taste; use varies on an instance-by-instance
basis.

Some people, for example, prefer European medicines for treatment of
illnesses of themselves and their children. Most individuals of this preference are progressive young men who have worked or lived in larger urban
areas. The scarcity of *dawa ya kizungu* during my stay in Mpala made
people like these uncomfortable. They said their bodies and those of their
children had become accustomed (*kuzoea*) to treatment with *dawa ya
kizungu*. If European medicine completely ran out and they were forced to
change abruptly to traditional medicines, these might fail to cure them or,
worse, make them ill.

Despite this, the vast majority of Mpala residents, most of these young

men included, are in fact eclectic in their choice among therapeutic
alternatives. People use anything that works, and do not, under most circumstances, make invidious moral or political distinctions between the two
medical technologies.

People are nevertheless averse to using both types of medicine on the
same day. According to current medical theory, such a mixture (*kuchanganika*)
of the two in the body could make one ill or kill one. People also say that the
priests and nuns of the old days would refuse to dispense European medicines to anyone who had used traditional medicines earlier that day.

Despite their usually pragmatic approach to such matters, people do, in
certain circumstances, make therapeutic alternatives into symbols of
political or moral choices. One such situation is the evaluation of people like
merchants, teachers and government agents, whose Europeanisation strikes
their neighbours as a way of giving themselves airs and belittling everyone
else. Another is the situation of local Jehovah's Witnesses (*Ba-Soswaiti*). To
be in good standing among them, one must give up recourse to divination,
and this is regarded as a significant measure of fundamental religious
difference.

DAWA YA ASILI

The alternative to *dawa ya kizungu*, *dawa ya asili* ('traditional medicine') is
also called by a number of other names. These are *dawa ya kinchi* ('medicine
of the land' or 'of the country'), *dawa ya kikwetu* ('medicine of our place')
and *dawa ya kishenzi* ('savage medicines'). The larger number of names by
which this medicine is known is indicative of its greater significance. Indeed,
each name can be said to reflect a different aspect of the way in which people
identify this type of medicine with themselves and with their land. There is
a way in which the very wryness of people's comments upon *dawa ya asili*'s
clumsiness and inefficiency is comparable to the high and affectionate irony
with which they regard their own more personal foibles and limitations.

Just as all adults have some knowledge of the European medicines
available in the environment, so does every adult have some knowledge of
traditional medicine. Beginning in youth with treatments of common ailments, knowledge of medicines increases with age and with the experience
of illness itself. Nursing one's children frequently provides a forum for
learning the uses of medicinal plants, and advising one's children on the
treatment of their children is a customary part of mature parent–child
relations. In general, the social lines along which therapy moves coincide
with the lines along which food moves; those whom one nurtures, one
treats.

In all cases, knowledge of medicines is the property of the knower.
Friends and kin may provide medicines free of charge and may also divulge
at no cost the names of the components contained in the formulae they

employ. Others, especially *wafumu*, usually charge a fee for treatment as well as for divulgence of the identities of the medicinal plants known to them.

Since everyone recognises the trees and plants themselves, what is esoteric about medical knowledge is specifically the knowledge of *conjunctions*: that is, the quantities and identities of herbal substances coupled with the means by which these are to be administered, and recognition of the illness that they cure. For this reason, when bringing medicinal plants to their patients, *wafumu* are careful to present them in such a way that clients are unable to identify them. Roots alone are brought, without leaves, and with bark removed if this is an identifying characteristic. Leaves are pounded and pulp alone presented, or dried plant substances are ground to powder.

A client who seeks to identify the medicines being brought him, or who attempts to advise the practitioner regarding his treatment, commits a serious breach of etiquette, and risks being dismissed from therapy by the *mfumu*. After successful treatment, however, the same individual (having paid for the cure) may invite the *mfumu* to his house, and, over beer, ask to be taught about the medicines used specifically to cure him, in return for payment of the fee without which the formulae would be ineffective.

An individual wishing to become generally knowledgeable of herbal medicines may enter into a similar relation with an *mfumu* or herbalist, usually connected by kinship. In such a relation, gifts of cloth, tools (such as hoe or axe) and livestock (chickens, ducks or goats) are given to the *mfumu* over a period of time. In addition, the novice offers his labour as part of his apprenticeship, and, following his mentor's instructions, searches for medicines in the bush initially without knowing the exact use to which they will be put, or the *vizimba* which accompany them.

Transmission of therapeutic knowledge is also an important part of the professional relations which bind practitioners to one another in a network of mutual support and sometimes rivalry. *Wafumu* who consider themselves less skilled will regularly seek the advice of colleagues more experienced and more successful than they. Though a relationship such as this may begin with per-formula payment, a more general exchange relation may develop over time involving mutual help, referral of clients, extension of hospitality, gifts of food, and the like.

Form and administration

Like its industrially manufactured counterpart, *dawa ya asili* takes its own distinctive forms. Starting from two primary types of component, *miti* and *vizimba*, formulae can be prepared in three different ways, and administered by ten different methods.

In KiTabwa, as in many other East Central African Bantu languages, the term *miti* is used to refer to plant substances in their capacity as medicines.

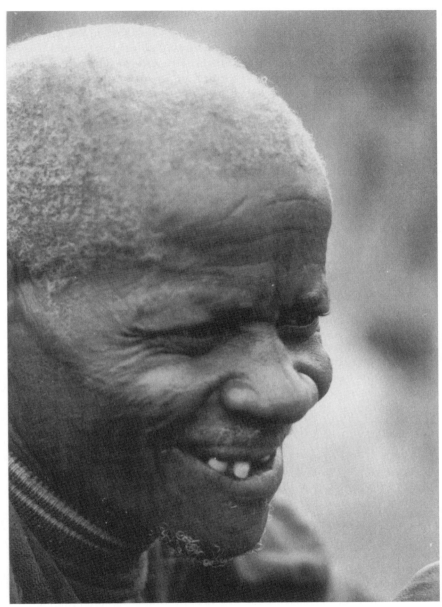

Figure 7.1 Abonamboka, Mbote herbalist

People would translate this into KiSwahili as *dawa,* and would use the word to refer specifically to the leaves, roots or bark of trees, and to the many different shrubs, plants and grasses which may be employed medicinally. During the course of my stay in Mpala, I recorded some 300 different names of *miti,* and collected for identification specimens of 230 of these.

People describe the archetype of the *kizimba* (pl: *vi-*) as being a piece of the dried, specific body part of an individual representative of a given species of mammal, which combination of context and creature has a fixed meaning that can be transferred to the patient or situation designated as its object. In practice this category also includes bits and pieces of birds, insects, fish and reptiles as well as human relics and artefacts, minerals, and even certain plant substances whose context makes them significant. There is no KiSwahili term for *vizimba.* I have recorded names and meanings of around one hundred and fifty.

A mixture of *miti/dawa* and *vizimba* is usually referred to by the term *dawa.* Practitioners say that this usage is meant to withhold from the patients even the hint of insight that might derive from reference to the presence of *vizimba.*

Combinations of these two components may be prepared in three different ways:

1. Infusions may be made by soaking *miti* and *vizimba* in hot or cold water. If hot, the infusion is usually allowed to stand until the water has taken on a colour the intensity of which is prescribed. If cold, the infusion is usually allowed to stand overnight.
2. Roots, leaves or the bark of plants may be cut into small pieces and dried in the sun, after which they are ground into a powder together with whatever *vizimba* are to be used. It is the powder which is then presented to the patient for use.
3. Roots, leaves or bark are cut into small pieces and combined with *vizimba.* These are placed on a potsherd (or in a little pot) and dry roasted until they are burnt to ash, which is then ground to fine black powder.

In all cases, the preparation of *vizimba* is the same. The practitioner cuts off from the small portion that is his stock a tiny piece of each *kizimba* to be used. These are set aside, and then added to the formula at the appropriate point during the process of preparation.

Once suitably prepared, medicinal formulae may be administered in many different ways. Each means has its appropriate therapeutic function, and reflects the logic of anatomy.

Foremost among the many methods of administration of *dawa ya asili* is the enema (*kuinamisha* or *kuinama*). In this technique, warm infusions of medicines are used as an intestinal 'wash'. For children a thin plastic pipette is inserted into the anus, and a small rubber bulb is filled with the medicinal solution, which is then injected into the rectum. Adults employ a larger (usually quart-sized) metal container, which can be suspended above them. The medicine is passed into the body by means of a thin rubber tube, which may or may not be attached to a small plastic pipette.

People often gloss the term *kuinamisha* with the French word *lavement*, and this usage correlates with the idea that enemas are methods of cleansing. People say that the 'fierceness' (*ukali*) of the medicine 'brings out the filth' (*kutosha uchafu*) of the illness, and thus cures the patient.

Though by no means considered clean, the faeces normally evacuated by a healthy person (called *mavi*) do not seem to be quite the same thing as the sodden stools eliminated by enema. The colour and consistency of the latter are often cause for discussion (they are described, not shown), should they vary from those of normal stools. In addition, the absence of *uchafu* during enema is also the cause for remark. Despite the difference between them, however, the *uchafu* and *mavi* do not seem to be sufficiently differentiated to warrant description of the former as the manifestation of a state of pollution or as an indicator of a generalised state of uncleanness.

The enema is the only therapeutic method that people also use prophylactically. In a manner reminiscent of the way in which doting new American parents are depicted as rushing out to buy a football helmet or toy typewriter for their child, so do doting Tabwa parents purchase tiny enema bulbs for their newborn offspring. Starting on the second or third day after his or her birth and continuing on a bi- or tri-weekly basis throughout his or her childhood, an infant will receive an enema of either plain warm water or warm water in which a small quantity of manioc flour has been mixed. Should he or she be feverish, have ochre-coloured stools, or show signs of lassitude and lack of interest in playing childhood games, the frequency with which the enema is given will increase until *lavements* are being given on a daily basis. Usually, an infusion made from the pounded leaves of the *mululuzia* tree (*Veronia colorata (Willd.)* Drake, also called *mululunkunja*) is employed at these times.

Adults do not routinely administer prophylactic enemas to themselves. They do, however, employ *lavement* if they feel the minor symptoms indicative of potential illness (when they 'think they're coming down with something', as we would put it). At this time, only warm water, or water mixed with flour, is used.[8]

While Tabwa medical theory defines enemas as an effective therapy because the strength of the medicine brings something out of the body, biomedical theory attributes the enema's effectiveness to the highly absorptive nature of the rectum. Medicines administered rectally often can be more rapidly and more completely absorbed than those administered by mouth (Steyn 1931: 631).

Dawa ya asili may also be administered by mouth in the forms of medicines that are drunk (*dawa ya kuniwa*) and those which are eaten. Formulae made up as infusions may be drunk by the patient. They go to the stomach, then move about the body, before leaving it in the form of urine. Medicine administered in this way cures abdominal illness because the snake of the stomach (*lombozoka*, *nyoka*) smells its odour (*harufu*) and settles down. Drinking, however, has only transient therapeutic effect, because of the rapidity with which the liquid leaves the body.

Purging and emesis (*kuendesha tumbo* and *kutapika*, respectively) are therapeutic techniques which are in some respect subsidiary to the enemas. The emetic/purgative is usually a few drops of the sap of a euphorbia species. This is drunk, in water, and diarrhoea and vomiting begin shortly thereafter. These continue until the antidote (*mutompololo*) of cooked sweet potato leaves (*matembele*) is administered.

This technique is used to bring out of the body inappropriately located substances of special tenacity, such as those deriving from sorcery (*ulozi*) or relating to chronic illness. It may be used to initiate a complex sequence of subsequent therapies, in this sense serving as something of a device for the effacement of previous history, or internal bodily states. In all cases, the aim is not putting something into the body, but the provocation of emesis and purging, which will either bring out the object (if put there by sorcery) whose presence is suspected or prepare the body to receive subsequent treatment.

Euphorbia are highly poisonous plants. People are well aware of the danger involved in employing them. They tell stories of suicides effected by deliberate consumption of excessive amounts of *kanoka* (*Euphorbia grantii Oliv.*). As a rule, only the most accomplished practitioners will undertake this therapy, and even they use a standard statement to inform the patient that if he dies it is not they, but his illness, which kills him.

Medicines which are eaten (*dawa ya kula*) can be prepared and administered in two different ways. Powdered medicines may be put in food, or infusions may be cooked into manioc gruel (*uji*) which is then 'drunk'. In either case, the medicine so consumed goes to a part of the abdomen different from that which receives liquid medicines. Formulae administered with foods stay in the body longer and therefore have a more lasting effect than liquid medicine.

Another method by which medicine can be administered is the steam bath. An infusion of medicines is heated until it boils. The patient then seats himself on a low stool, with the pot between his legs on the floor. He closes himself over the steaming pot with a cloth, and permits the steam to envelop him. The process is called *kujifunikila*, and is named for this act of 'self-enclosure' or self-envelopment.

The effectiveness of this method derives from the fact that it opens the 'holes' (*tundu*) which lie at the base of the hairs on the body. Through these, the 'poisons' (*sumu*) in the body are emitted in the form of perspiration. The medicines may then enter via the same holes.

Variations of this are smoke baths, used for ailments of the limbs, and the *lizuba*, used to correct infertility. With the former, powdered medicines are sprinkled on coals, and the affected limb is held under a fabric 'tent' in the smoke. With the *lizuba*, the steaming hot infusion is placed beneath the woman patient, who closes herself over it in such a way that the steam envelops her genital area. Inside her body, the *kisumi* smells the odour of the medicines and calms down, permitting the interior of her body to become suitable for conception. Smoke baths may also form part of the ceremony of 'throwing the person in the bush' (*kumutupa mutu mupori*), when they are used to fumigate the house, to rid it and its inhabitants of the avenging ghost which pursues them.

Two other methods of administering medicines are soaking and washing. With the former, the affected limb is soaked in a hot water infusion. The medicine enters the body by means of the holes in the skin at the bases of the hairs.

With washing, the infusion may be administered in two complementary ways. With the process called *kusukula* (meaning 'to cleanse'), the medicinal infusion is poured over the patient with the hands, starting with the head and working down the body. As with soaking, medicines enter the skin through the holes at the bases of the hairs. This method may be used for fever in children.

The second means of administering a wash is called *kusampula*, a term which has no other referent. With this method, medicines are flung onto the patient with a broom made of willowy twigs cut from a tree. The method by which the medicine enters the body is the same as with the process *kusukula*.

Working in a similar manner, but with longer-lasting effects, is the technique of applying to the skin medicines which have been mixed in the medium of castor oil. Prior to mixture, formulae have been dried or burnt, then ground to powder. Their mixture with castor oil means that they continue to enter the body as long as the formula remains on the skin. With water washes, in contrast, the activity of the medicine ceases as soon as the water evaporates.

Still another therapeutic technique is the administration of medicines by means of *machanjo* (sing: *chanjo*), small, superficial incisions made in the skin with a razor blade. Used in treatment of localised pain and swelling, these are usually made over the affected area, and ash or powdered medicines are rubbed into them. Only a limited number of such incisions may be made in one place if undue swelling is not to result. Medicines administered by this means go directly into the blood, and the release of blood from the incision is essential to the effectiveness of the technique. In addition, formulae so administered *never* leave the body, and it is for this reason that *machanjo* are often the devices through which protective medicines are applied. Injections are considered to be European medicine's counterpart of *machanjo*, and this is a reason why a single injection is often considered to be sufficient to cure an illness.

Massage (*kufinyanga*) constitutes yet another therapeutic means of administering medicines. With this, medicinal infusions and/or a mash of plant pulp is used to massage and manipulate the patient's body vigorously. The purpose of this often painful technique is both to cause the medicines to enter the body through the skin, and to cause the blood to move about (*kutembea*) within the veins. Massage also prevents or corrects stiffening and pains of the muscles or joints. This technique is prominent in the cure of 'paralysis' (*bulebe*), which is due to inactive blood.

The final method by which *dawa ya asili* may be administered is instillation. Medicinal infusions are made and instilled, drop by drop, into the eyes, ears or anus of the patient. In the absence of a European-style eye-dropper, a leaf may be bent to the shape of a cone, or a hollow reed may be filled with locally grown cotton (*pamba*). Both such devices are called *ntontonfwa*. This technique is employed for illness localised in the treated area.

These, then, are the many different methods of preparation and administration available to the practitioner of traditional medicines. Though the specific medicines employed may vary widely from person to person, the techniques are of fixed meaning and are known to all. Each method of administration has its own rationale, and there is a clear connection between therapeutic technique and the characteristics of the illness being treated.

Therapeutic relations

While *dawa ya kizungu* is exchanged under the rules of the marketplace and the money economy, *dawa ya asili* is contained in a network of customary rules which give form to the therapeutic relationship. This can be considered as a technology-specific subset of practices which are contained within the larger set of practices that govern the management of illness and make up medical culture as a whole.

In Mpala, a person is ill as much when he *says* he feels unwell as when his more physical behaviour indicates his withdrawal from customary roles. However, minor complaints do not cause substantial modification of social behaviour or expectations. People may continue to work as they always have, with verbal expressions of concern as their only marking of the presence of illness.

With somewhat more bothersome symptoms, an individual may begin self-medication. For adults this takes the form of self-administered enemas and the like, with *miti* frequently gathered and prepared by the patient himself in his spare time. Discussions of his ailment with friends will result in the generation of new ideas as to alternative medical substances, and, if the illness persists, these in their turn will be tried.

In response to even more serious or debilitating illness, kin of the sick person will suggest or bring medicines for use. Individuals doing so tend to be members of the patient's own generation or those senior to him. There may be discussion among the group regarding the correct plant substances to be employed, and the patient himself may make the final decision, if he is able. A young person might be dispatched to the bush to seek the plant, but would not administer it. This kind of collective problem-solving has been described by John Janzen (1978) as a function of the therapy management group. Such attention is part and parcel of the mutual concern which people say should characterise kinship relations.

Close friends of the patient *may* also bring or suggest medicines to treat him. In their case, however, this is a matter of considerable delicacy and is rarely done. People say that a friend would be under tremendous risk of accusation should the patient worsen after treatment with his medicines. Instead of spontaneously offering such substances, friends more often make their concern felt by visiting the patient, or helping with the therapy itself.

If the illness fails to respond to the various types of lay therapy attempted by the patient's family, it may come to be classed as problematic, following the characteristics outlined earlier. In this case an 'arrow' may be sent to a diviner/practitioner, either for divination or for straight herbal therapy or both. If divination is to be made, the situation will unfold as described above, with insight gained first into the social problem and then into the physiological one. If the 'arrow' is sent only for physiological therapy, the diviner may or may not dream to discover the nature of the illness.

In either case a visit is made to the patient, and a diagnosis is rendered on the basis of the patient's description of how and what he feels and the history of the illness. A small payment called a *kienda pori* ('of going to the bush') is made to 'cause the diviner to depart' (*kumuondosha mfumu*) for the bush to seek medicines.

Once gathered, the medicines are brought to the patient's home, disguised in such a way that the family cannot recognise them. The use is explained to the family by the practitioner/doctor, who may or may not demonstrate the technique.

One bundle is brought at a time, and the therapist visits the household at intervals to see how the patient is getting along. Ideally, the doctor should visit his patient every day, to ask him how he slept. If the patient is resting well, the practitioner knows his medicines are having an effect; if the patient has slept poorly, the doctor knows he must seek further until he finds the formula that works. In reality, as was observed in Kulimba's second illness, it is frequently up to the family of the sick person to pursue the *mfumu* and

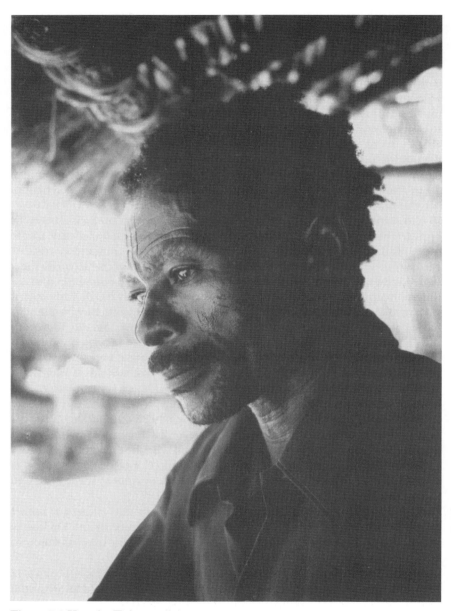

Figure 7.2 Kawele, Tulunga diviner

make certain of his ongoing attendance to their patient. In chronic illness, on the other hand, extended lapses between visits are not unusual, and are tolerated if the doctor has previously brought a sufficient supply of medicines.

After several uses (the exact number of which varies with the tree or plant), the 'fierceness' (*ukali*) of the particular items brought by the practitioner is spent, and further soaking results in a solution so weak as to be useless. When this happens, the exhausted plant materials are set aside, but not disposed of, by the patient's family. A Good therapist will quickly provide more medicinal plants if he has not already done so, so that treatment may continue uninterrupted.

The patient's family retain all used materials. They are returned to the practitioner at the end of the therapeutic relation. If the patient is not cured, 'to return to him his medicines' (*kumurudishia dawa yake*) is the polite way of informing a *mfumu* that his services are no longer needed, and that he is considered by the family to have failed. In such a case, a temporary impasse is reached. People say that the family must pay whatever the doctor asks for as a token in recognition of the trouble he has none the less taken on their behalf. For their part, practitioners say that they do not feel justified in asking for money if they have not had the satisfaction of cure. Actual practice reveals that both alternatives are in fact taken, depending upon the parties and the situation involved.

In either case, the doctor eventually receives the entire quantity of exhausted plant substances, and disposes of them as he wishes. He may either bury the substances in the ash heap (*kiziala*) or abandon them in the bush, throwing them away or leaving them at the foot of a tree away from where others are likely to pass.

It may also happen that after the original diagnosis/divination, treatment may result in partial remission of symptoms, but not complete cure. When the progress of the therapy appears to be stalled in this way, another divination may be made into the case, or oracular devices be consulted, to learn the cause of the hitch. It is customary for the diviner handling the case to make this secondary inquiry himself.

Finally, the patient's return to a state of health is marked by his or her return to work in the fields. This may be and often is done somewhat before all symptoms are totally gone, but, like the chill of spring when compared to that of autumn, symptoms remaining at the end of illness do not have the same meaning as the identical symptoms which were experienced at its beginning. After a lapse of several weeks or months, to ascertain that the illness will not, in fact, return, the patient and/or members of his family (his parents, maternal kin, spouse, etc.) will ask the practitioner to set his price for the cure.

Doctors are full of complaints about the ease with which they are forgotten by those whom they have cured. For their part, laypeople are fond of commenting upon doctors whose complaints (or other, more sinister abilities) are sufficient to undo their own handiwork, and cause recurrence of a former patient's illness, should this latter fail to pay up quickly.

In addition to the above customary relations among therapists and patients, as the illness unfolds there is also the more subtle effect of the occurrence itself upon the household in which the patient lives, irrespective of the particular medical technology used. The overall relation to illness of household members, including the patient himself, is one of gradual concession of increasing time and energy as the occurrence seems to demand more and more of these. In so far as is possible, a normal routine of housework, work in the fields, and visits to friends is maintained.

If it increases, the suffering of the sick person functions to curtail these, as household members restrict their movements to stay with the patient and to care for and comfort him. A man's wife may not go to her fields, so that her husband will not have to remain alone in the house. Her sisters may help her with manioc or firewood. Or she might simply be forced to leave him alone for a morning now and then, while she attends to necessary tasks. Increasing amounts of money, too, may be spent, as the family go from one practitioner to the next (including alternation between the two therapy types) seeking a cure of the patient's illness.

In one possible outcome, chronic illness may simply exhaust both people and resources to a point where further therapy appears out of the question. In such a case, the family will say 'we are tired' (*tunachoka*) and that they ought to 'just sit' (*kukaa tu*) instead of continuing to expend their time and money in a hopeless search for cure.

While minor illness indicates the proximity of *mizimu* to the sick person, this condition of chronic ill health, called *ubovu* ('unsoundness', 'rottenness'), is regarded quite differently. A person who is ill in such a way may be considered to have been abandoned by his spirits (because of an obstinate refusal to obey them), or to have been marked by sorcery. Indeed, the taintedness of this state is indicated by the idea that, when in it, a person has been hobbled like a goat (*kufungwa sawa mbuzi*) by the sorcerers, who intend to make of him their meat. Such a person is thus doomed to die and be eaten by them no matter what he does or where he goes.

Despite the brutal realism of this vision, and the readiness with which they return to it after a new disappointment, like everyone else in the world, people here are loath to give up any cause as completely lost. Long periods of simple toleration of an illness state will give way to renewed attempts should a new medical alternative become available. Even so, unless complete cure is accomplished, the weakened state of the chronically ill person becomes a part of the social reality in which he and his household live. In planning their lives and activities, people take into account the disability.

In the other possible outcome, the illness neither remits nor remains chronic, but becomes worse and worse. In such a situation, there is not only expenditure of increasing amounts of money and attention by the few, but there is also a widening of the group involved and an increase in the intensity of their involvement, as well. During the condition of critical illness (*ugonjuwa hatari*), members of the immediate household may curtail most of their outside activities, with those not immediately involved in treatment simply sitting and watching over the patient. Friends and neighbours may lend a hand in care, household maintenance or guardianship, and failure to appear at such a time is unequivocally indicative of ill-will harboured against the patient.

Finally, if the transition to death is made, all normal activities completely cease. Such maintenance functions as are required by the dead person's kin are performed by their *baendo* clan partners. The normal routine of housework and social life cannot be resumed for at least three days after the death, and usually is not fully resumed for much longer.

Dawa ya kizungu and *dawa ya asili* are the two major medical technologies available to people at Mpala. Each is distinguishable from the other by its form, its method of administration, and the transformations of which it is capable. However, both form part of a single medical culture, are managed by one overarching logic of use, and have place in one processual sequence that is the search for cure.

8

THE LOGIC OF A SUBSTANTIAL WORLD

It is an ethnographic commonplace that divination is the switch-point connecting illness to unfolding social relations. We take it as given that 'religion' and 'magic' or 'ritual' and 'symbol' will be among the devices employed in effecting cure, and that this is because, in the thinking of those with whom we study, the archetype of the 'natural' is the social, and there is little or no concept of the natural as such, particularly with reference to problematic illness.

Do we really know what we mean by this? Or is this commonplace a point at which we are blinded to a gap in our thinking because we maintain, in however attenuated a form, the idea that there is a lapse in the thinking of others? Much problematised of late has been this relationship between ethnography and mind; the complex interplay between the mind in the ethnography and the mind, so to speak, of the ethnography, the thought represented and the representation of that thought.

As we are now only too aware, ethnographies, like detective stories, are two tales told at once. There is the primary story of the reality constituted by ethnographic facts, and then the secondary story constituted by the construal of those facts. The latter can be an extension or correction of the former; it can explain or it can explain away. Choices between these two basic options or refined combinations of them are in part affected by the perceived strength and accuracy of the thought taken to be manifest both in the passive or inherited structures and in the conscious uses people make of them. Choices are also, and perhaps more heavily, generically conditioned; and this conditioning is part of what has undergone change as part of the disciplinary crisis of recent years.

Medical systems are particularly suited to the exploration of thought because they are so consciously held and managed, and because so much is at stake in their use. This strength justifies working with the grain of the thought represented, developing construals which take ethnographic facts as facts, and work to explain them rather than to explain them away.

In this light, constructions and definitions of the body which set the terms of medical practice must be seen as inherited and implicit answers to questions posed by the problem of the body. This is to say that the body is an intellectual problem in itself, even when it does not go wrong. The strength of this starting point would be followed through by the insistence that the medical system be fundamental to the study, and not taken as a manifestation of something else.

If medicine is not taken as allegorical of social structure, then, in developing our construals we do not ask 'What do they mean by that?', but rather 'What would the world have to be in order for this to be so?' That is, we track efficacy back to its literal, not symbolic, point of origin, and building our understanding out from there would allow us to create ethnographies that are also types of addition to or intervention in a philosophy, globally conceived.

In the context of Tabwa medicine, pursuing the question in this way allows us to refine our definitions of religion and magic, ritual and symbol. The terms as currently used become recognisable as no more than workable approximations of more subtle principles which themselves have place in a world whose properties are more complex than we might have imagined.

It is to the establishment of the properties of this world that the rest of this chapter is devoted. The following chapters build on it representations of the transfigurative and transformative processes through which human beings act to intervene in the course of life's events.

The best place to begin taking things seriously and explaining them in their positivity is with the body itself, because this terrain has already been covered in Part I. Consideration of the dimensions of the body began from the concept of the body undissected, that is, of a body with indefinitely defined internal space, and with indefinite capacities and capabilities. Such a body can be the habitat of other entities, whose presence is perceptible as subjective sensations, and it can be the site through which pass entities and objects deriving from the outside world. Illness is in the undissected body, but often not of that body. The undissected body in this respect does not in itself necessarily resist the numerous narratives that come, in time of illness, to be woven around it.

Further, the undissected body is also the heeding body. That is, it is a body whose response to circumstances is a heeding more akin to hearing than to the mechanical reactions of the biomedical body. As a consequence, it is possible to class the body with other types of subject which heed but do not speak. Goats, dogs and infants, like the heeding body, exist on the threshold of the social being, meeting the minimal requirements necessary to be regarded as a subject capable of social relations.

Seeing it in this light allows us to grasp that built into the body is a kind of uncertainty or hesitation. Perhaps the body, like a goat, dog or child, will simply refuse (*kukataa*) to respond. Bodily therapy, in all its clumsiness, thus becomes a kind of dialogue or interrogation made possible by a catalogue of illness terms and a set of medical practices. This is so, and people regard it as such, even when the illness is not problematic.

In problematic illness the heeding body, or the body as subject, becomes the body subjected to the will or intention of an unknown other. Divination operates to make contact with that other, to determine the other's intent, and to articulate the history from which the other's intention derives. Its message realised in speech, the other, now recognised, permits the body to heed medicines, and the person is made well.

Parts I and II were representations of the body as therapeutic subject. Here, we have already begun regarding the body as a therapeutic object, considering in Chapter 7 the types of bodily therapy available and the norms which govern their use. Further negotiation of the body as therapeutic object opens the way for understanding the wider world in which that body exists and by whose ordering principles all other things exist as well.

PROCESS AND PRODUCT

The undissected body exists in what I shall call a substantial world. This is a world in which the meaningful is united with the material at the level of substance itself. The capacities existing in the substantial world are clearly visible in the terms by which medical efficacy is construed, in the words used to describe its reality.

The capacity of a given medicinal formula (*dawa*), plant substance (*muti*) or animal substance (*kizimba*) to cure a given illness is referred to as the 'meaning' (*maana*) of that substance. My early attempts to discover the uses and therapeutic capabilities of medicinal substances were entirely non-productive when I asked about their strengths or what they did. Nobody had any idea what I was asking them. It was only when I noticed that people used the term 'meaning' to refer to the cause as well as the consequence of an event that I became sensitive to the relationship between event and meaning, and so could begin asking warrantable questions.

Knowledge of a medicine's meaning is crucial to one's effectiveness in the therapeutic situation. Ignorance on the part of the practitioner not only results in failure to cure, but may even prove dangerous to the patient. Following from this is the importance of the reliability of the person from whom one learns the meaning of a medicine. One must be sure of both their knowledge and their honesty. Practitioners in the area are linked to one another in relations of trust through which they learn new meanings.[1] With regard to medicines, the world of words creates the world of things.

As would be expected, causality in the substantial world differs from causality in a material one. The outward, visible sign which, in relations of material causality, serves only to mark the presence of the inner, invisible state can itself cause that state in the substantial world. The progress of the illness *ndege* ('infantile convulsions') to the illness *kifafa* ('incurable epilepsy') is illustrative.

Though a cause for concern, *ndege* is not an altogether uncommon illness among children. In fact, it is considered to be such an integral part of the almost universal childhood syndrome *kimbeleka* that the two are virtually synonymous; symptoms of one prompt therapy which includes treatment of the other. In its mildest form the illness is characterised by transient shudders, not unlike those of the *petit mal* seizures recognised by biomedicine. When a parent observes these, treatment is undertaken to prevent the occurrence of the more severe form in which the child's eyes turn upward and he stiffens with mild convulsions.

If the child falls to the ground during a seizure, foams at the mouth, and/ or demonstrates urinary incontinence, *ndege* 'is transformed' (*inageuka*) into *sinsa*, a more serious illness.[2] *Sinsa* is also the term applied to convulsions which occur in the presence of high fever. Its name is derived from the KiTabwa term *kusinsa*, meaning 'to cause to depart', and it is so called because its seriousness causes the family to set off at once for the diviner's. Symptomatically, *sinsa* is identical to *kifafa*, but it occurs in younger children, and its prognosis includes possible cure.

Should the victim of a seizure be older and/or the seizure be accompanied by faecal incontinence, with stronger, longer-lasting convulsions, *sinsa* is transformed into *kifafa*. Treatment undertaken at the outset of the illness has some possibility of success, but if more than six months has elapsed, cure is impossible.

In addition, after *sinsa* has become *kifafa*, the patient's family must take care that he does not fall into the fire. Should he be burnt during the course of a seizure, the patient's *kifafa* 'matures' and becomes totally incurable, thus completing the progress of the illness.

In all of the above cases the bodily events by which one stage is transformed into the next (urinary incontinence, age of patient, insensitivity to pain of injury, etc.) can be considered, biomedically, as fairly accurate *indicators* both of the severity of the seizures and of the likelihood that they are unconnected to other, more transient conditions. In Tabwa medicine, however, these do not simply mark the illness's progress from one stage to the next; they *cause* that progression. By the appearance of urinary incontinence and foaming at the mouth, *ndege* 'is transformed' into *sinsa*, just as immature, potentially curable *kifafa* 'is transformed' into its mature, incurable state by the patient's contact with fire. Thus, while the material world's causality organises the two entities hierarchically (that is, into (primary) cause and (secondary) effect) with the transformative force moving in one direction only, the substantial world's use of meaning as the (non-invidious) device linking the two permits the transformation to move in *both* directions.

The connection betweeen meaning and process, which is manifest in a medicine or a symptom as the change it can create in the body, is itself part of a wider order wherein entities, living and non-living, are constantly in transition. The progress is emergent from within the entity, and is the summation of processes not visible or perceptible as such. As it emerges, its existence and its specific state or condition are realised in outward, tangible manifestations; visible miniatures which coincide with the larger process and which are substantial renditions of it.

A medicine which captures perfectly the principle identifying events and processes in or with things is *ntentami*, which figures in the fertility formula to be discussed below. A *ntentami* is any tree which grows on top of another, and the word from which it derives, *kutentama*, has two meanings in KiTabwa. It refers first to the appearance of the new moon (*mwandamo* in KiSwahili) and also to the state of possession of Bulumbu diviners whose spirits mount (*kupanda*) them.

Working in this idiom, Nzuiba, a friend and healer, also makes use of *mupupukila* or *ntentami ya mawe*; that is, plants or small tress which grow directly on top of the large boulders which are often also the residences of spirits. He says this variety of *ntentami* is especially powerful because only rocks which are very old can be found with such things. They appear upon the rock at the time when its strength is declining. Just as a man's head puts forth grey hairs (*invwi* (KT) or *ndale* (KS)) only when his strength decreases, so does the strength of the rock go into the plants.

Through *ntentami*, we can understand objects as substantial renditions of events and processes in a world where everything is progressing and maturing all the time. Events are realisations or conjunctions of processes, while processes are continuous and imperceptible. Emergent from an unseeable within, processes, like events, become substantial as and in the material forms of the things to which they give rise. As substantial forms, these things are artefacts or seeds of the unseeable; they are the means by which both processes and events can be captured, grasped, held in abeyance, and then reproduced.

In Tabwa medicine this transformative potential of the substantial world not only determines illness, it also provides the means to treat it. The application to the body, through ingestion or other means of assimilation, of its outward, visible and manipulable signs can produce the condition which is the desired inner state. Medicines thus permit intervention in the body's hidden, processual dimension.

Fertility medicines (*viabiko*) are particularly illustrative of the way substantiations can be constructed and consumed and so come to redirect bodily processes. Couched in terms corrective of the illness, but also in terms of the desired state, they are miniatures of the bodily condition which their consumption will bring into being.

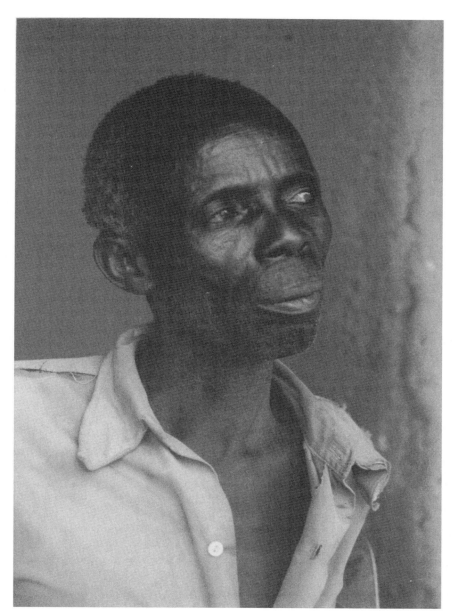

Figure 8.1 Nzuiba, Tulunga diviner

As a group, *viabiko* are used to achieve general ends. They are used to correct conditions such as 'dysmenorrhoea' (*nkazi*) which result in infertility; to induce conception; to protect pregnancy from the misfortunes of abortion or miscarriage; and to facilitate the easy delivery of a healthy child. They are employed only in case of problematic infertility and are not routinely administered. Each practitioner has his own medicines, which differ in their particulars from the medicines of his colleagues. Overall, however, many features are shared among them. Taken together, they form a brilliantly poetic substantiation of pregnancy and the way in which it ought to unfold. Below is one particularly complex fertility medicine, designed to induce conception after an especially prolonged period without pregnancy. It illustrates the workings of them all.

Description

Very early in the morning, the practitioner goes into the bush with a *mupapo*, the cloth in which children are carried. He goes first to the *musankati* tree (*Pseudolachnostylis maprounaefolia Pax var glabra* (Pax) Brenan, also called *kusakantila*). He climbs up the tree and then breaks off a branch, letting it fall to the ground. As he does so, he says 'My fertility was that which was placed above' (*kizazi kuangu kilikuwa kenye kutiwa juu*). The branch is put in the cloth and worn to the next tree, *bumpulukuswa* (*Flacourtia indica (Brum. f.)* Merr. sterile).

Roots of *bumpulukuswa* are dug, placed in the cloth and worn to the next tree, *lukobola* (both *Rubus pinnatus willd.* Sterile and two *Capparis* sp. sterile). Again, roots are dug, and put in the *mupapo*. The whole is then worn to the next and last tree, *muparamusi* (*Sterculia quinqueloba (Garcke)* K. Schum, also called *mutelempuza*).

Here the practitioner selects a root which 'comes out above' (*kutoka juu*), that is, on the surface of the ground. To the eastern end of the root, he applies *pemba* (kaolin) and to the west he applies *nkula* (powdered wood of the *mwenge* or *mukula*). As he applies these powders he says, 'You, my medicine, I pursue fertility (or a birth). It has been inactive for a very long time. Thus, I seek you. I seek fertility' (*Wee dawa yangu, nafuata kizazi. Kinasimama tangu muda murefu sana. Kumbe nakutafuta weye. Natafuta kizazi*). Then he cuts the root, first at the end spread with *nkula*, then at the end spread with *pemba*. He puts the resulting section of root in the carrying cloth and goes home.

At home, the practitioner evens off the ends of the *musankati* and *muparamusi* sections, so that they will stand upright. The *bumpulukuswa* and *lukobola* roots are split into slivers. The *bumpulukuswa* slivers are fastened around the section of *muparamusi* root, and the *lukobola* around the *musankati*. The *vizimba* of the backbone of the *mamba* (Gaboon adder) and of *tutumusi* are put in the centre of each of the two bundles. These are then taken to the home of the patient. At the patient's home, two pots are employed as containers of the bundles, each of which is stood upright in one of them. Cold water mixed with manioc flour is put into both. The pots are covered and are stored by the patient under her bed, with one at the head and the other at the middle.

Every morning the patient arises before sun-up. She uses a dipper to withdraw some of the medicated mixture from the first pot, being careful not to jiggle it or to disturb the bundle of medicines as she does so. She then cooks the solution and drinks the resulting gruel. In the early evening, she draws liquid from the second pot, at the middle of the bed, and prepares and consumes its contents in the same way. 'If her god permits, and if he is compatible with your *mizimu*, she will become pregnant' (*Mungu wake akijalia na mizimu wako, wakipatana, atapata mimba*).

Exegesis

The above formula is especially illustrative because it is meant for use in the treatment of 'fertility which is very inactive' (*kizazi kenye kusimama sana*). It differs from lesser therapies only in that it includes a larger than usual number of items which substantiate pregnancy.

In harvesting *musankati*, a branch of the tree is dropped to the ground from above. This movement from above to below is but one of a group of like actions which are employed in various fertility medicines. Other members of this group include a branch or twig seen to fall to the ground from any tree; a piece of meat which has been partly eaten by the patient and then stuck by her into the roof straw of her house to be removed two to four weeks later by the practitioner; a fruit of the *mufungulume* (sausage tree, *Kigelia aethiopica* Decne. sterile, also called *kivungilwa*), which has been shot off the tree with an arrow; and a branch from a *mupupukila* or *ntentami* tree (that is, from any tree which grows on top of another).

Such movement is identical to the movement of a spirit from the head of a dreaming woman to her body at the onset of pregnancy. Further, in a more abstract sense, the movement from above to below is one means of accomplishing an inversion of a principle of verticality which itself has meaning, and sets the terms in which drought and infertility are oriented. Reversing the distinction between above and below can result in both the cessation of infertility and the termination (through the use of rain medicines) of the dry season associated with it. In the medicine under discussion here, the fertility that has been 'put above', that is, held in abeyance, is caused to descend by the practitioner, so that its potential may be realised.

Using inverse means to arrive at the same end, other *viabiko* make use of the *lizuba*, a clay pot which has been moulded and fired in a single day, to administer medicine in the form of steam baths. Another pot of similar fabrication, the *lilindwe*, is employed to cause or prevent the onset of the rains through the careful release of columns of medicated steam which rise up to unite the above and the below. With the *lizuba*, the patient puts medicine and cold water into the pot, and closes the top with a large castor leaf, which is tied on with a long piece of dried grass. She pierces the leaf with her finger, making a single hole in the centre. The *lizuba* is then put on the fire to heat. When steam emerges from the hole, the patient removes the pot from the fire and arranges herself so that the steam rises over her genitals. Inside her body, the *kisumi* smells the medicine and becomes tranquil.

The means of gathering the final root, that of the *muparamusi*, make it substantiate another feature of the desired state of fertility, that is, the process of birth itself. The particular root selected is one which 'emerges above' and does not need to be dug out. By its position it substantiates the orientation along which space can realise time: the span of a day, the span of a month, the span of a life and the span of generations.

The *nkula* spread to the west of the root, the site of the first cut, substantiates the blood that is shed at the moment of birth, when the infant is separated first from its mother, then from its placenta. The *pemba* spread to the eastern, growing tip of the root is identical to that which is spread on the infant's end of the dried stump of the navel cord (*kishina*) after this has dropped off following birth. In conjunction with the practitioner's guiding invocation, his spreading the root with *nkula* and *pemba* makes of it a static substantiation of the transition that is birth.

Like the methods by which they are gathered, the means of preparing and administering them also make of these medicines realisations of pregnancy's significant features. First they are carried on the back of the practitioner in a position identical to that of the child whose conception they are meant to make happen. In addition, the bundles of slivers into which the pieces of root and branch are fastened are reminiscent of the bundles of firewood transported by women, and evoke the euphemism by which pregnancy is described as a 'load' (*mzigo*).

The positioning of the bundles, and the *vizimba* which these contain, are also significant, as are the circumstances under which the two pots are stored. The upright position of the medicine is suggestive of the vertical posture earlier noted as appropriate to a human being. The *vizimba* tucked into these make their substantiations fascinatingly complete.

The *kizimba* of the *mamba* (that is, the backbone of the Gaboon adder) substantiates the attributes of a snake, which lies remarkably still in the presence of humans. Consumed infusions of it affect the snake *kisumi*, which comes to lie still and so refrain from the internal movements which break up the blood that is coalescing into a conceptus.

The *kizimba tutumusi* is a red substance that people describe as a 'thing like dirt' or a hard, dry mushroom.[3] It is not to be found in the vicinity of

Mpala, but grows underground near the Lualaba river. Where it grows, it makes the earth pop up above it.

Tutumusi is a regular ingredient of medicines meant to bring good fortune and increase. It may also be planted in fields to improve the size of the manioc root crop. In the *kiabiko*, its meaning is similarly graphic and refers to the swelling out of the abdomen by the child which grows large inside.

The storage of the medicated bundles in pots which are covered and the interiors of which must be seen by no one[4] corresponds to the unseen, silent[5] and fundamentally secret onset and early stages of pregnancy. Similarly, the injunction against unnecessary jostling and movement as the water is being drawn duplicates the abdominal tranquility which is a prerequisite of successful conception.[6] Further, as noted in Chapter 7, administration of medicines in the medium of manioc gruel results in the retention in the body of those medicines for a prolonged period of time.

Finally, dawn and dusk, the two times at which the medicine is to be consumed, are also two of the times of day at which the spirits who are ultimately responsible for the success of the medication are most active among human beings. Dawn is the propitious time of day associated with the east and with the renewal of light and life. However, dusk also has its spiritual associations, because it is the time of day at which the dead antecedents of household members draw near to the house and may be addressed. It is also the time at which the new, next day begins. The placement of the two pots at the head and middle of the bed, and the consumption of medicines according to a corresponding dawn and dusk schedule, together give the condition of pregnancy cosmological position, and further underscore features of pregnancy outlined above.

Taken as a whole, then, the bundles of *miti* and the *vizimba* which they contain constitute a substantialisation of the meaningful in the material. Containing in themselves the circumstances which surround them (such as, the invocation made at the time of gathering and the methods of gathering, of transport, the means of administration, etc.), the medicines are the substantial versions of conditions which would mean conception and successful pregnancy. Since conception is the desired result, a first guess would be that the medicines consumed are substantiations of the conceptus itself. However, both the upright position of the bundles and the meanings of the *vizimba* they contain indicate that what they mean, and therefore intervene to cause, is the condition of the healthily pregnant woman, one whose body will soon grow large with child. The patient thus consumes a miniature version of *herself* as she will be; and it is a miniature operating on two levels. The first (the bundle) means the features of pregnancy as an entity, while the second (the *vizimba*) substantiates the physiological situation of the woman herself.

The above treatment makes it clear that the effectiveness of medicines lies, in part, in their capacity to contain, in substance, the process that is to unfold in the body after the medicine is consumed. As in the 'maturation' of an illness, the tangible realisation can mean the inner state. In this respect, medicines are the logical, artefactual outcome of an order founded upon the awareness of constant change, and the containing of a human body whose internal processes are accessible as miniature renditions of larger, sometimes external, events.

The causality by which medicines function is an ordinary part of the order of the substantial world. That is, it is totally amoral and operates apart from human intention, which merely makes use of it. While it is put to positive use in curative practice, it may also be used negatively by sorcerers. In addition, it can act entirely beyond human knowing, as when a patient unwittingly violates a therapeutic proscription.[7]

There is a respect, then, in which objects and events can be constituted as variants of one another in the substantial world. The union of the meaningful with the material entrains both the eventfulness of things and the thingfulness of events. In this world, present being is one moment of a process which is in some sense continuous, inscrutable and ineffable. Though this process can never itself be directly apprehended through the separate moments that are inchoate being, it can be grasped through the separate objects which are its products or artefacts.

In the substantial world the 'Problem of Meaning' does not exist in a form altogether comparable to that suggested by Geertz (1973b: 108), for whether or not order inheres in the process is not a valid question. Instead, the opposition appears to be between processes which are intelligible and those whose meaning is not *yet* clear. The process that is existence is an unfolding of something whose form is prefigured, just as the form of a plant, creature or person is both prefigured *and* unintelligible in a seed, egg or pregnancy. The meaning may take months – even years – to become clear; but it *will* eventually be so.

Though the existence of meaning is always presumed, its particular content can be perceived or comprehended only at certain points. Diachronically, such points are usually the conclusion of certain processes or of the more proximate phases of these.

Two of these are the moments of birth and death. The womb and the tomb are analogues, people say, beause both hide from view the individual they contain (*haionekani*, 'she or he is not visible'). When a hydrocephalic infant was brought through Mpala by his mother (who was making her way to Moba from Kalemie), everyone went to look. Coming away from there, men shook their heads and commented that, as they saw their wives walking about pregnant, they knew that what was inside was a mystery. One could never tell until its emergence exactly what would be born.

It is for this same reason that the social breaches formed by quarrels and harsh words uttered during pregnancy cannot be completely healed until after delivery has revealed their ultimate meaning. Thus it was in Kalwa's case that the indemnity she was due for the insults and threats she suffered from her irate neighbours could not be determined until the birth of her child demonstrated the exact extent of the harm their words and their anger had done her. Gestation, then, is a process whose outcome is in some sense prefigured, but whose ultimate meaning, whose prefigured yet uniquely individuated form, remains unintelligible until its end.

Turner (1967b: 202) has noted that death, for Ndembu, marks a similar conclusion of a process, and hence affords a comparable revelation of a period's meaning:

> The verb ku-fwa 'to die' contains in many contexts of situational usage the implication of 'summing up', of marking off a distinct phase or period of time. The meaning of a chain of events is condensed into it. There seems to be a close relationship, in the implicit philosophy of the Ndembu, between the uniqueness of a sequence of events or acts, such as the life of an individual, a court case, or the performance of a ritual, and the notion of death. Death is the punctuation mark that gives the series its idiosyncratic meaning and immortalizes it for thought.

Just as birth is the summation of the period of prenatal development, so is death the summation of the life to which birth leads. In Mpala, much of the grieving done by a person's principal mourners consists of eulogising his virtues and delineating the ways in which he will be missed.

One might suggest, as well, that the analogy between birth and death as points at which the process that is existence changes modes (or changes key) is the analogy which underlies alternation of generations. It is customary for people to name their children after their parents, and 'grandchildren', whether classificatory or real, are individuals to whom one has relations of absolute equality. As Mulombe put it, his granddaughters could enter his house, pound him on the head, and be on their way, saying 'this one is our *eternal* husband' (*huyu ni bwana yetu kwa milele*). Similarly, grandchildren may take immediate possession of or hold for ransom any item of clothing one mistakenly wears inside out. Grandchildren are also ritual mediators, participating in the creation of *misambwa* and in the offering of beer to *mizimu*.

It is arguable that this intensely equivalent relation reflects and puts to social use the intense, inverse equivalence between birth and death. Just as life itself lies between the two opposing strands of gestation and cessation, so does mature adulthood lie between the opposing generations of those whose strength is waxing and those whose power is on the wane. Since both moments reveal the ultimate meaning their processes contained, who is better suited to the actualisation of implicit, inchoate spiritual relations than those living in the shadows (youth and old age) cast by the moments called birth and death?

Turner's use of the term 'summing up' is quite felicitous, for a significant characteristic of the diachronic revelation of meaning is precisely this reduction of many partially analogous situational features to one, almost univocal whole whose significant features can be 'summed up', that is, condensed and abbreviated in expository prose. Such a moment is one of relative completion and resolution. It is as if all the harmonic movement of a symphony becomes condensed into its final chords. What is hidden becomes manifest, but is changed. It is reduced and simplified and loses some of its power in the process, if only because it has become something one has lived beyond.

Inversely, like summation, the 'condensation' of its meaning into the conclusion of a chain of events is, for BaTabwa, also a model of the process of maturation (*kukomaa*); only here, the power can be increasing. An illness is more intensely itself when it has matured. This intensity is in large measure due to the fact that maturity is an *artefact* or residue of the growth giving rise to it, and which therefore is, in some sense, condensed in it. It is this very intensity which results in the state's transformation (that is, resolution) and allows the 'mature' form of one illness phase to be called by another name, that of its postdrome. Further, in a usage that is not clear without these understandings of the fluid relations uniting process and product, people often define a postdrome as its prodrome, matured (*yenye kukomaa*).

The characteristic summations/condensations of processes' meaning/ strengths in their conclusions/products also figure prominently in the unfolding of *social* processes. Such a situation is found during the conclud-ing rites of the Ndembu circumcision ceremony, *mukanda*: the moment at which the *nfunda* medicine so necessary to future ceremonies' success is fabricated anew (Turner 1967b: 193).

It is also of some importance in the fabrication of the first eight *vizimba* employed in the *mwanzambale* amulet to be discussed in the chapters which follow. These are the most powerful of the *vizimba* employed. None is of animals, but all are derived from the revelatory climaxes, as it were, of stories; sequences of events which have had their outcomes; which have passed and which have so made the transition into narrative. They are taken from the points at which the hidden, ultimate meanings (that is, outcomes) of processes (that is, sequences of events) have temporarily been revealed. A person has climbed a tree and unfortunately fallen; a bit of the tree is taken. Someone has been killed by sorcery, has arisen to take his revenge and then been put to rest anew; a bit of his bone is taken. Someone has killed another then has been killed himself; and a bit of his bone becomes a *kizimba*, and so on. Such *vizimba* are like *nfunda*, where the ashes of the 'stations' of circumcision (such as, the novices' leaf beds, the harnesses with which their bleeding penes were held, the seclusion lodge in which they lived, etc.), contain a whole situation which has previously unfolded and come to relative conclusion or maturation. All are objects in which the past has been substantiated, made graspable as an object which can endure, unchanging, over time.

In such a circumstance, the occult destinies of the story's participants have become visible at its end. In objects taken from the scene at the moment of such resolution, the process is in some sense frozen for reactivation and use at a later time. It is this identity as pieces of a process that is both known and temporarily stilled that constitutes the affecting power of *vizimba*. By means of them, not only are past processes immortalised for thought, but future processes can be prefigured and preconditioned or determined as well.

With the eventfulness of things and the thingfulness of events thus made plain, the continuity of therapies from bodily to circumstantial is given its foundation not in symbolisations of the social order, but in the literal capacies of the order of the world. 'Magic' and 'religion' considered in this light become complementary processes, one transfigurative, the other transformative, which use complementary strategies of substantiation to make things of events – and complementary speeches of realisation; invocations to quicken events, making them grow out of things.

EVENTS OBJECTIFIED: WORDS INTO THINGS

The overlap between events and things, characteristic of the substantial world, makes logical a continuity of bodily and circumstantial therapies. Here, 'ritual' and 'magic' can be seen to be but different aspects or refractions of one therapeutic practice. Entirely continuous with interventions in bodily events, circumstantial therapies are interventions made through the body of the subject, but in the eventful life that body sustains. Locating them thus permits us to begin to refine our understanding of the two by taking as our perspective the practicant's point of view. We can begin by comprehending what people themselves mean by 'magic' and why neither such things as 'throwing the person in the bush' nor the creation of amulets (*erisi*) are magical acts.

MAGIC AND THE SCIENCE OF THE CONCRETE

Magic

People employ several different terms to refer to what anthropologists would describe as magical acts. Foremost among them is the term *manyele* (KS) or *mafii* (KT), which people gloss in French as '*magie*' (pronounced *mazii*), a translation that is very commonly known.

By *manyele* people are referring to the ability to effect astonishing transformations. These may range from acts of prestidigitation (such as were done for entertainment by several of the priests formerly resident in the area) to the incredible ability of sorcerers to fly great distances during the night or to raise the dead.

The term may also be used to refer to cunning or deceit. A person who 'goes around' or 'encircles' (*kuzunguka*) another by doing or arranging things outside the other's knowledge is one who has or who has used *manyele*. Finally, *manyele* may also be used figuratively to mean social-political cleverness, or the intellectual ability to control or manage a situation in such a way that circumstances unfold in one's own best interests.

Related to this is the word *viezia*, which is derived from KiLuba and specifically refers to theatrical events in which deception is employed to present an apparently fantastic phenomenon. Those who practice *viezia* dance about wildly, cutting their tongues and spitting them out with great flourishes and outpourings of blood. Close examination, however, reveals that the 'blood' and the 'tongue' are really just a mixture of roots held in the mouth, cut and spat out to create the desire effect. *Viezia* is thus a specific type of *manyele*, which has a circumscribed area of deployment.

Marifa (KS) is yet another term which occupies the same conceptual domain as *manyele*. It can be used to refer to 'a gift' (*don de Dieu*) or talent; that is, a special ability not derived from learning. More usually, however, it is used as a synonym for the cunning that is *manyele*. People deny the standard KiSwahili definition of the word as 'knowledge', though the word *kuarifu* (to notify) from which *marifa* is derived is both known and used.

The concepts signalled by the terms *manyele*, *viezia* and *marifa* point up the fundamentally political nature of knowledge in Tabwa society. Possession of knowledge is a marked state, as is the possession of a particular talent. It is a condition of which other people are aware, and is automatically associated with superior power over social and natural circumstances.

Central to the concept of *manyele* is the visual or intellectual perspective of the term. What distinguishes *manyele* from other transformations is neither the nature of the change itself, nor the mechanism by which it is effected, but the fact that the knowledge of its techniques and devices is esoteric.

People say that if a person performs an astonishing feat and you don't know how he does it, it is *manyele*. If he tells you or shows you how he does it, or if you yourself see how it is done, the act is not *manyele* any longer, 'because you all know'.[1] Similarly, *manyele* does not inhere in objects, but in consciousness. It is not a property of *vizimba* or medicines, but of the person using them.

That *manyele* inheres in consciousness is graphically expressed in the Tabwa concept of 'having eyes' (*kuwa na macho*). People say that ordinary mortals are 'blind' (*kipofu*) in the sense that they look at the world, but do not see it. In a similar fashion, people say that one can walk through the bush and see only grasses and trees, while to one's neighbour the same items are medicines which cure various illnesses.

Like the neighbour, sorcerers and *wafumu* (both Tulunga and Bulumbu) 'have eyes' in that they see things that others do not see. They will recognise their fellow adepts among a crowd of laypeople, and can detect the presence of sorcerers in a group or in the darkness just beyond the circle illuminated by firelight. They can also see through the illusion or deception of *manyele* to the technical reality behind it.[2]

Thus, the term *manyele* contains within its meaning two consciousnesses: that of practitioner and that of observer. *Manyele* can be said to exist precisely at the place where these two consciousnesses meet. Further, it is dissolved into mundane, albeit esoteric, knowledge when the two consciousnesses are united in their awareness of the technical realities underlying it.

Hence, the transformation that derives from such knowledge/ignorance is a transformation of the world through a transformation of the vision. Whether considered in terms of the 'front-stage' transformation that is *manyele* itself, or in terms of the overall change which gives one 'back-stage' (that is, esoteric) vision, the 'magic' is in the eye of the beholder, more than in the nature of the beheld.

Since magic or *manyele* exists within the invidious relation of knowledge to ignorance, operations that have been called magic in anthropological literature must be redefined so that their status is more accurately represented. Thus, there is nothing particularly magical in the workings of the circumstantial therapies below, even though the use of them is part of *manyele*. The therapy called 'throwing the person in the bush' employs such transformation to change the perception of family members held by an avenging ghost (*kibanda*). Similarly the fabrication of amulets operates, in part, on the perceptions of those encountered in the world by the amulet's owner.

'Throwing the Person in the Bush'

Technique

The therapy of 'throwing the person in the bush' (*kumutupa mutu mupori*) is the one employed in treatment of illnesses caused by a *kibanda*. A *kibanda* is the vengeful ghost of a person who was unjustly killed by the patient or his or her family through sorcery or other means; or it is the ghost of a dead infant brought into a household other than its own through an adulterous contact.

In either case, for the therapy of 'throwing the person in the bush' to be effective, the *kibanda* must be a person whose kin are unknown to or beyond reach of the patient's family. They are thus unavailable for more direct resolution of the problem, which would consist of payment of indemnity by the guilty followed by absolution of them by the deceased's kin.

Further, the patient must first recover from the illness which prompted the divination. His cure shows the willingness of the *kibanda* to be laid to rest by the therapy and in exchange for compensation paid to the Tulunga *mfumu*. Bulumbu diviners may not perform this type of circumstantial cure. Contact with the *vizimba* necessary to its performance, as well as to the *kibanda*, drives off or destroys their spirits.

Finally, all members of the concerned individual's household and/or kin group must be available for the therapy, for the *kibanda* is attached to all of them. Those for whom treatment is not undertaken not only remain at risk themselves but may recontaminate their treated kin when next they come in contact. Due to the unseemly nature of the ways in which a *kibanda* is acquired, this therapy is usually done in secret.

At 3:00 p.m. on the day appointed for the cure, the practitioner meets

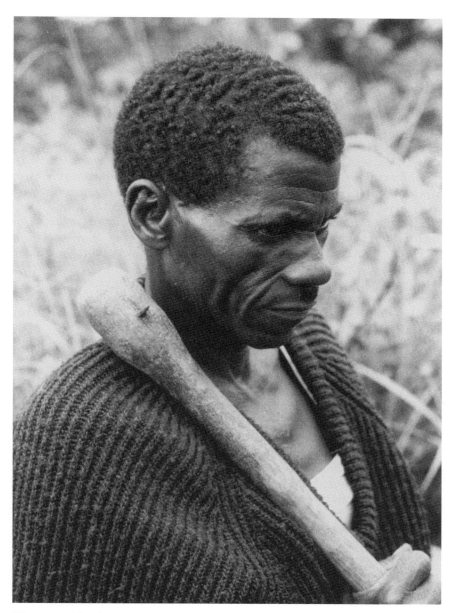

Figure 9.1 Mumbyoto, Tulunga diviner

with the family at his home, and has with him all the *materia medica*
necessary to its performance. Though these, like the technique, may vary
from diviner to diviner, the combination outlined below is illustrative of the
type. Plant medicines (*miti*) may be a stick of the tree *mulungi* (*Strychnos
innocua* Del. sterile) or roots of the *musankati, banda* (*Rhus vulgaris* Meikle
sterile), *kalongwe* (*Dalbergia nitidula* Bak. sterile) or *kibanga* (*Heeria
reticulata* Bak. f.) trees, as well as the central stem of the *kizime* plant (aloe
sp.). The *vizimba* employed may be *kapondo* (a piece of the bone of an
outlaw) *mwikuliki* (the rope of a suicide by hanging), *nzima* (a melanistic
serval), *kinyanto ya tembo* (the sole of an elephant's foot) or *likala* (charcoal).

The practitioner removes his shirt, rolls up his pants and wraps a white
cloth around his waist. He spreads another white cloth on the ground before
him, and on this he lays out the therapy's ingredients. He also places there a
small pot (*kikaya*, literally 'potsherd'), filled with water. In the middle of his
forehead, he rubs a small red spot of *nkula*.

He then takes the *kizime* plant, and hollows out its stalk. After this, he
cuts a tiny piece from each of the *vizimba* to be used and sets them aside.
Next he has his clients cut all their fingernails and their toenails. These are
combined with a bit of hair cut from the widow's peaks of the clients as well
as with a pinch of dirt taken from the place on which the clients' shadows
have fallen.

Into the hollowed-out stem of the *kizime* plant, the practitioner then puts
the one-*likuta* coin that has been the 'arrow' (*mshale*) sent him by his clients
when the work was requested (*kazi*). On top of it, he places a piece of
charcoal (*likala*) taken from the client's own fire. After this, the fingernails,
toenails, hair and 'shadows' of the clients are put into the stem, and are
followed by portions of each of the *vizimba*. Last, scrapings from each of the
medicinal roots are inserted, and the remaining pieces of root are split and
put into cold water in the little pot (*kikaya*).

Finally, when all is thus prepared and the sun is low in the sky, the *mfumu*
takes the *kizime* stalk and the liquid medicines and, dressed normally,
carries them to the bush. There, at the base of any tree, he digs a small hole
and lays the filled *kizime* stalk in it. Alongside the hole, he places the pot of
medicated water. He then returns to the village and waits until night.

Well after dark, at around 9:00 p.m., the hour at which most people are
preparing to go to bed, he tells the family that the work is ready. He asks
them for food, saying he is hungry (*unipatie kitu, nasikia njaa*). His clients
give him a chicken and a length of white cloth. If there is no chicken or only
a small one, they may give him 50 *makuta*. They will also give an additional
zaire for each person to be treated along with the patient.

Taking these things, the practitioner tells the family he is carrying away
their *kibanda*. He then begins to prepare himself for his trip to the bush by
licking a burnt and ground version of the same medicines (including

vizimba) as above. These are stored in a small antelope horn called a *kilambo* (from *kulamba* 'to lick') and pinches of them are also rubbed onto the forehead and the soles of his feet by the practitioner. These precautions will protect him from the *kibanda*'s wrath as he approaches it.

Once prepared, the *mfumu* goes to the bush in advance of his clients, to make ready the site. He carries with him the *kilambo*, the stick of *mulungi* wood, and, if he has one, his *mukia* or empowered fly-whisk. He undresses himself at a little distance from the site, then lays the *mulungi* stick on the ground in front of the pot of medicines and the hole containing the *kizime*, placing it so it lies like a threshold across the path of his approaching clients, between them and the pot. With his back to the tree, the *mfumu* then awaits his clients.

When they arrive, the clients disrobe on the opposite side of the *mulungi* stick and, nude, step across it to the site, where they stand before the *mfumu*. After all have made the crossing, the practitioner sprinkles each with the previously prepared medicated water, using his *mukia*. During this time, the clients must not speak a word, but the *mfumu* invokes both the *kibanda* and his own *mizimu*. He tells the *kibanda* to lie down (*kulala*) and to stop harming his clients through illness because they are now unrelated people (*watu wa bure*) against whom it has no claim. The *mizimu* are called upon by the practitioner to bring success in the endeavour, so that the *kibanda* may be laid to rest, and trouble his clients no further. As each person is sprinkled he arises facing away from the *kikaya* of liquid medicines and the hole containing the *kizime* stalk.

When all have been cleansed, the practitioner himself steps back across the *mulungi* stick. From the end of the *kilambo* he licks some of the burnt medicines. Following his example, each of the clients steps over the stick and is given a bit of the burnt medicines to lick. After each person consumes the medicine, he immediately starts for home without dressing, looking back or speaking. Ultimately, only the practitioner remains behind in the bush.

After all his clients have departed, the *mfumu* buries the *kizime* stalk in the hole in which it has lain. He there inverts the pot, dumping the liquid medicines over the nearly filled-in hole, and pressing the *kikaya* down over the spot. He takes up the stick of *mulungi* wood and starts back to town, also without looking back or speaking.

When he arrives at the house of the clients, he does not call out the usual request for entrance ('*Hodi?*'). Instead, he simply takes the stick of *mulungi* wood and knocks on the door with it. Hearing his knock, the people call out 'We're inside' (*tumo*). The practitioner then throws the stick up onto the roof and enters the house.

Once inside, the *mfumu* takes powdered but not burnt forms of the same medicines, and mixes them into a paste with castor oil. His clients take some of this from his hands, and rub it over their faces and heads. Other, dry powder, he throws onto a fire lit in the house for this purpose, so that medicinal smoke permeates the area. This concludes the therapy and the *mfumu* leaves. He may not see his clients again that night. If all goes well, weeks or months will pass with no further deaths or serious illnesses occurring in the family.

Processes

The aim of this therapy of 'throwing the person in the bush' (*kumutupa mutu mupori*) is the establishment of a discontinuity between the practitioner's clients (that is, the patient and his family) and the *kibanda*. Both the plant medicines (*miti*) and the animal substances (*vizimba*) employed are directed to this same end.

Of the six *miti* employed in the particular formula under discussion, four are trees or plants whose names contain some of the meanings involved in the discontinuity desired. The name *kizime* is related to the term *kuzimisha* ('to cause to be extinguished'). The plant is a member of the genus Aloe and is also used in the treatment of burns. In former times the grave sites of twins were marked by the planting of *kizime*, because it sprouts anew after the burning of the bush. In this context, the extinguishing power of *kizime* causes the *kibanda* to 'lie down' (*kulala*), and also substantiates the death and rebirth by which patients are separated from their former, compromised state.

The name *kibanga* is the near-homonym of *kabanga*, the east (that is, the direction from which the dead return to be reborn), and of *kubanga*, 'to speak to' or 'to interact with'. Hence, like the *kizime* stalk, the root of *kibanga* also means auspiciousness and rebirth after death. The name of the tree *banda* is connected to the term *kibanda* , and is employed in all therapies and medicines whose aim is protection from avenging ghosts. Finally, the tree *mulungi* conveys a situation that is rightly directed, for *kulunga* in KiTabwa is 'to set in order,' or 'to arrange (things) in a straight line'.

One of the two remaining plant medicines employed to 'throw the person in the bush', *kalongwe*, also plays a part in the fabrication of the protective amulets called *mwanzambale*, to be discussed below. It is also commonly used as a sitz bath in treatment of *kidonda tumbo*, an illness involving the entrance of cold winds (*pepo*) into the body via the rectum, the symptoms of which resemble those of spirit (also called *pepo*) possession. The other, *musankati*, may be used in the fabrication of the medicines which give Tulunga diviners their power, and figures in the fertility medicines discussed above.

The meanings (*maana*) of the *vizimba* reiterate the point. The piece of charcoal (*likala*) is the very substance of fire extinguished, and the small piece of melanistic serval (*nzima*) pelt conveys the same meaning in another form. *Mwikuliki*, a piece of rope used by a person to hang himself, serves to bind the *kibanda*, to restrain its actions. This *kizimba* may not be employed, for example, when one is trying to cause a ghost to arise and take revenge upon its killers because it thwarts one's efforts. Finally, *kapondo* is a tiny bit of the bone of an outlaw. It is meant to kill those against whom it is directed in the same way as the *kapondo* himself killed people during life.[3] In this context, it will lay to rest the *kibanda*.

Collectively, the hair, fingernails, toenails and 'shadows' of the clients are called 'the soul of the person' (*rho ya mutu*). By a process of abstraction resembling synecdoche (part-for-whole substitution), but literal and not figurative, clients' lives are both miniaturised and essentialised. Thus abstracted, clients can be transfigured in their being, at least in so far as the object of the medicine, the *kibanda*, is concerned.

By means of the medicines that substantiate these meanings, the clients undergo microcosmically realised and macrocosmically enacted processes of death and rebirth. People say that the burial in the bush with *vizimba* which mean extinguishing and death makes *kibanda* believe that the people have been killed by it. In addition, the plant medicines also function to 'extinguish' or reverse the conflict out of which the vengeance came.

The techniques employed also reiterate the idea of transformative discontinuity. Patients are made to traverse the stick of *mulungi* wood, are washed with medicated water, abandon their usual clothing, and must not look back or break silence. They thus 'die' only to be reborn, as we all are, naked and speechless.

Finally, the *mfumu* himself also occupies the medial space between the living and the dead. His fee is the compensation due the *kibanda* in restitution of the wrong done it during life. The payment of this is the jural counterpart of the discontinuity therapeutically accomplished by 'throwing the person in the bush'.

Protective Charms

Protective charms or amulets (*erisi* (KS)/*makana* (KT)) are fabricated in response to several different sets of circumstances. They may be the *pièce de résistance* of a group of therapies. They may also be made and worn in response to illness or misfortune, especially if these are diagnosed as being of human origin (that is, sorcery). Shopkeepers and merchants may obtain them for general protection of their health, well-being and goods, both on the road and at home. People may put them in their fields as protection (*makingo*) from thieves. Other, simpler charms may be fabricated and worn to prevent the recurrence of certain illnesses, especially the childhood diseases of *ndege* ('convulsions') and *kibende* ('diarrhoea'), as well as the more serious syndromes of *wazimu* ('insanity') and *kifafa* ('epilepsy').

No matter what their purpose or the circumstances of the fabrication, however, all *erisi* are but differing varieties of the same thing. They all employ the same types of substance, and are based on the same principles of operation. The discussion and analysis below, which will be of *mwanzambale*, one of the more complex and controversial types, will therefore illuminate all such amulets.

Form and techniques

An *erisi* is composed of a combination of plant medicines (*miti*) and *vizimba*. The *miti* are green or dried roots, and leaves which have been ground into powder, while the *vizimba* are tiny fragments of mammals, fish, insects, birds, reptiles, human beings, human artefacts, artefacts of specific situations, and minerals.

In a protective charm such as the *mwanzambale* to be discussed here, the fingernails and toenails of the persons to be protected are also included, as are locks of hair clipped from the widow's peak and nape of the neck. Dust gathered from the place where the shadow falls and blood taken from shallow incisions (*machanjo*) over the sternum made with a razor blade are mixed in as well.

As a rule, the *miti* and *vizimba* are prepared by the Tulunga practitioner in advance. They are brought to the client's home ready, and with all distinguishing features removed, so that their identity may remain secret. It is the clients themselves who clip their fingernails and toenails and hair, and it is they who gather the dust covered by their own shadows. All of these things are presented to the practitioner upon his arrival.

The collection of ingredients is then inserted into two different containers. The larger container, which remains in the house, is a clear, glass medicine bottle, such as the bottles in which injectable penicillin is packaged.[4] In addition to this is a small cloth or leather pouch, worn on a string about the neck. Instead of the small pouch, the dried body of the *kafwabubela*, a large black weevil with red dots, may be emptied of its usual contents, filled with medicines and worn, placed in the mouth or kept at the head of the bed.[5]

No matter what the container, the method of filling it is the same. Layers of plant medicines and animal substances are alternated. First, root scrapings are inserted, followed by green leaves of other medicines which have been pounded into pulp. These are then followed by a layer of *vizimba*. At the middle of the container are placed the fingernails, toenails, hair clippings, and 'shadows' of the clients. These are surrounded above and below with layers of *vizimba*. The final layer inserted is always one of *miti*. Included in the bottle as means to close the house to misfortune are bits of straw taken from the thatch hanging over the front and back doors.

Once all the medicines have been tightly packed into the bottle or pouch, the *erisi* is closed by sewing it shut with needle and thread. The pouch itself is sewn, while the bottle has a cloth sewn around it. It is at this time that the invocation activating the *erisi* and determining its function is made by the practitioner as he works. Finally, the incisions are made over the sterna of the clients, and the ends of two needles are covered with the blood. These are then stuck into the bottle, one pointed up and the other down. A copper wire is wrapped around the neck of the bottle, and it is attached to the head of the bed by this means. Strong nylon string is attached to the smaller amulets, and these are worn around the neck by each of the clients.

Contents and processes
As with other aspects of medical practice, the actual ingredients of any given *mwanzambale* will vary both from practitioner to practitioner and from time to time. Each *mfumu* knows the meanings of and/or possesses only a limited number of *vizimba*, and, though each may conscientiously attempt to expand his knowledge through conversation with his colleagues, clients arriving at any particular moment will receive an *erisi* containing only those *vizimba* that are both known to the practitioner and available to him at the time. People say that it is this, along with the differential strengths of their *mizimu*, that accounts for the varying powers and success rates of *wafumu*. The contents listed and explained below are of a *mwanzambale* prepared for Allen Roberts and me by a noted local practitioner on 28–9 October 1975, after a series of inexplicable fevers and a nightmare had caused friends and neighbours to insist that I seek some protection from my hidden enemies.

The *mfumu* with whom I worked had travelled to other areas both to learn his art and to practise it. He was possessed of more *vizimba* than any of the local practitioners who were my friends and teachers, and, during his stay at Mpala, a number of them went to him, seeking to increase their knowledge and their stock of these substances. He was believed to be a sorcerer, who had the power to kill with his medicines, if he so chose. He was not, however, believed to be in the process of ensorcelling someone at the time, despite the fact that at least one person was overheard as he approached the practitioner to request the medicines necessary to kill an enemy.

According to its fabricator, this was a 'first-class' (*première qualité*) *mwanzambale*, because it contained some forty-odd *vizimba* and *miti*. These and their exegeses are listed here in the order in which they were added. I was told that people who might come to 'test' (*kupima*) the strength of their medicines against mine (that is, to attempt to kill me through sorcery) would find my *erisi* contained medicines of every kind.

1. *Kabongo kimuti ya mutu.* A stick that someone uses to strike another person who is consequently knocked down. Thus, if someone comes to do something bad to you (*kutenda vibaya*), perhaps he himself will have an accident. He will be hit and will fall, and blood will begin to flow. Perhaps he will break a leg.

2. *Mikankalwa* (KiLuba). The handle of a hoe which has split or broken while being used. If a person comes up to hit or do something to you, he will be without self-mastery (*hajiwezi*), and will be vanquished (*ataanguka yee mwenyewe*).

3. *Muhunde.* This is a *kizwa* (or *kibanda*); a man who has died and arisen (*kufufuka*). Perhaps *walozi* ensorcelled him; they begin to see him again. They then must go to a very great doctor (*docteur*), to cause him to lie down (*kulalisha*) again. After laying him down anew, they kill his power and make a *kizimba*. Thus, if someone comes to do evil, it will make him have this trouble himself.

4. *Muti kuliangukako mutu.* A piece of wood from a tree that a person has climbed of his own volition, fallen from, and died as a consequence of the fall. If someone comes to do evil to you, perhaps he will then go to his field or climb a tree and fall, or somehow have another bad accident.

5. *Kapondo.* A man who was alone; who had left a town such as Moba or Kalemie (towns near Mpala) without company and walked along by himself. People seized him and killed him. Then the great ones of long ago would take part of him as a *kizimba*. When mixed with other *vizimba* it means that if you are alone, and someone comes to test (*kupima*) your *dawa* (that is, to measure themselves against you), they will see you as though you were no longer alone; as though you were many people together.

   (Note: *kapondo* is also the name applied to an anarchic bandit who travels the countryside setting fire to the houses of chiefs, or killing people for no other reason than the sheer enjoyment of the confusion that results. Other meanings of this *kizimba* stress that it kills in the same way that the *kapondo* himself did.)

6. *Manzi.* The *kizimba* of men who have killed each other (*kuuana*), or of a snake which first bites and kills a man and then is killed itself. Because blood has been spilt, this is a very strong *kizimba*. Its meaning is that a person will not be able to throw medicines upon you or harm you. He will either do nothing or, if he does achieve something, will get trouble himself (*asara*). If someone harasses you (*kuchokoza*), he himself will have an accident.

7. *Mutu aliyekufa musala.* A person who has died all by himself, perhaps of fatigue while travelling. He died *bure-bure* (literally 'nothing-nothing'), that is, without precipitating illness or incident and without company. If someone tries to harass you, he himself will die thus.

   (Another formidable practitioner says that the precise term for this is *mumba wa musala*, and that it refers literally to a person who has died of hunger. It is said that people died this way not infrequently during the post-independence wars and rebellions, and could be found sitting or lying by the side of the road where they had died. *Musala* is also the term used to refer to a barren woman who has never had a menstrual flow.)

8. *Kinkenke* or *kekete* (KiLuba). A person who dies suddenly (*kwa lafla*). The truly great practitioners of long ago would take something from the body of such a person. Anyone harassing the owner of the *mwanzambale* will die suddenly in the same manner.

9. *Ngwezie*. The black mamba (*Dendroaspis polylepis*).

10. *Mamba*. The gaboon adder (*Bitis gabonica gabonica*).

11. *Mpili*. The common African puff-adder (*Bitis arientans arientans*).

12. *Mulolo*. Another variety of snake.

13. *Kapiyono*. Another variety of snake.

The *vizimba* of these snakes both serve to make the medicine very 'fierce' (*kali*) in a general sense, and mean the poisonous snakes which might do one injury. All the snakes are put in the *erisi*. If you get the *vizimba* of five or so and the rest are missing, it doesn't matter. If you are missing *ngwezie* and *mamba*, the two most deadly types, however, you are lacking the crucial elements.

14. *Uso la mbogo*. Bone from the forehead of the buffalo.

15. *Uso la simba*. Bone from the forehead of the lion.

16. *Uso la tembo*. Bone from the forehead of the elephant.

17. *Uso la chui*. Bone from the forehead of the leopard.

As with snakes, these *vizimba* form a cluster which substantiate but a single meaning. When your enemies see your face, they will feel fear, as if you were one of these large and frightening animals, and they will therefore leave you alone.

18. *Milima*. A small pebble from each of the larger, named mountains. Whereas you were a small person before, you will now be seen to loom large, as a mountain does. The mountains are things of God himself (*Mungu mwenyezi*), because this is the origin (*asili*) of the world. If you beg the mountains they will respond. So though you are little, now you are a big person.

19. *Nkaka*. A bit of the scale of the pangolin. When this is combined with the other things in the *mwanzambale*, people won't come around you as sorcerers (*walozi*). When they go to put their *dawa* in your house at night, it will just remain as such, inert.

(Note: Scales of the *nkaka* have the general meaning of driving off, and are used for such things as keeping predators from the area where one is sleeping in the open, keeping other fishermen from making a good catch, etc.)

20. *Ngozi ya mamba ya maji*. The skin of the crocodile. Through the use of this, nothing can enter your body. 'Indigenous medicines' (*madawa indigine*, meaning sorcerous formulae) may not cause you pain or illness because they cannot penetrate your skin.

21. *Musipa wa mbogo*. The vein or nerve in the neck of the buffalo.

22. *Musipa wa tembo.* The vein or nerve in the neck of the elephant.
    Both of these *vizimba* have the same meaning, one that is shared by the
    kizimba of the neck vein of any large animal. With these, though others
    look at you with an idea of attack, they will instead only lower their
    heads (*kuinama*) as these animals do.
23. *Kababo.* A kind of insect, like a bee, which flies with great force, and
    passes one making a whooshing sound. It can bang into a tree, and die
    doing it, but it leaves a mark on the tree.
24. *Shafu.* Red army ants.
25. *Matembo.* Wasps.
26. *Minao.* Another sort of stinging or biting insect.
    All of these little insects are fierce (*kali*) and they bring their fierceness
    to the *erisi*, to harass (*kuchokoza*) whomever threatens one. Perhaps a
    snake will awaken and bite him, if he comes to do anything bad to you.
27. *Kisiki ya njia.* A stump in the pathway which stands up. Just as people
    who are passing and who are not careful may trip over this and fall, so
    the person coming to do you harm might fall himself. Perhaps he
    himself will get sick and die.
28. *Popondege.* The bat.
29. *Jicho la nzima.* The eye of the melanistic serval (*Felis serval*).
30. *Jicho la mbuzi.* The eye of a goat.
31. *Lubangu la kipofu.* The stick with which a blind person guides himself.
    The meaning of this cluster of *vizimba*, substantiated as much by each
    individually as by all together, is that if someone comes to your house to
    do you harm, he will be as one blind, and will not see you.
32. *Kichwa cha kwale.* The head of the francolin quail.
33. *Kichwa cha sungura ya pori.* The head of the bush rabbit.
    When these two animals are in the bush, they hide themselves so well
    that it is very difficult to see where they are or to hunt them. Thus, it will
    be very difficult for bad people to see or find you. You will be a person
    who protects himself completely.

In addition to the 33 *vizimba* outlined above, the *mwanzambale* also contained a number of plant medicines (*miti*). These were:

1. Roots of the *ndale* (probably *Swartzia sp.* sterile) tree (also called *kabigi*
   and *kilonde*). This tree is called the 'elder of the medicines' (*mzee wa
   dawa*) by some, and it a crucial, non-substitutable ingredient in *kalunga*
   horns.
2. Stump (*kisiki*) of the *mubanga* tree (*Heeria reticulata* Bak. f.). Its
   meaning is as above.
3. Stump and roots (*mizizi*) of the *mulama* tree (*Combretum molle* G. Don
   sterile). The *mulama* makes any affair (misfortune or conflict) concerning you remain as one, so it will be a failure (*itashindwa*). The *mulama*

acts like a magnet (*chalamata*) pulling the matter down, keeping it compact, so that it does not unfold and overwhelm one.[6]

(*Kulama* in KiTabwa means 'to care for', and is glossed by the term '*kutunza*' in KiSwahili. This word is used to refer not only to the process of curing, but also to the act of preserving something from harm or the dangers of ordinary wear and tear.)

4. Roots of the *mukute* (*Psorospermum febrifugum* Spach. var. *febrifugum* sterile). This also closes off the affair, so that it does not become too complicated or dangerous.

5. Roots of the *banda* (*Rhus vulgaris* Meikle sterile). This also figures in the composition for the therapy of 'throwing the person in the bush' and is used in other protective compounds and ceremonies as well.

6. Roots of the *lunfunga* (*Ziziphus abyssinica* A. Rich. sterile and *Ziziphus mucronata* A. Rich. sterile). This is another tree which is found in the 'throwing' and other protective therapies. Its name, containing the term 'to close' (*kufunga*), is what it means here.

7. Roots of the *kingoma* tree. The roots or stumps of all of these trees are scraped, and the scrapings are all mixed together. They are used in combination with the following items.

8. Roots of the *kalongwe* (*Dalbergia nitidula* Bak. sterile, also called *kafisia*). Scrapings of the root of this tree also figure in the therapy of 'throwing the person in the bush' as well as in the *nsipa* medicines used to draw a large number of residents to a village.

9. *Mupindi wa njia*. A root which crosses the road, so people must step over it. This is a common ingredient of protective amulets. Perhaps the person who comes to do one harm will trip over it on his way, and decide to return home.

10. Green leaves of *mukute*. The new leaves from the end of the branch are taken.

11. Leaves of *kifumbe* (*Philiostigma thonningii* (Schumach.) Milne-Redh. sterile). Again, the green leaves which grow at the end of the branch are taken. Commonly known in English as camel's foot, this tree has leaves which, people observe, fold like a book. With the use of *kifumbe* the affair will fold or lie down, and not cause one trouble.

12. Leaves of *musie* (*Grewia molle* Juss., also called *musha* and *musia*). The leaves of this tree make the affair slippery (*inaterezeka*), so that it does not stick, but easily comes to a successful conclusion.

13. Leaves of *kifubia* (probably *Antidesma* sp. sterile). If an affair is 'awakened' (*iamuke*) against you, if conflict begins to cause you trouble, or if 'they' come to ensorcell you, nothing will happen. The affair (*maneno*) will remain indifferent, without power (*itabakia tu hivi-hivi*).

In an ordinary *erisi*, the *mfumu* said, *miti* would be present only as leaves. Roots were used here because this was the stronger charm of *mwanzambale*.

Nevertheless, the greenness of the leaves is important, for their liquid is the 'blood' of the amulet. Dried leaves may not be used, nor can the final combination be permitted to dry out. Like a human being, a *mwanzambale* without 'blood' (*damu*) is a dead thing. To prevent drying, I was to add a bit of kerosene to the mixture from time to time, to maintain its strength.

As can be deduced from the individual meanings of the various *vizimba* and *miti*, the purpose of the *mwanzambale* is the active protection of its owners. It is the very nature of this activity that makes the *erisi* a controversial one.

The *mfumu* who prepared it was very careful to specify that the *mwanzambale* would cause injury to befall only those who had come to injure me. Indeed, the understanding of *mwanzambale* generally held by laypeople is that it exactly reflects in intensity the harmfulness of the medicines used by another. If he seeks to ensorcell you with serious illness, he, too, will fall seriously ill. As Mumbyoto put it, if you die, they will find him dead when they return from burying you. But if, on the other hand, he decides to try curing himself by removing his medicines from you, he will recover as you recover.

Nevertheless, the entire first category of *vizimba* is *prima facie* evidence of sorcery, because the items are derived from the deaths of human beings, and therefore constitute a kind of profit based on others' diminution.[7] It is these which give *mwanzambale* its exceptional strength.

Further, the capability of the protective device includes a capacity to kill. The fact that one may not think about a specific person when making the objects, or name a given enemy when activating the device, seems to many people to be ethical hair-splitting. In general, the more bellicose the person (whether due to character or to situation), the less inclined is he to regard *mwanzambale* as sorcery; and everyone acknowledges that there are some situations which warrant its use no matter who one is.

The possession of *mwanzambale* is always kept secret, however. People say this is because advertisement of its presence in a house is like an open invitation to all sorcerers to come and test the strength of their medicines against it. Unspoken, but never far out of mind, is the possibility that possession of such a thing, reflecting, as it does, the very social incompatibility that motivates sorcery, might cause the accusation of *ulozi* to return upon oneself.

VIZIMBA AND THE SUBSTANTIAL METAPHOR

Though the above description and exegesis of a *mwanzambale* and its contents depicts a fairly complicated charm containing some 33 different *vizimba*, this series by no means exhausts the stock of *vizimba* potentially available to the *mfumu*. During the course of my study I learned of approximately 150 different *vizimba*, each of which had as its meaning (*maana*) a single feature or characteristic.

This specificity of meaning contradicts depictions in the literature which make amulets seem as tales told by idiots, 'full of sound and fury, but signifying nothing'. Indeed, work with practitioners makes one realise precisely how little *erisi* can be described as being composed of 'snail shells, beads, and such other odds and ends as the *mufumu*'s fancy dictates' (Beattie 1963: 39).

Vizimba can be organised into *erisi* whose overall purposes vary widely. In my discussions with practitioners, I learned of formulae whose aim was to draw people to a village, so that it (and consequently its chief) might grow great and important (called *nsipa*); formulae to excite affection in the heart of the object of one's desire; formulae to bring luck in business or commerce; formulae to make one invisible; formulae to increase one's skill at stealing; and formulae to improve one's success rate in hunting or fishing.

As with the *mwanzambale* noted here, each formula itself consists of a combination of *vizimba* which all have the same tone, as it were. That is, their meanings all fall into the same or similar categories. This is a reflection of the poetic, proliferative character of the system based on meanings, one in which elegance is by no means defined in terms of efficiency or simplicity of argument. On the contrary, as with poetic forms, the very strength of the *mwanzambale* lies in its consistent reiteration of a single principle through the use of differing, concrete images; images which are repetitious but not redundant. In this respect, such a complex charm is akin to a work of art.

People say that the meaning of a *kizimba* inheres in its nature as such. When alive or in its mundane context, the animal or object held no such meaning. Though the meanings attached to particular *vizimba* are naturalistic in reference; they are, in fact, conventional associations. No one knows where they came from, and everyone agrees that it is impossible for an individual to invent a new *kizimba* through the observation of an animal's habits or appearance. The use of a *kizimba* whose meaning is undisclosed is as unthinkable as the administration of pills contained in an unmarked bottle.

Further, with *vizimba*, the entire meaning is present when even the smallest portion of the actual object is employed. Most of the stock of *vizimba* in the possession of local practitioners are pieces too small to be recognised by sight alone. The portions actually employed in the fabrication of *erisi* are hardly larger than a grain of rice or coarse sand. This is especially true of the human *vizimba*, which are very valuable and so are frugally employed.

Vizimba may be used more than once. Valuable ones may have a string tied around them, so that they can be pulled from an infusion in which they might be soaking and hung to dry until the next use. Or they may be inserted in a niche made in the middle of one of the plant medicines, so that they can be dug out and carefully set aside while the infusion is being employed. Their active principle is thus unquantifiable and immaterial. *Vizimba* are the absolute union of being and meaning. As such, they are not subject to the inflation of the symbolic and must be exactly themselves and nothing other. It is impossible to expand one's stock by transferring the meaning of one *kizimba* to another, or to a neutral but more easily obtainable substance.

In these respects, *vizimba* differ markedly from *miti*. With *miti*, the strength of the medicine follows directly from the quantity of the plant substances used. In addition, the 'odour' (*harufu*) of the medicine decreases after the roots or leaves have been used for a time, and thus necessitates their replacement. Hence, in contrast to *vizimba*, active principles or substances of *miti* are material and quantifiable even when they are used for what they mean.

Indeed, *vizimba* epitomise substantiated meaning. Each *kizimba* can be described as a material realisation of the process or event captured in what it means. Equally, they can be regarded as that event or process essentialised by its bonding with a meaning in a substantial form. When combined in an *erisi* with the abstracted essence (soul) of a person, *vizimba* transfer to that individual's being (bodily and social) characteristics derived from another domain. This process resembles metaphor, but is not a figure of speech; instead, it is a transfiguration of being.

Since they constitute substantialised fragments of processes, it is not surprising to find that *vizimba* themselves are considered as the precipitators of change. Hence, my friend Kalulu, when asked to explain the relative significance of *vizimba* and *miti*, said that the two were like gunpowder, wadding and bullet. The *vizimba* are the gunpowder and wadding which speed the bullet on its way, and without which the bullet will never find its mark, no matter what its own strength might be. Similarly, Richards describes the Bemba variant, *fishimba*, as 'an activating principle' without which medicines are ineffective.

Despite their intimate connection to both the representation and trans-formation of outcomes, however, *vizimba* are to be distinguished from that other affecting device, the ritual symbol. Unlike ritual symbols, as defined by Turner, *vizimba* cannot be divided into ideological and orectic poles. They make no particular reference to and are not associated with the principles of the society in which they are found; and they have no visual features or attributes which connect them to emotionally charged bodily states or products.

In addition, *vizimba* are uni- rather than multi-vocal in character. Though one animal may have more than one use in *vizimba*, each *kizimba* from that animal has one meaning and only one meaning regardless of the multiplicity of contexts in which it may appear.

Thus, rather than being the prompters of contemplation, *vizimba* can be said to be precision tools of transfiguration. They are effective regardless of whether or not their presence is known to the actors who are their objects.

Their purpose is not the provision of a desired, generalised transformation of a social state, but change in a particular situation which has been disordered through conflict, illness or misfortune.

METAPHORIC STRUCTURES OF TRANSFIGURATION

Vizimba function only when brought into proximity with the human objects they are to transform. This association is accomplished partly by the invocation essential to the functioning of every *erisi*, and partly by the simple, mechanical positioning of *vizimba* and their object, the person, in one place, the enclosing cloth or leather pouch.

In such a context the human's being is abstracted and essentialised in his fingernails, toenails, hair, blood and 'shadow'. Together, these items constitute 'the soul of the person' (*roho ya mutu*), and this term of reference helps us understand how to think about a process of part-for-whole representation by virtue of which people may intervene in unfolding reality at its source.

Fingers and toes are two of the portals of the body. Poisons and medicines set as invisible snares by sorcerers may enter the body through the digits and travel to the torso via the long bones of the arms and legs. Part of the administration of many different types of protective medicine consists of the cutting of shallow incisions (*machanjo*) in the skin over the knuckles of fingers and toes. Medicines are rubbed into these, and thus form a transverse line which 'cuts' (*kukata*) or obstructs the path of the noxious substance. Similar incisions 'cut' the path of such substances at the joints of the limbs. Fingernails and toenails thus lie on the very points where the individual's internal and external environment meet.

Another portal of the body is the space in the middle of the top of the head (*katikati ya kichwa* (KS)/*luboziabozia* (KT)). Medicines thrown onto one by sorcerers may enter one's body at this point. It is also the place from which the soul leaves the body at the time of death. The clippings of hair taken from the widow's peak and nape of the neck mark two points lying on an invisible line which crosscuts that descending from *katikati ya kichwa* into the body. By means of this intersection the head is 'closed' (*kufungwa*) to outside dangers.

The shadow of the person is joined (*kuungwa*) to his soul (*roho*, life or breath) and can be seen as something of the soul's external extension. The dead have no shadows, and the soul of a person may be stolen by stabbing his shadow with a magical stick or cane.

Blood, too, is the soul of a person. If it is lacking in sufficient quantity or if it fails to move about the body properly, the person dies.

These particular items thus serve to frame and to substantialise the intangible entity which is the person himself. When they are present in the *mwanzambale*, they miniaturise the whole human being. By means of such representation, the person is abstracted from the totality of his mundane existence, and his essence is made manipulable in ways that are not otherwise possible.

Vizimba and the 'soul of the person' may be combined and recombined in whatever way one chooses. Hence, the *erisi*, potentially a mechanical, microcosmic model of the world in all its infinite variety, permits the possible management of reality in ways which are exceptional but by no means unnatural. While *miti*, *vizimba* and *roho ya mutu* together give their processual structure to the world fabricated through their use, they cannot in themselves bring about transfiguration as act. This is done by the metonymic process of invocation (*kusemelea* (KS)/*kulandila* (KT)), to which we will turn our attention in Chapter 10.

RELIGION AND REALISATION

In the context of medical practice, religion becomes visible as the type of circumstantial therapy employed when an illness is diagnosed as being due to a spirit. Like the therapies just considered, religion involves the realisation of events in things; the substantiation of the meaningful in the material. However, the events thus substantiated and the relationship of substances to them are entirely complementary to those we have just seen. This complementarity is one of two differences fundamental to the distinction made by people themselves between 'magic' and 'religion'.

As has been noted above, spirits which may make a person ill are divided into two groups, *mizimu* and *pepo*. The former are those of a person's antecedents and family members who, after death, continue to protect him and generally to nurture him, while the latter are a class of spirits who have never been human, but who are sent by *mizimu* to confer specific benefits. In theory, the illnesses caused by spirits are not fatal, no matter how gravely ill the patient may appear; and death or permanent disability is sufficient grounds for abandonment of this diagnostic hypothesis. Further, spirits tend to cause illness in those situations where there is intrafamilial tension, often involving failure to fulfil familial obligations adequately.

Msambwa

The establishment of a *msambwa* is the least complicated type of religious circumstantial therapy which may be undertaken. It is initiated after divination into the cause of an illness or other misfortune or is begun in response to instructions received in a dream.

The first step in the establishment of a *msambwa* is the brewing of beer that is both an oracle and an offering. Though in content and method of fabrication the beer is identical to *kibuku*, ordinary corn and millet beer, it differs from *kibuku* in that it is dedicated to a particular antecedent by invocation at the time the grains are soaked and their germination process set in motion. The identity of the antecedent is determined through divination, and by virtue of the dedication, called *kupupa* (KT) or *kutambikia* (KS), the beer becomes an oracle through which the will of the antecedent is made known. If the beer ferments properly, the antecedent has conceded that it is, in fact, she or he who has caused the illness in question, and has also agreed that a *msambwa* ceremony should be performed. Beer which sours (*kuchacha*) instead of 'ripening' (*kuivia*) means that the antecedent named in the invocation is not responsible for the illness, and that a *msambwa* established in his name will therefore do no good.

When the beer is ready, the person notifies his joking clan (*baendo*), and/ or his real or classificatory father's sisters (*shangazi*) and grandchildren (*wijukulu*),[8] that they should participate in the celebration and aid him in the establishment of his shrine. Most of the beer is drunk amidst dancing and singing, but a little of it is set aside for therapeutic purposes.

In the afternoon, near dusk, one of the above types of person takes the loop of beads or the bracelet or empty tin can that is to be *msambwa* and rubs it with crushed, green *lugangani* leaves (*Ocium basilicum* L.). While this is happening, the person for whom the shrine is being established speaks to it, saying 'Now you are so-and-so. Let us go about together' (*Sasa upo fulani, tutembee pamoja*). The small portion of beer that has been set aside is then either passed about to be drunk by all, or poured into a small hole hollowed in the ground at the side of the house, from whence it is sucked up by the guests. After the shrine has been established, the person is expected to make to it occasional small gifts of money from the profits he receives through fishing, hunting, beer making, rice growing, etc.

In general *misambwa* derive from the larger, less differentiated pool of dead antecedents (such as M, MM, MMB or siblings) who were the person's close kin. Though these may be invoked by him in time of need, and remembered by him with small offerings of beer and the like, they are addressed as a group. One names all the antecedents one can think of, and concludes by addressing as a collectivity all antecedents whom one cannot then remember.

While a *msambwa* is part of this more general group, people say it is stronger because it has manifested itself more vigorously through illness, misfortune or dreams. It has thus singled itself out for substantiation and thereby become bound to the person by the specific set of obligations outlined above.

Bulumbu

In contrast to *misambwa*, *bilumbu* are spirits which have never existed in human form. There are two types of these, possessing and non-possessing spirits, all of which originated in Lubaland. The possessing spirits arrived in the area of Mpala during the thirties, gradually displacing another kind of possessing spirit which came from the Bemba, and becoming assimilated into a pre-existing system of belief in *ngulu* spirits of the land. The non-possessing spirits arrived sometime later, possibly as late as the early fifties.

Both types of *bilumbu* are acquired only after illness, misfortune and/or dreams have been divined into by specialists. Divinations may be made by either Bulumbu or Tulunga diviners, and the non-possessing spirits may also be prepared by either type of *mfumu*. Possessing *bilumbu* can be 'put in order' (*kutengeneza*) only by Bulumbu adepts. Both types, however, are sent by the *mizimu* (KS)/*mipasi* (KT) mentioned above, who are said to be the hierarchical superior from whom their power ultimately derives.

The arrangement of a possessing spirit is undertaken after it has been determined to be the cause of the problematic illness. To this end, an adept is contracted and a nighttime, public performance takes place. Drums are beaten and the assembled throng are led in the singing of Bulumbu songs by the adept, who is posssessed at the time. If all goes well, the patient, (or, sometimes, his representative) is 'mounted' (*kupandwa*) by the spirit, which then states its name and the benefits it has come to confer, be these fertility, success in hunting, knowledge of medicines, etc.

With the exception of spirits which have come to divine, and which are called regularly to mount their human vehicle (*kapondo*) for this purpose, *bilumbu* come only in time of crisis, spontaneously possessing their human consorts in response to illness or misfortune. At these times, they make pronouncements upon the actual situation. The diagnostic aspects of their statements may resemble divination and may include the naming of the medicines to be employed for cure.

Non-possessing spirits are of several different kinds, each of which takes a different form and which has a different meaning. These are as follows:

1. Mukalaye–Kiungu. This joined pair of spirits consists[9] of two spirals of beads sewn onto a small piece of cloth. Mukalye is the husband, Kiungu (literally 'pot') his wife. They are manifest in dreams as Europeans and cutomarily wear white. They are associated with the blessings symbolised by whiteness and generally protect and confer fruitfulness (especially fertility) upon their human consorts.

2. Kabwangozi. This spirit is made of a split, pear-shaped seed onto which beeswax (*bupula*) is pressed and studded with the red seeds of the *minkeke* vine (*Arbus precatorius L.* ssp. africanus Verdc.).[10] Kabwangozi is a dog (*kabwa* means dog, in KiTabwa), and appears in dreams as such. He is the punishing agent of Mukalaye, and it is he who is dispatched by Mukalaye to bring illness. It is said that a person who has already acquired Mukalaye and Kiungu can be certain that Kabwangozi is sure to follow. Together, the three constitute the most prevalent non-possessing spirits in the area of Mpala.[11]

3. Mwilambwe. This spirit takes the form of a tiny carved canoe and

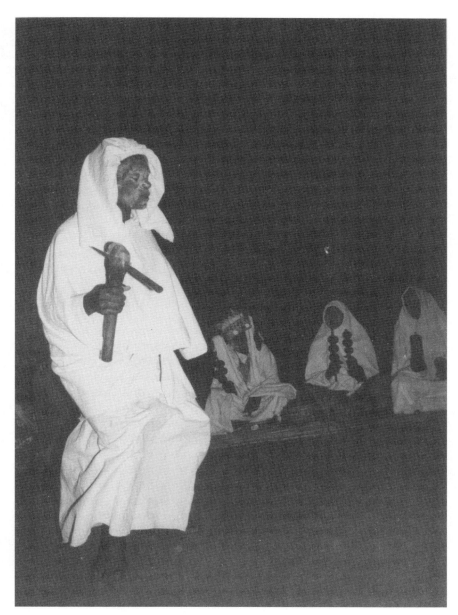

Figure 9.2 Bulumbu diviners in practice

paddle, and appears in this way in dreams. Mwilambwe confers general fruitfulness, but is especailly associated with water, near where his house[12] is built when possible.

4. Mwamba. This spirit takes the form of an arch moulded in clay. In dreams it is a rainbow or the crossing of two streams filled with water of only ankle depth. Like the preceding spirits, Mwamba confers general benefits. Very few people in Mpala have this, however, as it tends to follow the other spirits, coming only after they have already arrived.

5. Kakuji. This is a small carved figure. Its form in dreams and the benefits it confers are obscure to people at Mpala, who say it is most often found to the north, around Kalemie. Indeed, it was at Kalemie that the *kakuji* spirits I encountered were acquired.

Despite their very evident difference, *bilumbu* share certain characteristics among themselves and with *misambwa*. All of these substantiations are similar in their simplicity. The containers which hold them may be small cans (in the case of *misambwa*), small baskets (as with non-possessing *bilumbu*), or larger, *mputo* baskets (in the case of possessing spirits); but on no account may these containers hold anything other than the spirit, a bit of *pemba* (kaolin), and the few coins given to the spirit as offerings.[13] Neither *visimba* nor *miti* may be near them.

In this respect, they may all be described as iconoclastic forms which shun both explicit images and the implicit imagery that is the meaning (*maana*) of *vizimba* and other medicines. Relations between human beings and *mizimu/mipasi* or *pepo* take the form of specific communications made through either the medium of speech (in dream or possession) or the medium of illness (as symptoms).

An awareness of the very reliance of religion on speech is crucial to a proper understanding of the more profound differences between *mizimu* and sorcerers as aetiologic agents of illness, and hence to the differences between 'religion' and 'magic'. Speech is the normal mode of relations between human beings and *mizimu/mipasi*, and this mode is dependent upon the maintenance of a certain social distance. Persons who have been made 'to feel' (*kusikia*) illness because 'they have no ears' (*hawana masikio*) to hear the requests of their dead antecedents are said to have 'been approached' (*kukaribiwa* or *kujongewa*) by their *mizimu*, who do not speak during this period of discontinuity. With the establishment of a *msambwa* or *bulumbu*, proper relations, with their appropriate distances, are restored. Speech is resumed and the illness remits.

Thus, because illnesses caused by *mizimu* are manifestations of temporary alienations in a system normally characterised by communication and nurturance, the assumption is that the illness cannot terminate in death or permanent disability. However, *mizimu* do kill sometimes, as was the case in certain instances occurring during my stay. In addition, one *bulumbu* possessing spirit, *mutumbi* ('aardvark'), may also kill by causing its human vehicle to engage in self-destructive acts. Such deaths, however, are only the exceptions which prove the rule. People see them as especially severe punishments for extreme obstinacy in the face of repeated warnings.

When *mizimu/mipasi* or *pepo* are aetiologic agents, therefore, death can be said to be *contained* by communication. It is not only theoretically excluded as a possible outcome of spirit-derived illness, it is made meaningful even on the infrequent occasions when it does occur. The meaning which is attributed to such illness and/or death serves only to connect proximate moments to ultimate rules and circumstances, and thereby provides insight and/or enlightenment by which people can modify their lives, can learn.

When sorcerers are the aetiologic agents, the opposite is true. Non-communication is the normal mode of relations with a sorcerer (*mulozi*). People illustrate this when they cite a KiTabwa proverb which says 'Oppression of heart. If he treads upon you with his foot, he will raise it' (*Ngilika mutima. Akuilike kulu wakakuilula* (KT)/*Kukandamiza roho. Akikandamiza muguu kuinua* (KS)). To it they attribute two meanings.

First, they say it means that if a sorcerer sets his heart against you (illustrated with a motion of squeezing the hand), you will surely die, because a sorcerer never relents. With others, if one quarrels, after a month or so of bad feeling, the affair will be finished. But with a sorcerer, you will never again be on speaking terms, and he will not be content until he sees you dead.

Second, if, by chance, you should have the misfortune to quarrel with a sorcerer, it is better to fight with him physically, and thus to provoke arbitration. By this means, the matter will be settled, and the sorcer will not remain with anger in his heart. Otherwise, communication between you will cease and his grudge (*chuki*) will end only with your death. When you die, the sorcerer will be the first to arrive at your funeral and foremost among the grave diggers and mourners, just so he can be rid all the more quickly of seeing your face.[14]

Since non-communication is the norm, a person who fails to visit an ill neighbour, friend or relative, or one who begins to avoid the patient's family (or to avoid making eye contact with them) during the time of his illness, is very likely to be suspected of sorcery (*ulozi*) in the case.[15] It is said that if he speaks or jokes with members of the patient's family, the sorcerer will feel compassion for his victim's sufferings (both the pain of the patient, and the losses suffered by his family) and will then relent. The maintenance in the mind of the intention appropriate to the magico-medicinal formula employed is essential to the working of any amulet (*erisi*), whether sorcerous or not. To relent is, therefore, to undo or withdraw the medicines. Thus, by not speaking to the object of his *dawa* a sorcerer ensures the sancity of his murderous impulses, and, hence, the effectiveness of his medicines.

When an illness has been diagnosed through divination as being due to sorcery, there is no direct course which can be taken to undo it. Unlike Azande social rules, Tabwa etiquette provides no means by which the person responsible for the illness can be approached and made to withdraw his maleficent influence.[16] To accuse someone openly of sorcery prior to the death of the victim and subsequent divination is to violate the law and to risk imprisonment.[17]

The only alternative possible for laypeople is called *kupiga mbila*. In this, a senior member of the patient's family stands before his house at dusk and at dawn, and shouts veiled accusations of sorcery for the entire community to hear. Subtle reference may be made to the identity of the sorcerer, and the *mbila* usually concludes with a request that the affair, whatever it may be, be settled by the usual channel, rather than through sickness. If the patient is lucky, the sorcerer will hear the appeals, feel ashamed and relent.

Diviners (*wafumu*), whether Bulumbu or Tulunga, are said to have another alternative at their disposal which they sometimes employ on behalf of their unknowing clients. Those practitioners who are themselves sorcerers (*walozi*) can meet with their 'colleagues' (that is, other sorcerers) during their nocturnal dances, and prevail upon the sorcerer in question to relent. By this means the healer will appear to have cured his patient in the usual fashion. Then, when he is paid for his work, he will split the proceeds with the sorcerer.

The lack of communication which is the prevailing mode of relations with sorcerers is also reflected in the types of illness caused by these aetiologic agents. Illnesses which are deadly or permanently disabling are the result of sorcery, as are those which are 'unintelligible' (*haijulikani*) and those which fail 'to hear' or 'to feel' (*kusikia*) medicines. Thus, deaths suffered as a consquence of such illness and such a cause are meaningless, and people who have died in this way are said to have died 'worthlessly' (*alikufa bure*).[18]

In contrast, then, to illness and deaths derived from *mizimu*, those derived from *walozi* can be said to represent death at its most uncontained. People see and depict it as death in its most relentless form, having as its aim nothing other than the reduction of a human being to the meat which the sorcerers hope to exhume and eat. Without an underlying context of communication and nurturance to give it meaning, death from sorcery contributes nothing to the development of insight or human understanding.

RELIGION AND TRANSFORMATIVE METONYMY

Sapir (1977: 4) defines metonymy[19] as a process which 'replaces or juxtaposes continuous terms that occupy a distinct and separate place within what is considered a single semantic or perceptual domain'. Thus, it involves the substitution of one 'cause' for another, as in the substitution of cause for effect, container for contained, instrument for agent, agent for act, etc. (Sapir 1977:19–20). Based as it is upon shared domains, metonymy emphasises or foregrounds the idea of 'wholeness', and its totalising function complements the specifying actions of part-for-whole synecdoche and of metaphor.

The therapeutic processes by which *misambwa* and *mikalye* spirits are created[20] resemble metonymy in their manner of transforming circumstances. At the time of the invocation ('Now you are so-and-so. Let us go about together'), the loop of beads, bracelet, or small disc of beads stitched in a spiral comes to embody the spirit for which it is named. Container thus substantiates contained. Further, in the same invocation, this realisation is juxtaposed to the human being for whom it is created. The whole that is their association is thereby foregrounded, and, by this very process, the reality surrounding them is changed.

Of subtle brilliance here is the commentary on religion and metonymy that is contained in the act of rubbing *misambwa* with *lugangani*. As the Latin name (*Ocinium basilicum* L.) indicates, this plant is an African variety of wild basil, and when crushed its leaves give off a strong odour. This smell is offensive to *pepo*, and, so when rubbed on the head, the leaves of *lugangani* drive off a possessing *bulumbu* spirit; a useful device when it has become a nuisance to its human consort. In the context of *misambwa* it can be said to perform a similar function, serving to create between spirit and person the distance appropriate to speech. Thus, the metonymic transformation of religious circumstantial therapy paradoxically foregrounds or emphasises the wholeness of human–spirit relations precisely by enacting the *space* around which the totality is formed.

Something similar occurs with the arrangement of *bilumbu* possessing spirits. Here, it is the spirit itself which states its identity by pronouncing its name and the benefits it comes to confer. After such pronouncement, the spirit is housed in a small round basket within the large *mputo* basket, and takes the form of the *mulako*; that is, either a small loop of beads or the smoked dried head of the chicken which is sacrificed at the time of the ceremony. Thus, the statement of identity which is the metonymic means by which relationship is established between *pepo* and *kapondo* (human consort) is precisely that by which the spirit is made to distance itself from the patient's body and instead become substantiated in the mulako.

Metonymy and Roundness

As a shape, roundness has many associations in cosmology. Among its multiple meanings are containment, cyclicity and horizontality. Of significance here, however, is the form it gives to metonymic transformation as this exists in religious circumstantial therapy.

All of the most prevalent religious entities (*misambwa, mikalaye* and *bilumbu*)

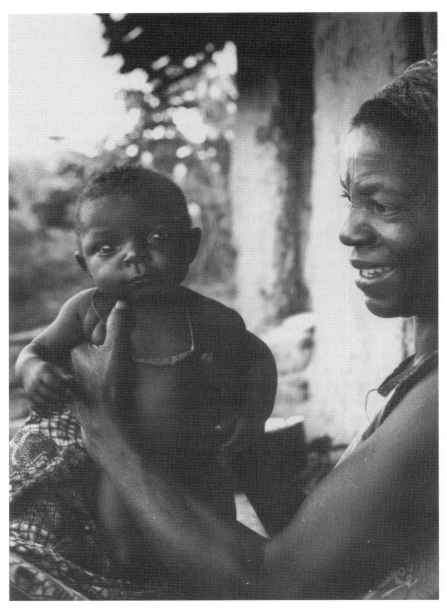

Figure 9.3 Mumba, Bulumbu diviner, and her daughter

use the circle or spiral. *Misambwa* are basically bracelets of metal or plastic or are empty tin cans; *mikalaye–kiungu* take the form of complementarily directed spirals; and *bilumbu* are realised in the loop of beads that is the *mulako*. In addition, the spiral plays an important part in the geometric motif used in the *nkaka* headdresses of Bulumbu diviners, where it is called the 'eye' (*jicho*).

The circle and the spiral can be said to represent visually the metonymic process that is religious circumstantial therapy, as well as the ultimate inscrutability and ineffability of the relation to which it gives form. The circle, like the bracelet or can of the *msambwa*, and the *mputo* and *mulako* of the *bulumbu*, is defined as much by the empty space within it as by the material substance which curves round the outside. In this crucial respect, it is a graphic version of the totalisation by which spirit and person are united in a single conceptual domain, united precisely at the moment in which, and through the means by which, they are separated from one another. The concentric rings that are the *mulako* in the small basket within the *mputo* underscore this point, and also constitute a medial form between the static circle that is *msambwa* and the dynamic spiral that characterises *mukalaye* and the 'eye' of *bulumbu*. As such, it has a character appropriate to its status as the substantiation of the *pepo* at rest.

As a form, the spiral can be described as the active variant of the circle. It can be said to represent the inscrutability of godly action in Tabwa cosmology, for no matter how deeply one goes into it, the centre of a spiral always recedes before one. Thus, people's statements of how *mizimu/mipasi* are able to effect their transformations are verbal encirclings which can only encompass but not exactly describe the process. The spirit 'becomes angry' (*anakasirika*) and illness ensues directly. The spirit 'responds' (*anaitika*) to human pleas, and benefits are directly conferred. One can approach no further, and in contrast to those of magic, the actual mechanics remain unknowable, or cannot be said even to exist as such.

In addition, the spiral can also be said to represent the transcendent nature of the godly. *Mukalaye–kiungu*, two counter-clockwise spirals which run into each other, demonstrate the inner fullness and processual activity that are the essence of the substantial world; its infinity. The two constantly turning spirals, male and female, which generate each other from the central points within each, thus graphically represent or, in fact, realise the infinity that is the continuity of generations, of life holding death in abeyance.

In a comparable fashion, the spiral that is the 'eye' of the Bulumbu practitioner's *nkaka* headdress is closely identified with the active spirit's superhuman powers. As we have seen, the eye is something which projects outward and is associated with mastery. When possessed, a diviner's spirit may 'see' (*kuona*) sorcerers invisible to others and may be aware of events and medicines whose existence lies outside of ordinary human knowing.

Thus, in the medical context, aetiologic agents such as *mizimu/mipasi* or *pepo* give rise to religious circumstantial therapies which are designed to restore normal communications between human beings and their spirit mentors, and thereby to cause the illness to remit. The establishment of *misambwa, mikalaye* and *bilumbu* is a metonymic act, which is reproduced in the circular and spiral forms which characterise the spirits themselves.

Taken together, then, and placed in the context of medical practice, the two types of circumstantial therapy that are 'magic' and 'religion' can be seen as two complementary approaches to the substantiation of events and of the agents which cause them. Here, we have considered the material, manipulable objects of which the two therapies make use; a bonding of meanings or words with things. This union can be said to create a heightened transfigurative or transformative potential, a capacity held in abeyance by the passive objectivity of the thing. It is through two complementary types of invocation that this potential is quickened, released for realisation in and as a future.

10

FUTURES REALISED: EVENTS OUT OF THINGS

INVOCATIONS AND METONYMY

The preceding discussion of the varieties of circumstantial therapy has given attention primarily to the devices of substantiation these therapies employ. That is, we were considering the objects in which processes, events and agents are realised, and the complementary methods by which this realisation takes place.

First among these are the complexes of contents and techniques that structure the ceremony called 'throwing the person in the bush' (*kumutupa mtu mupori*) and that constitute the substance of the *mwanzambale* amulet (*erisi*). Complementary to this are the means by which *misambwa*, *mikalaye* and *bilumbu* are established and the emblematic forms in which the being of each type of spirit is realised.

Speech is the transformative act by which these structures are quickened and directed towards the future. Speech takes the form of invocations, and by means of them people unite differing realms in the creation of a single domain. In keeping with their distinction at the level of objects, people distinguish two different types of speech, called *kupupa* (KT) (or *kutambikia* (KS)) and *kulandila* (KT) (or *kusemelea* (KS)), respectively. This distinction between invocations is the further basis on which 'religion' and 'magic' may be differentiated.

Kupupa is employed in circumstantial therapies we may gloss as religious. The invocation describes, and by the process establishes, relations between a human being and a non-human mentor. This type of invocation involves the dedication of a given substantiated process to a specific *mizimu* (dead antecedent) with the request that the spirit employ the process unfolding within that substance to make manifest its intentions. The one most often offered is *kibuku*, corn and millet beer.

Thus, people say, one might return from a divination session at which a specific *mizimu* has been named and, while wetting the grains, dedicate the beer to that particular antecedent, saying, 'If, so-and-so, if it truly is you who is bringing this illness, let the beer mature' (*Kama, fulani, kama kweli ni weye, mwenye kuleta ugonjuwa huu, pombe ikomae*). One may similarly employ the process that is one's own ill body, specifying that the *mizimu* cause one's recovery if it is truly that *mizimu* who is causing the illness with which one then suffers. In either case, the answer is the same: successful outcome (potent beer, remission of illness) is an affirmative answer while failure is a negative one.

People say that in former times, beer-drinks were given in honour of *mizimu*, as libations were poured out and chickens offered to them. An adult might brew beer and invite his classificatory grandchildren (*wijukuu*) to drink it. Each would contribute around five *makuta* and would drink his fill. The coins would be placed in the centre of the floor and later would be used to buy a chicken for the *mizimu*. Similarly, one might invite people over to drink beer and dance in the dead antecedent's honour. All of these ceremonies were called *kupupa ka kufu* or *kupupa ka muzimu*.

People say that with *kupupa*, one 'gives' (*kupa*) to the *muzimu* the substantial medium (*kapupo*), be it beer or one's body. As a consequence, the outcome of the process that the medium does or contains becomes a clear communication of that spirit's intent regarding a particular situation. As the *muzimu* has done in the medium, so will she or he do in the more general circumstances. As her or his intent has been made manifest through the process of the medium, so shall it become manifest through the process of unfolding events. It is this structured specificity of relations among human, spirit and medium that distinguishes *kupupa* from its complement, *kulandila*.

With *kupupa*, the invocation's metonymic action specifies as it totalises. In the first part of the invocation ('If, so-and-so, it is really you who is bringing this illness'), a statement of situation is made. In it, there is reference to a particular spirit, and to a relationship which might exist between that spirit and a given person at a given point in time. The evocation of this specific relation and the particular significance it causes to inhere in the outcome of the process together make of the medium a domain shared by the person and the spirit. With the statement of intention ('let the beer mature'), the offered medium (*kapupo*) becomes a miniature rendition of the situation in general. Thus, though the human and spirit realms are fully and relatively permanently connected via the *kapupo*, the connection has immediate bearing only upon the unique process and particular beings invoked. This stands in marked contrast to the metonymy of *kulandila*, which totalises as it specifies.

Kulandila or *kusemelea* literally means 'to speak to', and this type of invocation takes different forms. If one calls upon all one's *mizimu/mipasi* by naming each one individually, or by citing them collectively, or by simply crying out (for example, 'Don't let this happen!'), the act is *kulandila*, people say. The fact that one may have asked for a specific outcome is not relevant to the definition of the invocation.

This is because reference was made to many spirits, and not one in particular. Though a positive response is affirmative, an unsuccessful outcome is less than a negative communication because one cannot know which of the spirits was responsible. The act remains *kulandila* even when one presents the *mizimu/mipasi* with offerings of beer, money or food.

The form of *kulandila* more commonly referred to by the term is the description given at the invocation of the 'arrow' (*mshale*) being sent to the diviner. In this, the entire set of circumstances surrounding the divination is outlined. Each one of the many possible causes of sickness is mentioned (such as theft, adultery, quarrels with neighbours, murder, sorcery, jealousy of others, etc.) and is told to reveal itself to the diviner should it be the actual cause of the illness. Without this, the divination could not possibly be successful.

The most elaborated form of *kulandila* is the invocation made by the *mfumu* at the fabrication of the *erisi*. People say that such invocation is absolutely essential to the effectiveness of any amulet. It 'matures'[1] (*kukomesha*) the charm, which would otherwise remain an inert collection of *vizimba* and *miti*; a mere object; something incapable of effecting transformation. As Luvunzo and Kalulu put it, an *erisi* without invocation is 'worthless' (*ni bure tu*); 'it is without meaning' (*haina maana*).

In its complex wealth of detail, *kulandila* forms the complement to the very simple form of the *kupupa* invocation. In fabricating the *mwanzambale* whose contents were described and discussed in Chapter 9, the diviner made lengthy invocations for both Allen Roberts and me. These were spoken into the amulet as the *mfumu* made it. His words were thus mixed into the ingredients, and were packed with them into the containers. His words also were part of the stitching with which he secured each small protective bundle. Made on 28 October 1975, one is excerpted at length here:

> Now *mwanzambale* ... does not play with a person. He of the bad heart who comes to harass those of Mr Roberts, for that one, the consequence is his business. But that person who only passes by, he has no reason to worry. Those who come in the night, or who harass (*kuchokoza*) by day, and he of bad things, he himself will come into difficulty (*kukwaa* or *kukwala*). *Mizimu* will be put in here, little animals, little snakes, mountains, trees, *bahunde* [avenging ghosts], all are in here. *Wamanzi* [mutual murderers] *bayembe* [ghosts], all are in here. Those of anger, of anxieties, all are in here.
>
> Good. We begin to close matters (*maneno*) with the whole body. Bad things in the country, evil sorcerers, bad people of the territory, those who start out even at night, they are not able to get them, to ensorcell those of Mr Roberts. It will do no good. An evil person won't do anything. He will fail.
>
> We close a bad thing. An animal, like the lion, if they walk in the

bush, that the lion miss them. Things like crocodiles, hippos, they will be unable to do anything. Or a snake, or a bad fish, or the bad wind of a river or lake, such as that which comes from the hills on the other side [that is, Tanzania], or those spirits/winds (*pepo*) at Tembwe, Mugandja, Kiai, and all other mountains, we close all of them.

They must travel about well, either in their boat, or in the boat of another person. Or in their boat, en route, if police, or runaway people (*batombosha*), bandits attempt to trap them, seeing them and thinking, 'Surely, to go to all Europeans, those of this sort must have something worth taking', it won't work. If they see them, just to see them, only the work of liking (*kazi ya mapenzi*) will come.

The policeman also, or the soldier of every country, if it is a country where they will go to travel, if it is Tanzania, if it is any place at all, America or Europe, Africa or Asia, all are thus. They are able to walk about only well. In short (*basi*) they have nothing bad done to them.

[Here he twice blew sputum onto the amulet.]

To be received well. On the road they are visited by health. All bad winds/spirits, if it is related to peregrinations (*matembezi*); if it is sorcerers, if it is God, a bad mountain and all mountains [are contained] only within (*mpaka humu*).

A person has a bad heart (*rho mbaya*). He intends to start off thus, with a knife. ... He goes and says 'Let me stab him' (*nimuchome*), ...

He goes and says 'Let me stab him'. The perpetrator's soul becomes indifferent (*mweusi*, 'black'). Or he takes up a spear, intending 'That I go do this to him', ... or he takes up a gun, thinking 'That I shoot him with a bullet', the person's soul is indifferent. He takes up a bow and arrow or any other thing at all; if he takes it in his hand, he, here in the world; a stone is a stone, water is water, poison (*sumu*) is poison in his hands.[2] Or if he leaves it in a bag, before arriving there at the place of doing his deed, his soul is indifferent.

Perhaps he will start off with the thought 'Let me steal from him. His valise will contain wealth.' Arriving there, his soul is different. The means of stealing fail. He is doing such thoughts, now he forgets and returns home. If it is night he does not go to steal from him at night. He won't be able to.

Or if a person sees them and wishes to use thunderbolts (*radi*, that is, lightning that strikes the ground), lightning can't do a thing. Or a animal, or a snake or the apparition (*mwjiza*) of a dead person, nothing will be able to do a thing, not even a little. The thing is closed inside (*ndani*).

We request (*tunaomba*, to supplicate or beg) only fondness (*mapenzi*). Even sorcerers will only like them. There is no sorcerer who will say otherwise (*ya kusema namna gani*). Even a person can act only to like them.

Chiefs like them, and the elders who had the titles of before (*mbele*), they must like them; such as those authorities, even the President ...

Good. When his mouth speaks, it is heard before others'. Or even before requesting work of important Europeans who are of America or any country they must respond at once.

The work is finished.

We request fondness. His male counterparts like Mr Roberts, they like him; and if he has work involving travelling; they will all like him.

This is the amulet of Mr Roberts.

[Here he spat again upon it.]

Good. We are finishing.

We close all, we meet all in here. Even all bad men will become slippery (*kuterezeka*, that is, become easy-going). And at the house he the bad person or sorcerer won't be able to do a thing, not a bit. A thing that can afflict (*kutesa*), it will begin to pass.

And all the mountains and all the bodies of water ... rivers, lakes, ... all types of animals ... We close all cunning/magic (*manyele*) evil in the world, all who are met in the path the bad thought – 'let me kill the European' – let him not be with this thought. Or a person whom a bad individual sends now – truly he will forget – his evil act misses. Or whatever kind of thing that is sent, it misses, it comes out before, or it fails to fire, nothing more. Or that he have that thought, that his only thought be affection. If he [Allen Roberts] has bad words, a conflict there, at the place of doing him harm, with countless people (*watu wangapi*), to drive him out (*kumufukuza*), they say instead 'You lacked this' (*ulikosa hii*, that is, 'you erred in such-and-such a way'). They just explain and the affair is finished.

This person and all bad things we close here. This business with the lake Tanganyika, bad winds, winds which bring illness, or which bring people with bad thoughts, we close in here. Mountains of this place, of all countries of the world, all mountains, we beg with God.

In its elegant completion, this invocation allows us to see most clearly the attributes of *kulandila* invocations. Like *kupupa*, *kulandila* consists of two elements which are of the utmost importance to the working of the *erisi*. Though indissoluble in the act, they are separable for the purposes of analysis. They are the statement of situation, by which the world is put into the *mwanzambale*, and the statements of intent, by which the *mwanzambale* is put into the world.

The *kulandila* invocation is spoken as the *mfumu* stuffs with *miti* and *vizimba* the small leather pouch that his clients are to wear and/or packs the little, clear glass bottle that is to stay in the house. As he speaks, he cites all the features of the natural world – mountains, bodies of water, trees, bush animals, snakes and fish. Many of the significant inhabitants of the social world are also described in both their negative and positive aspects – people in authority, police, soldiers, thieves, sorcerers and vagabonds – as are some of the circumstances of potential danger encountered during the course of one's life. This is the statement of situation, and it is the verbal counterpart of the large variety of *vizimba* simultaneously employed.

As substantiations of outcomes, actions or processes, the *vizimba* form the structure of the *erisi*, which the invocation makes complete. This is to say that the re-presentations in *vizimba*, as individuals and as clusters, are sketched, as it were, in dotted lines; five types of snake instead of all types, four sorts of stinging insect instead of all sorts, and so forth.

The statement of situation in *kulandila* totalises these specifics, referring to them in such a way that they encompass, in fact, nothing less than the entirety of their categorical counterparts which have been miniaturised in *vizimba* for the purposes of the *erisi*. In this manner, the *vizimba* cease being specific re-presentations of the individual animals, insects, people and situations from which they derived, and instead become substantiated representatives giving command over whole categories of possibility.

As Luvunzo put it, the invocation 'matures' (*kukomesha*) the *erisi* so that the tiny fragment of a lion that the amulet contains becomes 'like a whole lion' *(kama simba mzima)*. Thus, through his speech, the *mfumu* links the substantial world of the present with the future world he is fabricating within and by means of the *erisi*. What was one lion in life becomes all any lion might mean by virtue of its substantiation in the domain of *vizimba* and its passage back into life through speech. Through the statement of situation, the world of possibilities is put into *mwanzambale*, but it is placed there piece by piece.

Through the statement of intent, the complementary process takes place, and the *erisi* is placed in the world. Even as the *mfumu* cites each item in the miniature world of the *erisi*, he also specifies the actions that pertain to it. This is what defines the function of the amulet, what quickens it and makes it 'go'.

Mwanzambale can be distinguished from sorcery only by this statement of intent, since many of the objects and circumstances it contains as *vizimba* are deadly in themselves. At the proximate level on which they operate, *vizimba* are subordinate to the human consciousness which employs them. They can be ordered to attack others aggressively as easily as they are told to protect their owners, and they will respond as readily. The functional amorality of its contents is one of the reasons why many consider this charm to be of questionable ethical status.

People say that an amulet of any sort will fulfil its purpose only for as long as its owner maintains the fixity of her or his will. When she or he has an amulet made, a person must 'tighten' (*kukaza*) or 'dry out' (*kukausha*, also meaning 'to stiffen') her or his soul (*rho*). Any loosening of will (*kuregeza*) automatically results in a weakening of the power of the *erisi* itself. Under such circumstances, a charm cannot be expected to function successfully.

The two parts of the *kulandila* invocation thus operate complementarily, and in a fashion that is the inverse of what obtains in *kupupa* invocations. The statement of situation forms the counterpoint to the *vizimba*. It delineates a series of features and circumstances which together form a miniature of the world, but a model which is weighted according to the *erisi*'s specific contents. The statement of intent activates that miniature world, and creates a relation of analogy by which the charm acts within and upon the larger life of which the *mwanzambale* is itself a part. By means of these complementary processes, microcosm and macrocosm come to contain one another. They are thus in the relation of exquisite and inextricable proximity which permits complex transformations to take place.

LOCUS OF TRANSFORMATION

Both *kupupa* and *kulandila* invocations function to foreground the common domain uniting the medium of transformation (whether *kapupo* or *erisi*) and the world. This domain is nothing other than reality itself, that combination of substantial objects with their particular, situational meanings which exists both inside and outside of people's perceptions and thoughts and in terms of which people live and act. It is in one aspect or another of this domain that the transformations resulting from circumstantial therapy, whether 'religious' or 'magical', takes place.

Just as they make complementary use of the processes of specifying and totalising, so do *kupupa* and *kulandila* prompt changes whose loci in reality are complementary. With *kupupa*, religious circumstantial therapy specifies as it totalises. Its statement of situation foregrounds the common domain of person and spirit, while its statement of intent creates 'mouths' for the words of others (antecedents, spirits) by giving particular meaning to the results of specific processes. Human speeches are requests for revelation of the spirit's or ancestor's intent; the resulting action is communication.

One might say *kupupa* is initially or outwardly metonymic, but secondarily or inwardly metaphoric. The changes which *kupupa* prompts take place in the substantial aspect of reality; in the beer being brewed, in the sequence of events unfolding in the body or elsewhere. Their significance derives from the identification that can be made between the events unfolding in the substance and events which will subsequently unfold in the life. The smaller is made to mean the larger thing.

On the other hand, with *kulandila*, circumstantial therapy totalises as it specifies. Its statement of situation delineates a large number of specific identifications between the macrocosmic world and the miniature *erisi*, while its statement of intent foregrounds the common domain uniting amulet and unfolding circumstances. Human words are instructions to subordinated entities, and human intention becomes the outcome of future, unfolding events.

One might say that it is initially metaphoric and secondarily metonymic. The changes which *kulandila* prompts take place in the realm of coincidence and of meanings attached to the substantial elements of the world, hence to appearances. They take place, therefore, in that delicate domain of possibilities, where chance meets fate and where the slightest shift at its outset can radically alter the outcome of a sequence of events.

Vizimba, as we have seen, metaphorically transfigure the way the owner of an *erisi* appears to others. The invocation which is their counterpoint commands the transfiguration of the thoughts of those who might wish to do the owner harm. Both these changes are encompassed in the idea of *manyele*, as a fabricated, significant difference between the realities of one person and another.

That the characteristics contained in *vizimba* are presumed by people to transfigure the substantial appearance but not the fundamental being[3] of the person is amply demonstrated in a simple invisibility formula described to me by Nzuiba. In it are combined *vizimba* of the faeces of the aardvark (*mavi ya mutumbi*), the pelt of the melanistic serval (*nzima*) and a piece of white porcelain plate.

The aardvark faeces are used because they are customarily buried by the animal and are therefore only very rarely seen. *Nzima* contributes that animal's ability to conceal itself successfully, an ability which is facilitated by its dark colour. The white plate is likened to a blank, unblinking stare.

According to Nzuiba, when used, the formula enables one to enter the houses of others and steal from them. If the people see you, they will be thunderstruck, so to speak, and will simply stare at you without blinking or moving.

While they are thus immobilised, you complete your work and leave. As you do so, the observers/victims start, as if suddenly awaking from sleep. They are aware that they have seen someone, but can't think who it might have been. When people ask them if they know who just robbed them, they reply that they can't identify the thief.

Thus, while one is materially perceived, you and your intentions or actions are not *recognised* as such. You are, for all intents and purposes, invisible.

Mwanzambale, like any amulet, affects its transformations in a manner similar to this. It is the way a person substantially *seems* to others to be, more than what she or he fundamentally is, that is changed by the *erisi*. Thus it is her or his meaning which is modified.

By the term 'meaning' I am referring to the intangible features of a person's being that none the less constitute significant aspects of her or his identity. Such features are part of what others may know or think they know of her or him, and knowledge of these features governs, at least in part, the interpretation of her/his past and present behaviour as well as expectations of her or his future activities.

Indeed, the 'soul of the person' (*rho ya mtu*), which is placed at the centre of the *erisi* as fingernails, toenails, hair, 'shadow' and blood, is in part the substantiation of this personal meaning. Through its representatives, the soul can become the object of direct transfiguration. As personal meaning, the soul is an entity abstracted.

By *rho* people refer to both the literal 'breath' that is synonymous with life, but distinguishable from the body, and to the equally intangible fixity of capability, outlook and motive that they presume to underlie the transient, changing interactions of social life. It is the latter which was considered in Kiabu's history as personal identity, and is here glossed as personal meaning.

By thus working its changes upon the unique meaning an individual has for others, *mwanzambale* has as the locus of its transfiguration the consciousnesses of people other than those for whom the amulet was made. This locus, implicit in the meanings of *vizimba*, is made explicit in the invocation which states that the bad intentions of evil people shall be transfigured when these persons come into contact with the amulet's owner.

The *kulandila* invocation vocalises these complex relations which include the fact that the owner is completely identified with the amulet, and thus himself becomes not only transfigured, but also transfigurative. The *mfumu* defined this identification when he explained the meaning of the two needles whose immersion in the client's blood and insertion into the medicine-filled bottle marks the completion of the *erisi*'s fabrication: 'If a person comes to harass my body … they will stab themselves as with thorns. I am *mwanzambale*. In short, I hide myself within this bottle and its meaning is that you will also hide your body in that little space.' Thus, in being identified with the amulet, its owner also comes to take on its properties. These include the ability to transfigure either the consciousnesses or the fates of others without even the necessity of oneself being aware of causing such changes. As they come into contact with the *mwanzambale*–person, individuals either forget their intention to do him harm, have their plans and/or instruments rendered ineffective, or cause injury to themselves if they persist in their evil ways.

Such transfigurative capacity becomes a property of the amulet's owner, functions apart from his conscious direction or will, and is not directed towards any particular person. These are the features which its defenders say distinguish *mwanzambale* from sorcery. As the *mfumu* said when he made it, with *mwanzambale* 'the one of the trap, we trap' (*tunamutega mwenye mtego*). The amulet makes the person into a metaphysical, metaphorical trap, set to spring shut only upon those who step into it, and to close with a strength exactly commensurate to that of the trapped person's intention to injure.

MUNGU NA MITISHAMBA

This description of *kupupa* and *kulandila* makes clear a complementarity of structure and function uniting while distinguishing the two. 'Religious' circumstantial therapy is iconoclastic and simple in nature and, through *kupupa* invocation, functions to bring into specific relation a unique individual and a particular spirit. This kind of therapy thus specifies even as it totalises, asserting a relationship in and to one life, but taking possession of the whole of it. *Kupupa* has the material aspect of reality as the locus of the transformations it affects, although its objects are not gifts as much as they are physical receptacles for metaphysical communications.

In contrast to this, is 'magical' circumstantial therapy; 'throwing the person in the bush' and *manyele*. Each of these is iconophilic and complex in nature. Through *kulandila* invocations, *manyele* outlines a great number and variety of particular identifications and thus delineates a world. Hence, it totalises even as it specifies; and it has the meaningful, immaterial aspect of reality as the locus of the transfiguration it effects.

As a device to help us comprehend the logic of 'magical', circumstantial therapy, we can consider *manyele* as the establishment of a series of metaphoric identifications by means of which a metonymic totality comes to exist. This relation is the result of a proximate determining will.

While the complementarity of the two types of circumstantial therapy (iconoclastic and iconophilic) is thus quite clear, there is a larger sense in which the interrelation between the two is considerably more complex than this. Each type can be placed so as to extend and to illuminate the other.

People indicate this when they cite the proverb '*Mungu na mitishamba*' in discussions of illness and curing. The literal meaning of the phrase is 'God and medicine-field' (or 'tree-field') and people give it two complementary interpretations.

Some say the phrase means that even though one invokes one's God (*Mungu wako*, that is, one's *mizimu/mipasi*) and requests cure, one is not going to be cured by God alone, without the aid of medicines (*miti*). Quite the contrary; one must dig roots as well as pray if one wishes to recover.

Complementarily, other people say the phrase means that all possible knowledge of medicines will not effect cure if one's God is not also willing that one be healed. In both cases the 'medicine-field' is the bush where one goes to gather medicinal plants, and people say that medicine is like food, something provided by God so that people may grow and prosper. Culture thus encompasses even the wilderness of the bush.

Though this is not emphasised in *kulandila* invocations, people say that the ultimate outcome of any medicine or *erisi* depends upon the willingness of one's *mizimu* to grant one's wish. *Mizimu* and their determining power are connected to one's life situation through one's will; and that situation also includes one's will and one's relation to the *mizimu*. If one slackens in one's determination to effect a given transformation, or if anger (*asira*) obstructs one's willingness, say, to be cured, the *mizimu*, too, must slacken their resolution. Medicines cannot possibly be effective under such circumstances. Inversely, neglect of *mizimu* and their needs can result in their refusing to aid one, despite the permanence of one's own intent.

Thus, if the fabrication and use of medicines and *erisi* constitutes human action to change and human transcendence over the limitations of a given reality, the awareness of the greater will of the *mizimu* constitutes human acceptance of the necessity of limitation. People will say of an unfortunate death that it would not have happened had it not been willed by the victim's *mizimu*, and in theory this is true even for cases of death by sorcery. They also state the inverse, saying that no matter how terrible the illness, one will not die if one's God does not wish it so.

Further, the inextricable association of *Mungu* and *mitishamba* in one sense represents the human awareness of the duality of ultimate and proximate. In this, one is conscious of the fact that the ultimate outcome of any situation is unknown, just as the (ultimate) will of the *mizimu* can be known only in and through the unfolding of events. Yet for this ultimate will to have concrete existence, it must be connected to or substantiated in a situation by a series of proximate acts which delineate its meaning, and which are themselves actively unified and bound to the ultimate by a proximate will.

The ultimate and the proximate thus form contexts for each other. In the long, ultimate view, the proximate takes on its true meaning, while the ultimate has no existence apart from the proximate's substantiation of it. Separated, both are without sense. Meaning without context and context without meaning are both forms of absurdity. It is in this way that *Mungu* and *mitishamba* extend and augment one another. The analytic illumination by each of the other's character is demonstrated in Figure 10.1.

In this figure are illustrated the relations among people, their *mizimu*, their medicines/*erisi* and their situations. The figure is based upon the balanced complementarity of 'religious' and 'magical' circumstantial therapies, and an examination of it reveals features of each that might otherwise remain obscure.

As their placement in Figure 10.1 indicates, the power and significance of such non-human beings as *mizimu* and *bilumbu* are best understood when it is recognised that they themselves *are* transformation. The inscrutability of their transformative capacity derives from the fact that their intention is deed; that they are, in some sense, pure process. If they are angry with an

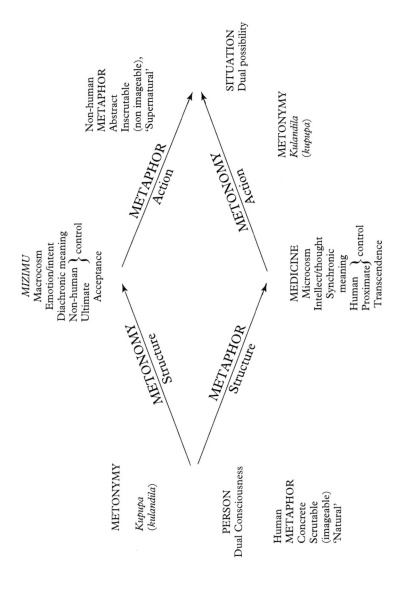

Figure 10.1 Complementarity of circumstantial therapies

individual he immediately becomes ill. If they feel mercy toward him, he is blessed. Thus, the attitudes of spirits have as their unmediated substantiations the events unfolding in reality. Hence, one of the functions of 'religious' circumstantial therapy is the establishment through speech of a substantial medium, within which these abstractly effected, but materially realised, transformations can take place.

Mizimu and *pepo* effect their transformations without themselves changing or departing from their realm. This fixity and otherness of nature is represented at the establishment of the relationship by the intervention of various intermediaries through whose agency human and spirit interact. Thus, with *bilumbu* the *kitobo/kapamba* of the diviner interprets the pronouncements of the spirit to the assembled throng and, most importantly, communicates these to the *kapondo*, the spirit's human vehicle, who was not conscious during the time the spirit spoke. Those receiving a *mikalaye* or other *bulumbu* spirit similarly have *kapamba* assistants, whose responsibility is the reception of the spirit's emblems and their fires.

Misambwa are likewise established through the mediation of those archetypal complements, the 'grandchildren' (*wijukulu*) or joking partners (*baendo*). Finally, *mikalaye* spirits punish not by changing their essentially beneficent nature, but by dispatching *kabwangozi*, the punishing dog.

For the purposes of this analysis, we can assign the label 'metaphor' to the actions of *mizimu* and *pepo* if not to these non-human beings *per se*. They are transformative while themselves remaining unchanged and removed from visible reality. Communication with *mizimu* is thus the actualisation of words which are made to emerge from the inchoate processes offered them by means of the net of speech thrown over (that is, spoken around and into) these.

Inversely, the structure of an *erisi* (amulet) is nothing other than a substantial, fabricated version of this abstract metaphoric power, an actualisation through meanings. Where *mizimu*, *pepo* and the dead (*wafu*) have the infinite variety of the material world's objects and events through which to make manifest their will, human beings, for their part, have a finite number of *vizimba*, which may be combined and recombined in an endless number of ways, then universalised through invocation, so that they constitute a miniature of reality.

Via this microcosm, human beings exert a proximate control over the movements of objects in the substantial world and over the consciousnesses of others. They thereby direct the unfolding of social and natural events, affecting the course and outcome of life itself. Hence, one of the functions of 'magical' circumstantial therapy is the establishment of a metaphoric structure through which the future can take shape.

'Religious' and 'magical' circumstantial therapies can thus be described as inverse opposites using processes like metaphor and metonymy in complementary ways. It is therefore not surprising that human intent (*nia*) should be the pivotal point through which people and *mizimu* (and other non-human beings) are connected in the active, realised form of their relation. Just as the *wafu* stand as directors and sources of ultimate meaning in relation to the macrocosm of human reality, so do human beings stand as directors in relation to the microcosm of human reality that is the *erisi* and that includes the person himself. Human transcendence as 'magical' circumstantial therapy thus takes the same form as godliness and, in so far as they are able, human beings control life by standing as god in relation to themselves and their world.[4]

People indicate their recognition of this identity when they state with wry humour that a sorcerer is God, or God's 'younger brother' (*mulozi ni mungu, ama mdogo wake*). This master of medicines is godly because he does things to one's body of which one has no idea. Like God, he puts illness inside and yet leaves no lesion or other sign of intrusion. Further, his medicines enable him to live forever; one is always amazed to hear a sorcerer has died. Finally, a sorcerer may cure those who were moribund, whom one thought would surely die.

Despite the inverse identity between human and non-human transcendent power, however, human godliness remains proximate and limited. When I suggested to Mumbyoto that *mwanzambale*'s strength lay partly in the fact that it was a microcosm (*kadunia*, literally 'little world') of all possibility, he, without batting an eye, replied that it was 'not a microcosm of great endurance; for, if they like, they will kill you all the same' (*si kadunia ya kuendelea zaidi; sababu wakipenda, watakuua vile-vile*). Though proximate success is all that is necessary in a proximate world, people are conscious of the fact that even this relies on ultimate will. As Lukwesa put it, 'even a sorcerer begs his god' (*hata mulozi anamuomba mungu wake*) for success in his wicked acts.

In our final conceptualisation of the intricate interrelation between 'religious' and 'magical' circumstantial therapies, we can depict an almost endless series of micro-within-macro-within-microcosms; analogous worlds which contain differing versions of one another, fitted together like so many concentric circles. At the centre would be the imagined worlds that would be contained in the 'thoughts' of the microcosmic person represented by hair, fingernails, etc., and made whole in the process of invocation.

The next ring would be the microcosmic person himself, who is in turn contained by the world of the *mwanzambale erisi*. This is itself contained by the real situation, which is in turn contained and controlled by the will or imagination of the *mizimu/mipasi*. Containing all of this is the self-consciousness of the human being, whose imagination stretches from micro-cosmic to macrocosmic limits to make sense of the events of life, and meets himself in them innumerable times.

This form of concentric rings is ultimately nothing other than a stable rendition of the spiral; it is a synchronic representation of infinity. As such, it is related to a number of other forms of infinity in Tabwa cosmology. Among these are the *mpande* shell, whose concentric rings represent the infinity of chiefly continuity, and the 'belt' (*mukaba*) worn by successive inheritors of a given name, which thus represents the continuity of kinship.

Finally, this model of infinity also has a counterpart in the birth of a girl child. During labour, one of the midwives sits behind the naked mother, squatting much as the mother herself does and supporting the mother by holding her between her legs. She is thus in some sense giving birth to a mother who is in turn giving birth to the child. If the child is a girl, she contains within herself yet another generation, and BaTabwa, matrilineal, make delighted note of this when they comment that 'if you give birth to a girl you give birth twice' (*ukizaa mtoto mwanamuke unazaa mara mbili*).

NOTES

BY WAY OF AN INTRODUCTION

1. An Anglophone example: as we were descending towards the anthropology building on the University of Cape Town's campus, a friend and colleague there, fluent in but not born to English, suddenly paused, glanced down, and asked 'Now are these steps or are these stairs?'

CHAPTER 1 DIMENSIONS OF THE BODY

1. This will be evident in the discussion of bodily therapies in Chapter 7.
2. 'KS' indicates the term in KiSwahili and KT the KiTabawa term. English terms are in quotes because they are glosses, rather than translations. Even where the physiological structure indicated is the same, its functions are sufficiently different to warrant this qualification.
3. The same KiSwahili term refers both to the brain and to bone marrow.
4. The association of the *safura* or spleen with pathological conditions is quite in keeping not only with the observations made in the field, but also with those of biomedicine. De Gowan and De Gowan (1971) indicate that the spleen may radically increase in size, becoming as much as forty times larger than normal in the presence of certain illnesses, among them malaria and measles (1971: 486–7). In vivax malaria infections the spleen may become sufficiently enlarged to be palpable by the end of the second week of an attack. In children suffering chronic infection, the spleen may become enormous, extending into the pelvis.

    With chronic cases of *kimbeleka*, the spleen is frequently visible at a time when the child appears most anaemic and listless. Clearly, in experience, the *safura* grows great at the blood's expense. Splenic rub, as well as internal congestion, may account for the shortness of breath often seen at this time.
5. Two cases of this illness occurred during my stay. Tests made in the village showed the patients to be suffering from diabetes, with excreted sugars accounting for some 2 per cent of their urine. People also have an illness category *ugonjuwa wa sukari* ('the illness of sugar'), which is the term used in hospital diagnosis of diabetes.
6. I have seen a number of cases of *mududu*, and the visual progress of the illness conforms to this image. According to the Merck Manual, inflammation in osteomyelitis is frequently of the marrow, which expands as the infection progresses. In addition, the pressure within the bone of the pus emitted during the course of the illness contributes to its splitting. In Zaire, even in those cases where the inflammation is of the tendons rather than of the bone itself (a condition also called *mududu*), the infection may become such that the flesh of the finger splits or a number of small holes open up, which resemble the holes made in trees or posts by burrowing grubs and woodworms. The pus produced

by such infection is rapidly destructive of cartilage; and my experience has been
that loss of the use of the joint is always the result of *mududu* illness, regardless of
whatever other outcome it might have.

7. The apical ancestress of a lineage may be called *shina* or *kishina* as well as
mamazizi.

8. Though it might be so among Zulu (cf. Ngubane 1977), digestion is not a model
for spiritual or ritual transformations. On the contrary, there are important
respects in which digestion is the archetype of the specific and the mundane,
while the role of significant transformer is exclusively reserved to sexual
intercourse. While they exercise normal care with reference to their diet, people
are not overly concerned with balancing internal equilibria by means of
controlled food consumption (as are, for example, the Lele, cf. Douglas 1975).
In a manner reminiscent of comments of BaBemba (Richards 1969: 54)
regarding spoiled meat, an acerbic old soul once told me that anything one did
not vomit after eating could be counted as food. Similarly people justify the ideal
of sharing by saying that it is unreasonable to deny food to someone, especially a
child, because, ultimately, 'food is just shit in the bush' (*chakula ni mavi mupori*)
and therefore not an object worthy of such selfishness.

9. People see this process in the hen's egg. The white is the male part, while the yolk
is the female. Fond of riddles, they jokingly ask themselves why it is that, given
the male/female, bones/flesh division, one often sees in flocks many chickens
whose feathers are identical to the rooster's.

10. The transformation is also called 'to give water to the child' (*kumupa mtoto maji*),
a term which plays upon the double meaning of the word 'water', often employed
as a euphemism for semen.

11. In infants and children, the visible symptom of this is the mucosal rectal prolapse
of biomedicine. Such a condition often accompanies illness in children whose
nutritional status is marginal. *Kidonda tumbo* often appears simultaneously with
other illnesses. It is, however, a separate disease entity, which has its own
secondary symptoms and its own treatments.

12. Despite the fixity of its symptoms, *buse* is not always regarded as a true illness.
People justify this view on the grounds that there is no curative treatment, only
this prophylactic one.

13. Such grasses and their method of illumination also have meaning, which is
discussed below.

14. The formation and significance of such substances are discussed below.

15. Pleasure or the expression of affection through sex have become an increasingly
important part of marital relations as more and more young people select their
own spouses. Freedom of choice is now universally accepted, though people in
their late thirties and early forties may have married by arrangement.

16. Cunnison, in his study of the Luapula peoples, describes the form taken by this
ceremony in that area (1959: 90–103).

17. In this repect the body as subject resembles goats, dogs and children, which all
share the characteristic of being able to hear without being able to speak. Like
adults and children, goats and dogs when stolen and killed are able to return as
avenging ghosts (*vibanda*), and indeed may be instructed to do so by their
embittered owners. The *vibanda* of goats and dogs are sometimes the causes of
repeated deaths of a household's children.

18. With these syndromes, contact with an adulterous spouse/parent (*mililo*) or with
his partner (*nsanga*) results in a dangerous reduction in the bodily integrity of
members of the adulterer's household.

19. The form of infantile diarrhoea sometimes caused by excessive conjugal inter-

course during the late stages of pregnancy.

20. *Mikia* are antelope-tail fly-whisks, elaborately decorated and filled with the medicines which make them into one of the power-objects at the Tulunga diviner's disposal. A *mukia* will contain particular *vizimba* which are closely associated with fire and transformations. In addition, for his medicine to be effective, the diviner must drink no water during his trip.

21. Most bundles of such grasses are simply pulled up from alongside the road. However, it is perhaps because they do not constitute a noticeable (or 'marked') feature of the landscape – a specific point past which people move – that this characteristic is not *explicitly* part of their meaning.

22. In a similar fashion, people may begin a 'new' fire with matches or by friction. This may be seen as the establishment of simple discontinuity – disjuncture without the destruction of what is past.

23. A full description of the techniques employed in the fabrication of medicines is outlined below.

24. Hot water can be seen as the material bridge uniting the cultural analogues of fire and coitus. A wife who desires sexual relations with her husband indicates this by heating water for him in the evening, so that he may bathe in it. Similarly, it was formerly the practice after intercourse to heat water in a small marriage pot and for the wife to cleanse her husband using it (cf. Richards 1956; Cunnison 1959). Lack of such a pot and warm water was what rendered adultery especially dangerous. Another wifely duty is the preparation of the hot water with which the husband bathes every morning.

25. People refer to the normal, spotted individuals of this same species by another name, *libalabala*. They are aware, however, that the only difference between the two, as animals, is in coloration; and have observed that spotted and melanistic individuals may be found in the same litter.

26. *Kapondo* is a particular sort of outlaw who travels from village to village setting fire to the houses of chiefs from the simple satisfaction of seeing the disorder the fire creates. Such a person may also stand in the peripheral darkness and kill those who rush to extinguish the blaze. When caught, the *kapondo* may be burnt, making the *kanfitwa* type of *kizimba* noted above; or he may be struck dead by a blow to the head with an axe. Purists such as Kalwele say that this latter type is the only true variety of *kapondo*, because the large number of people involved in the burning of *kapondo kanfitwa* dilutes its power as a *kizimba*. In any case, *kapondo* is the most important *kizimba* contained in a Tulunga diviner's horn.

　　In 1966, two youths sought to rob the office of the chief Kansabala, who then resided at Kiobwe, a day's walk from Mpala. To distract the populace, they set fire to the chief's house, and stole the cash box under cover of the disorder which followed. However, they were caught and were burnt alive by the villagers on orders of the chief and one of his advisors. Their relics were still being employed by Tulunga practitioners at the time of my field stay.

27. This is a distinct state of being or phase in an illness occurrence. Marked by the physiological phenomena noted above, the stage *mugonjuwa hatari* also has its social characteristics. These include the notification and gathering together of distant kin of the patient; final efforts in seeking treatment (if the case is not considered hopeless); visitation by local friends and neighbours; and nightly vigils of an increasing number of people. Paradoxically, such increased activity appears to be both the community's greatest moral effort that a person not die, and the start of its preparations for the person's death.

28. Kibawa is also the residence of a Bulumbu spirit of the same name: one of the most important of the possessing types. BaTabwa indicate that long ago people

made pilgrimages to the cave, to have disputes settled or to learn the reasons for misfortune. In the cave, though they could see nothing, people would hear all the sounds of village life, and they would be addressed by their deceased kin, whose voices they would recognise. The spirit Kibawa himself would make the pronouncements and predictions.

29. For a description and analysis of the form of the *msambwa* shrine and the process by which it is created, see below.

30. The two can be seen as inverse analogues of one another as well. As the place for the transformation of blood into human, the womb is nature contained in society. As the place where the body decomposes, the grave is society contained by nature.

31. The dead are conscious of their dependence upon the living and take care to remind the living of their obligations by appearing to them in dreams. A person who is not remembered is ridiculed (by the other dead) for poverty.

32. In discussions of dreams, particularly those in which one's *mizimu* appear, people are quick to note that one never sees *mizimu* except in times of conflict or stress. If one has 'many thoughts' (*mawazo mengi*) on the ills of the world, or if one has just quarrelled with kin or spouse, one is likely to be visited in dreams by a dead antecedent who either wishes to be remembered or chides one for one's quarrelsome nature (*ugomvi*). On the other hand, if one has spent the day at a beer-drink singing and joking with kin and friends one will cheerfully stumble home, fall into bed happy, and sleep without dreaming a thing.

33. As noted above (p. 60), the term *pepo*, which has 'wind' as one of its meanings, is also used to refer to spirits, usually those of the land that are called *ngulu*. In addition, the soul of a dead person who is not yet buried is also called *pepo*, and can enter the body of a child who is given an enema in the village before the burial has taken place. Following a similar logic, it was formerly the practice to refrain from administering enemas at noon and at dusk, as these are the hours during which the spirits of dead persons are most active. The entrance of such a spirit into the body of the child exacerbates the illness or results in death. Mothers are currently somewhat less concerned about the dangers of the noon hour. 'What is one to do', they ask, 'if the child has a high fever?'

34. Not without some irony, people say that in the old days, death was such a rare occurrence that people would come from miles around to view the body in amazement. Funerals took a week and only mature people could attend, not silly adolescents. Everyone would quarrel over who would get to wear the best clothes. But these days, so many people die that it is no longer amazing; and a funeral that lasted a week would have few guests because of the others so closely succeeding it.

CHAPTER 2 THE DISORDER OF THINGS I

1. I worked with one group of laymen, two *wafumu*, practitioners with divinatory powers (one Tulunga, one Bulumbu), and one herbalist who did not divine.

2. Requests for the similarity uniting the whole group were meant to offset a tendency towards classification through diadic pairing. In this an illness might be classed with a particular group because it shared a feature with one member of that group, which member had itself been classified on the basis of another, altogether different, but individual feature of its own.

3. In the act of classifying, the criteria took the form of the reasons given for the unification of certain illnesses into a particular group.

4. Though the site of appearance is the same for all of these diseases, they are not

developmentally related to one another. The grouping into which they are formed therefore cannot be said to employ existential criteria.

5. Despite its visual resemblance to one, this is not a taxonomic chart, and it is to be noted that the two systems are, in fact, quite different. The criteria for groups and subgroups in Table 2.2 are *features* around which the groups are formed. They do *not* show terms of increasing generality by which such groups might be called. The illness marked with an asterisk may be classed in more than one way. The openness of this system, compared to a taxonomy, is part of its function, and serves its own purpose.

6. Though some of the larger boils can be exceptions to this, they are none the less classified with their lesser kin.

7. I have seen a number of cases of *mbavu*, and, in all of them symptoms included not only cough, chest congestion and rib pain, but also severe headache, thoracic, abdominal and lower back pain, constipation, and loss of appetite. In two cases there was also profuse sweating at night, and in several others coughing of blood. However, none of the second set of symptoms figures in the description of the disease. Had they done so, it would have had to have been reclassified as *mkola*, with its far more negative prognosis.

8. Kilimamboka even included 'keloids' (*loni*) in his subgroup of swellings which do not emit pus, though others refused to do so, and, in fact, refused to class this phenomenon as an illness, because it is painless and besides, 'you went and invited it' by seeking the decorative satisfaction of which *loni* is sometimes an unfortunate side-effect.

9. Kilimamboka classed this with other members of Group IIIa, because like them, 'styes' are not treated medically. Luvunzo and Kalulu classed 'stye' with non-itching eruptions.

CHAPTER 3 THE DISORDER OF THINGS II

1. These spirits appear to have come from the Luba area to the north and west of Tabwa. Non-possessing spirits are the same as Luba *bavidye*. Possessing spirits have been assimilated into an older group of indigenous land spirits, *ngulu*, relations with which have also changed in recent years.

2. This, and all other mammal identifications were made through the use of Dorst and Dandelot's *Field Guide to the Larger Mammals of Africa* (1969).

3. 'Possession' does not mean a psychic state of complete dissociation such as one finds in shamanism. 'Possession' appears instead to be the adoption of an alternative identity, that of the spirit. Though the adoption is quite complete, in terms of behaviour, the consciousness of the possessed individual is nevertheless not only aware of minor aspects of the environment, but even acts as the director of the *mise-en-scène* while the *kitobo/kapamba* has the role of stage manager.

4. It is an interesting reflection of the equalitarian principles upon which present Tabwa society is founded that *mizimu* are said to respond equally to the complaints of junior and senior lineage members. As my friend Katato put it, 'even a child must have his justice'; and *mizimu* might afflict a mother's brother for wronging his sister's son.

5. It is this division, as well, which characterises old age, and which people see as one of ageing's greatest burdens. People are also very aware of the effects of long-term, incapacitating illness upon the consciousness, which becomes more and more consumed by purely physiological concerns as the illness becomes increasingly serious.

6. This transfigurative capacity of speech is realised in its most condensed form in

the fact that, at death, a person's voice becomes light or goes into light. Encrypted here is a conjunction between the integrity of speech and discernment of sight, which elsewhere appears as the identification of knowledge with identity-as-being; that is, knowledge which implicates the bodily being of the knower as well as the identity of the known.

CHAPTER 4 THE DEFILE OF THE SIGNIFIER

1. The names of all individuals who figure in this and the following case histories have been changed to protect the privacy of those who shared their experiences with me. Since most of the people on whom the histories are centred are friends of mine, and since illness is a time of crisis and concerned questioning, I myself am present in some episodes as an active participant.
2. Kaputa was one of several people who gathered and dried the medicinal plant specimens in my collection.
3. One hundred *makuta* (singular, *likuta*, abbreviation 'k') equals one zaire.
4. This was the diviner Polombwe, who also figures in Kiabu's case (Chapter 5) and Kulimba's (Chapter 6). He was famous for the roles he had earlier played in the detection of sorcerers in Mpala and Kapanza villages.
5. For example, if he and a group of companions committed some infraction only he would be caught.
6. Before beginning his work, however, the diviner asked specifically about Kalwa's relatives, demanding of Kaputa the reason why they were not present.
7. This particular diviner placed the pot on the fire with his hands. Another practitioner, however, said that this should be done with the feet.
8. *Nkula* here represents the bloody or deadly aspects of human life, and *pemba* the white, bountiful or beneficent aspects.
9. Placing *nkula* on the centre of the forehead, at the location of the mental activity of sight, is said to put blood in the diviner's eyes (*kuweka damu mu macho*). It shows he has no relatives or friends among men and is prepared to tell the truth, even if it is deadly, no matter whom it affects.
10. This particular diviner conducted his seance without letting the water actually boil, though it was quite hot. I have attended other sessions at which the water repeatedly came to a full, rolling boil during the questioning.
11. This gourd contains the same ingredients as the *kalunga* horn itself, and is the place in which are seen the circumstances in question at the divination.
12. Many people consider this to be mere theatrics, designed to convince the client that the diviner is really seeing into their affairs. They say that the fact, however, is that he has had his insights the night before in a dream and at the session is only reciting what he saw there.
13. It is customary for such a story to be told at the outset of the divination. Kalwele says that one can give such a story at the time the arrow is received.
14. Here, my recollection of what was said differed from Kaputa's. His version is discussed at an appropriate point below.
15. At the time I felt this was a test of Kaputa's truthfulness. A diviner who thinks his clients are wrongfully resisting his truths may challenge one of them to plunge his hand into the boiling water to retrieve the *lukusu*. Only an innocent person may do so. I believed the diviner thought Kaputa would expect the *lukusu* to burn him if he were lying, and so would involuntarily flinch, thus revealing himself.
16. *Mukulaye* and *kabwangozi* are two of the types of non-possessing *bulumbu* spirits prevalent around Mpala.

17. At the death of a married adult, the person's spouse must pay indemnity and be cleansed of the death by the deceased's family. This is done by marking the centre of the forehead with *pemba*.
18. This would be done by means of the ceremony of 'throwing the person in the bush'.
19. If *wazimu* lasts for six months, it is considered incurable. This case would be doubly so, owing to the refusal of the woman's affines to remove the ultimate cause of the illness.

CHAPTER 5 ILLNESS AND PERSONAL HISTORY

1. I have reserved commentary for the end of this history because my points refer not only to its component episodes but also to the case as a whole.
2. Because of its size, Mpala offered a greater number of therapeutic alternatives both biomedical and 'traditional' (*ya asili*) than did many of the smaller lakeside villages.
3. The next village north of Mpala, some two miles away.
4. Illnesses of the consciousness, such as 'lunacy' (*wazimu*), 'epilepsy' (*kifafa*), and 'infantile convulsions' (*ndege*) can sometimes derive from inappropriate proximity of human and spirit (*pepo*). Urination is an indication that the spirit has removed itself from the body and/or that the strength of the illness is weakening.
5. This is not entirely true. *Ndege* is a serious illness, and people treat it very much as though it is potentially fatal.
6. Divination into death is called *mululubululo*, and costs substantially more than the ordinary divination.
7. This same person also divined into Kalwa's disturbing visions(Chapter 4), and into Kisile's daughter's illness (Chapter 6).
8. This was an exceptionally high price and reflected both the reputation of the diviner and the significance of the divination.
9. The sex of the person is not marked in the third person pronoun in Swahili, and in looking back at my notes I realise I never learned this diviner's gender.
10. A reaction such as this can sometimes occur after the administration of certain traditional medicines. As is noted below, the small and large intestine are highly permeable to medicinal and toxic plant substances.
11. Kneading involves the fairly strong-handed grasping and pulling of limbs, and the forceful squeezing of muscles. This is sometimes part of the treatment for certain illnesses, and is rather disagreeable to the patient, against whose pleas for gentleness the family must harden their hearts. When one has been kneaded by sorcerers during the night, one awakens the next day feeling as though one has not slept a wink. You are tired, not refreshed; you feel aches and pains in your limbs; your neck is stiff; and your outlook is generally gloomy.
12. Called *kupiga mbila*, this practice of shouting threats to people who are vaguely described but not named is a customary response to sorcery.
13. He had recently lost another wife, who had died in childbirth six weeks before. As his involvement with Kiabu preceded his first wife's delivery, the husband was held doubly responsible. He was made to pay to his affines 50 zaires, as well as goods.
14. Early in my stay, Citoyen Katumpwe very generously offered to examine and treat free of charge anyone whom I brought to his clinic. He gave instruction regarding the diagnosis and treatment of common illnesses in Mpala, and the appropriate channelling of patients in Kalemie. He is the hero of this piece.
15. There are parts of the description which follows that may seem to the European

reader to range from melodramatic to shocking. They are included here only to show the difficulties which were encountered by rural dwellers if they chose the hospital as an alternative.

16. This type of packaging is common for injectable medication and such a form would be especially representative of European medicine (*dawa ya kizungu*).

17. Dr Mwendy would not have been able to find anything amiss, had the illness been caused by sorcery.

18. Also called *kutekuna*.

19. Such dreaming is called *kuzozota*, and constitutes a perception of sorcery, indirect in that the sorcerer substitutes the faces or persons of others – often one's best friends – for his or her own.

20. I know this group to have included other friends of mine who, at that very moment, were *themselves* coming to Mpala with reports of conflicts involving sorcery.

21. This is an idealisation of the norm. It is quite usual however, for the chief, like the local diviner, to take the most conservative and passive position possible with reference to suspicions and accusations of sorcery.

22. *Nzunzi* are small figurines carved by sorcerers, and activated through medicines, which can be sent, invisible, to steal or kill.

23. These are also representatives or signs of spirits, specifically of *kabwangozi*, the dog accompanying *mukalaye*.

24. Snakes are one of the forms taken by the *ngulu* spirits, and have been assimilated into *bulumbu*.

25. The syndrome *tumbo kupanda* ('the abdomen mounts') is characterised by the sensation of abdominal fullness. Patients with *tumbo kupanda* often also complain of constipation, epigastric pain, and lack of appetite and weakness, though they are not part of the illness description. *Tumbo kupanda* frequently follows another major illness. Late in my stay I found it to be the result of a deficiency of vitamin B1 (thiamine). Treatment of only one or two days resulted in the dramatic remission of all symptoms, which is characteristic of thiamine deficiency.

26. Her husband's salary had not been paid in several months; looking into this was the reason for his trip.

27. People are quick to note the highly legalistic approach taken by diviners to situations such as this. Even if the person whom one suspects of sorcery is, in fact, a sorcerer, and even if this person has caused illness to one on another occasion, if he or she is not specifically responsible for the particular illness into which one is divining, the diviner will not name him or her.

CHAPTER 6 ILLNESS AND LOCAL HISTORY

1. As defined by V. W. Turner in his *Schism and Continuity in an African Society* (1957).

2. This name, as well as those of lineage members currently living, has been changed.

3. While the lineage group blamed neighbours who had been accompanying Mbwisha at the time of her death, others in town said they had done it themselves, to put her soul into the motor, and thereby ensure the success of their transport business.

4. Like names, clan identities have also been changed.

5. Other significant illnesses struck more distant members of the lineage, but affected the local group only mildly and are not discussed here. Insignificant illnesses affecting members of the group are also not discussed.

6. The diviner in this case was none other than Polombwe, renowned (or notorious) for his pivotal role in several celebrated cases. The same practitioner divined into an early case of Kaputa's, and into the death of Kiabu's daughter.

7. It is customary to use the third person plural in this circumstance to indicate that one has no idea whatsoever regarding the identity of the culprit(s).

8. Kiondwa, Kulimba's mother, seemed unimpressed with this particular treatment, as *mululuzia* is a very common medicine, frequently used by mothers in treatment of infantile skin diseases, as well as in treatment of fevers.

9. In the days immediately following our return and the recounting of the story, the *mfumu* failed several times to visit Kulimba and bring her new supplies of medicines to replace those whose strength had been spent. During this time, Kisile visited the diviner daily, to remind him of his promise. On one day the *mfumu* himself was ill, requiring an injection by the local dispensary's nurse; on another, he was called away to divine into the current *cause célèbre*. Both the interruption of treatment and the persistence of Kisile are characteristic of traditional medical practice (*dawa ya asili*).

10. Kulimba's parents had become involved in a case of sudden death when they stopped at a beer drink on their way home from the initial divination into their daughter's illness. They spent several months awaiting resolution of the matter in another village, two days' walk from Mpala. The case against them was dismissed.

11. The lesions were very reminiscent of *Pitoriasis rosea*, a self-limiting viral disease, whose biomedical progress is similar to that of Kulimba's illness.

12. If its dried umbilical cord touches an infant's genitals when it drops off, the child will be rendered impotent/infertile. The practice of tying a cloth over the sex organ is meant to prevent such an accident. In ordinary circumstances, failure to do this would be tantamount to sorcery.

13. This was the same day as Kisile and Kiondwa visited Polombwe to inform him of Kulimba's recovery and to ask his price. In fact, I went from one session directly to the other.

14. I obtained permission both from Matipa, Kibambo's husband, and from Kipetele, Mitwele's husband. This was one of the first divinations I attended.

15. Such a repudiation of an unborn child is itself sufficient to cause miscarriage.

16. This ignorance, as well as ignorance of etiquette, also caused me to commit several *faux pas* in this instance. Among these was asking if I might not attend the divination. Two years later, when I did find out that others' divinations are not a fit subject for polite conversation, I assumed that everyone had grown so accustomed to my gaucheness that there was no point in changing.

17. In addition, it also provides insight into relations among diviners, and the effect these have upon the outcome of divination.

18. Several months later, Kisile told me that Kipetele and Mitwele had determined to divorce during the pregnancy itself. Their parents, however, had prevailed upon them to remain together until the birth of the child, so relations could end on an amiable note.

19. A normal pulse is 70–90 beats per minute.

20. Many say that a drop or two of this is sufficient medication for adults. Cases of 'serious irritant poisoning with fatalities' are reported by Watt and Breyer-Brandwijk (1962: 407). Verdecourt and Trump describe the poisonous principle as euphorbon, a mixture of two alcohols, but say little is known about it (1969: 50–2). The symptoms they provide correspond very closely to those manifested by Bulela.

21. The sarong style in which Kibambo wore the cloth she swept in the dirt was itself

indicative of her state of mourning for mother. During this period women maintain symbolic bare-chestedness by refraining from wearing blouses and simply wrapping their skirts around their chests under the armpits.

22. People are well aware of the fact that, at least with the first type, it is the element of potential truth which gives this joking its special (and especially amusing) quality. One's *mwendo* might actually *be* a sorcerer, but in the context of the relationship she or he would have to take the accusation as a joke.

23. Though providing carbohydrate energy, *uji* is almost completely lacking in other nutritional value, from a biomedical point of view. In addition, patients are usually unable or unwilling to take as much of it as they should. Prolonged illness with extensive reliance upon this food usually results, therefore, in considerable wasting of the body. Rural farming conditions and irregularity of availability of produce contributed greatly, in my opinion, to certain basic inadequacies in nutritional support during illness, despite the quality of nursing care.

24. Violent episodes of 'lunacy' *(wazimu)* are the only exception to this general rule. In these instances, the person may be constrained for their own and for others' safety.

25. Due to their temporal proximity and their thematic interrelation, Episodes Six and Seven will be described separately, but discussed together.

26. My specimen of this was so poor as to be unidentifiable. Kisile described this as being 'large *kanoka*', which might make it a species of euphorbia.

27. This is described in Chapter 1, p. 61.

28. In discussing it later, Masele and Kisile said that part of the problem lay in the nature of the illness itself. Had it been one where the child lingered, they might have been motivated to try again, perhaps with greater sincerity and success, to terminate their conflict. As it was, because everyone saw the child was moribund, nobody made the effort.

CHAPTER 7 BODILY THERAPIES

1. In fact the world of artefacts and lifestyles is divided into the two broad categories *kizungu* and *kinchi* (of the land). The European pole of the duality is now completely disengaged from Euro-Americans themselves, and has come to include those Zairians who lead an urbanised, upper middle- and upper-class life. The opposition is situationally sensitive, as well. Urbanised Zairians may define themselves as *kinchi* when opposing themselves to Europeans. Rural dwellers may define their use of matches and kerosene (instead of fire sticks and fish oil) as *kizungu*. Indeed, the present moment is regarded as *kizungu* when contrasted to the days 'of long ago' *(ya zamani)*. In the light of this, it should come as no surprise that all practitioners of European medicines are Zairian.

2. Without the help of Allen Roberts this practice would not have been possible. He not only recorded the information that arose during the clinic's session, but helped to maintain the records we kept of individuals' treatment; and, above all, he organised our life in such a way that the bulk of the cash income from his grant could be spent on medicines.

3. Shortly after leaving the area, I received word of a cholera epidemic brought into the city from Kigoma, Tanzania. Through correspondence with the US Consulate at Lubumbashi, I learned that the railroad company undertook control of the outbreak through vaccination of Kalemie's population of 150,000. They did not, however, also vaccinate residents of lakeside villages, and I was informed that hundreds died, including at least 25 adults at Mpala.

4. My personal experience with practitioners contradicts this assertion. In discussion,

I found them to be quite specific about the quantities of medicines to be employed. Bulela's was the only case of one brought close to death by a practitioner's error, though several others suffered shock from self-prescribed overdoses.

5. The following general description is based directly upon the experiences of the various individuals whom I took with me to Kalemie for treatment. The only modification I have made is the removal of myself, so to speak, from the situation.

6. The trip to Moba would be substantially less complex from certain points of view. The town is really only a large village; it is within the same zone as Mpala; and it is considerably closer than Kalemie. The problems of obtaining food and lodging, and of paying hospital fees (as well as the price of medicine), are identical to those obtaining in the larger city, however. In addition, though the town of Moba is on the lake itself, the hospital is on top of a mountain which rises above it; a distance of two hours' brisk walk for a healthy person, virtually impossible for a sick one.

7. Ova of both *S. Mansoni* and *S. Haematobium* were found in Mpala residents' urine and stools. A dose of 25 mg/kg/day orally in divided doses for 7–10 days is considered effective against both types of fluke.

8. So important is the therapeutic value of the enema that my friends were astonished to hear that I had managed to become over 30 years of age without ever in my life having had an enema.

CHAPTER 8 THE LOGIC OF THE SUBSTANTIAL WORLD

1. Knowledge of medicines is, for the most part, orally transmitted. Written description of treatment is considered by many to be inadequate. This is not only because written formulae are accessible to anyone who can read, regardless of character or temperament; but also because a written description must fall short of the experience of explanation, demonstration and practice that is the totality of apprenticeship.

   Certain practitioners are nevertheless inclined to commit their formulae to paper. In some cases, the small school notebook in which medicines and treatments are outlined constitutes part of the inheritance which will be left to succeeding generations; in others it is a device by which new cures learned from colleagues may not be forgotten. People are fully aware of the fragility of oral knowledge over time, and the loss to the community of various therapies is one of the principle topics of conversation at the funerals of renowned specialists.

2. While these symptoms change *ndege* to *sinsa* in theory, in practice, as with the illness *mkola* ('tuberculosis'), the consequences of the change are such that people are reluctant to apply the more serious term.

3. I have seen *tutumusi*, but was unable to identify the substance. Nor was I able to obtain a sample for subsequent identification.

4. Nzuiba says he does not approve of the storage of liquid medicines because they might become contaminated. He uses powdered medicine into which he mixes ground *kizimba* of the *geogeo* or chameleon, 'so that the patient may not know' (*asijue*) what she is taking.

5. As with this, self-administration of other *viabiko* must be done in silence, which duplicates the unmarked, non-verbal qualities of pregnancy's onset.

6. In health, women should feel nothing during the course of the menstrual cycle, and the menses themselves ought to last only three days each month. As a rule, women do not announce the onset of pregnancy even to their intimates until several months have elapsed. In addition, it is considered very bad form and

(because of sorcery) extremely dangerous to make a general announcement of the condition, or to indicate the onset of labour. Ideally, these things are merely observed; and the model for correct conduct at birth is that one's neighbours will note with surprise that one is no longer pregnant.

7. One uneventful year after her first attack, the child of a good friend was again stricken with *ndege*. No one could imagine why the illness had returned. However, it was finally determined that when eating at a relative's, the child had been served food that had been prepared in a clay pot that had previously been used to prepare chicken. This food cannot be eaten by persons afflicted with 'convulsions' because of the similarity between the seizures and the motions made by a chicken when dust-bathing.

CHAPTER 9 EVENTS OBJECTIFIED

1. Like the Kaguru to whom Beidelman showed photos of European circus aerialists, BaTabwa deny that such skill derives from 'mere practice and training' (1963: 61, n. 3). When a group of travelling acrobats passed through Mpala with their displays of pole-balancing, abdominal strength and other feats, everyone insisted that the men were not really performing the acts we had all paid to see. What we were *really* watching, people said, was a goatskin, not a man, magically balanced on the end of that pole. The acrobat himself was really standing on the ground, at the pole's base.

2. It is not only that they *can* see; but that they cannot *avoid* seeing it. Thus, with the case of the acrobats mentioned above, it was generally known (that is, it was more than believed) around the village that all the locally recognised sorcerers had been chagrined to find that they had paid to see only a goatskin atop a pole, and they would have demanded the return of their entrance fees, but for the fact that this would have exposed them.

3. *Vizimba* such as those of *kapondo* and *mwikuliki* are considered to be in themselves objects of sorcery, and possession of them is the reason why Tulunga diviners are sorcerers *d'office*.

4. Richards (1935) describes the similar use of such bottles by practitioners of the *Bamucapi* witch-finding movement which passed through Bemba country in 1934.

5. The significance of *kafwabubela* lies in the fact that it will be seen and found by some, while it is overlooked by others. Thus, if a group of you are standing together talking, only one of you will look down and actually see it, even though all or any of you might have.

6. In an almost classic example of why one should never second-guess one's teachers and how one unconsciously does so nevertheless, I had automatically assumed that a magnet would *attract* affairs (conflicts, etc.), whereas everyone else in Mpala automatically understood the meaning noted above.

7. This is why they may not be handled by Bulumbu practitioners, whose spirits will not tolerate proximity to such *vizimba*, but will flee.

8. A person has joking relations not only with all members of his *baendo* clans, but also with his real or classificatory 'grandchidren'. These people also have special ritual obligations. In their joking capacity they are all classed together as *watani*.

9. As with *misambwa* the emblem is the spirit itself.

10. The spirit is formed in a manner nearly identical to that of the hyena of the Ndembu diviners (see Turner 1975).

11. The migration of these spirits is indicated by the fact that Mukalaye has only recently arrived at the southern end of Lake Tanganyika. On a trip to Molilo

near the Zambian border I found that the chief there had only recently aquired a *mukalaye*. Kiungu was unknown to people in this area, as were the other non-possessing spirits outlined here.

12. Mwilambwe's house is a three-pronged tree branch, set upright in the ground, onto the three prongs of which is put a conical straw roof. The houses of Mukalye, Kiungu and Kabwangozi are erected alongside the main house. Such houses are not essential to the fabrication of the spirits, however, and are of little relevance to our discussion.

13. The *pemba* may be seen as materialised benediction, because of the associations between whiteness, fruitfulness and general good fortune. During seances, a favourite tactic of Bulumbu spirits is emptying out their baskets to show the audience that they contain no medicines.

14. Those analysts who find it hard to conceptualise the existence of such intense hostility need only think of the type of relation which can develop when radically opposed personalities and temperaments are harnessed together in the daily contact of work situations.

15. This becomes a self-fulfilling prophecy when, knowing the pre-existence of hostility, a person avoids situations in which there is likely to be confrontation. Foremost among these, of course, are the home of the patient and the paths of his kin.

16. Crucial here is the point that, unlike witchcraft, sorcery is made and therefore premeditated.

17. This is in part because Zairian law, like the Belgian colonial law after which it is patterned, does not recognise sorcery as a crime, but makes divination the criminal act. However, because they result in (as well as reflect) the total social incompatibility of two persons, such accusations are considered as being as serious in their divisiveness as the act of sorcery itself. They are 'sorcery of the mouth' (*ulozi wa kiniwa*).

18. This usage is so prevalent that to say someone died 'worthlessly' is almost as much as to say that he was ensorcelled.

19. In his seminal article on the subjects of magic and religion, Luc de Heusch (1971) suggests a 'rediscovery' of Frazer's considerations of metaphor and metonymy and the correspondence of these to two differing structures of subordination. Metaphor is the magical form of communication, one in which the human being is superior to the thing invoked. Metonymy, on the other hand, is the religious form of communication, one in which human beings are supplicants.

   In his discussion de Heusch describes what he refers to as two complementary metonymic functions. By these he means both part-for-whole substitution and the substitution of container for contained. Here, however, I shall follow the somewhat more precise definitions of Sapir (1977), who defines part-for-whole substitutions as synecdoches, and reserves metonymy for other relations based on shared domain (such as cause for effect, agent for act, etc.). Further, the distinctive structures of subordination do not seem to find an exact correspondence in any brute distinction between magic and religion.

20. Called *kusimbula* in the case of the former and *kutengeneza* in the case of the latter.

CHAPTER 10 FUTURES REALISED

1. In this respect speech becomes one of a paradigmatic set which includes those other agents of maturation: fire and sexual intercourse.

2. That is, it remains its substantial self, and does not become what will turn out to have been a cause of one's misfortune.

3. By this phrase I mean to include the idea that, in the logic of the amulet, the subject's materiality is changed in some way, but is not fundamentally transformed. The person's body becomes capable of sustaining the illusions or appearances described. This view takes seriously the identification of the amulet with the body and vitality of the person for whom it is made. Persistent bad luck reflects the same logic and is said to be 'in the flesh' (*mumaongo*) of the person.
4. De Heusch makes a similar point in his discussion of Bantu magico-religious thought (1971).

BIBLIOGRAPHY

Abrams, M. H. 1973. *Natural Supernaturalism: tradition and revolution in Romantic literature*, New York and London: W. W. Norton.

Althusser, L. 1971. 'Ideology and ideological state apparatuses' and 'Freud and Lacan' in *Lenin and Philosophy and Other Essays*, New York: Monthly Review Press.

Antze, P. and M. Lambek (eds). 1996. *Tense Past: cultural essays in trauma and memory*, New York and London: Routledge.

Appadurai, A. (ed.). 1986. *The Social Life of Things: commodities in cultural perspective*, Cambridge: Cambridge University Press.

Appadurai, A. 1995. 'The production of locality' in R. Fardon (ed.), *Counterworks: managing the diversity of knowledge*, London and New York: Routledge.

Appadurai, A. 1996. *Modernity at Large: cultural dimensions of globalization*, Minneapolis and London: University of Minnesota Press.

Appiah, K. A. 1992. *In My Father's House: Africa in the philosophy of culture*, New York: Oxford University Press.

Arnold, A. J. 1981. *Modernism and Negritude: the poetry and poetics of Aimé Césaire*, Cambridge MA and London: Harvard University Press.

Arnold, D. 1993. *Colonizing the Body: state medicine and epidemic disease in nineteenth-century India*, Berkeley, Los Angeles and London: University of California Press.

Asad, T. (ed.). 1973. *Anthropology and the Colonial Encounter*, London: Ithaca Press/ Atlantic Highlands NJ: Humanities Press.

Asad, T. 1986. 'The concept of cultural translation in British social anthropology' in J. Clifford and G. E. Marcus (eds), *Writing Culture*, Berkeley, Los Angeles and London: University of California Press.

Asad, T. 1991. 'From the history of colonial anthropology to the anthropology of Western hegemony' in G. W. Stocking (ed.), *Colonial Situations: essays on the contextualisation of ethnographic knowledge* (History of Anthropology, Vol. 7), Madison: University of Wisconsin Press.

Asad, T. 1997. 'On torture, or cruel, inhuman, and degrading treatment' in A. Kleinman, V. Das and M. Lock (eds), *Social Suffering*, Berkeley, Los Angeles and London: University of California Press.

Baker, Jr, H. A. 1987. *Modernism and the Harlem Renaissance*, Chicago and London: University of Chicago Press.

Bakhtin, M. 1984. *Problems of Dostoevsky's Poetics*, Minneapolis: University of Minnesota Press.

Bakhtin, M. 1986. *Speech Genres and Other Late Essays*, Austin: University of Texas Press.

Barker, F., P. Hulme, and M. Iversen (eds). 1994. *Colonial Discourse/Postcolonial Theory*, Manchester and New York: Manchester University Press.

Bascom, W. 1975. *African Dilemma Tales*, The Hague: Mouton.
Bayart, J.-F. 1993. *The State in Africa: the politics of the belly*, London and New York: Longman.
Beattie, J. 1963. 'Sorcery in Bunyoro' in J. Middleton and E. H. Winter (eds), *Witchcraft and Sorcery in East Africa*, London: Routledge and Kegan Paul.
Beauvoir, S. de. 1993. *The Second Sex*, London: Everyman's Library.
Beidelman, T. O. 1963. 'Witchcraft in Ukaguru' in J. Middleton and E. H. Winter (eds), *Witchcraft and Sorcery in East Africa*, London: Routledge and Kegan Paul.
Bennett, J. 1988. *Events and Their Names*, Oxford: Oxford University Press.
Berman, M. 1983. *All That is Solid Melts into Air: the experience of modernity*, London and New York: Verso.
Bernal, M. 1987. *Black Athena: the Afroasiatic roots of classical civilization, vol. 1: the fabrication of ancient Greece 1785–1985*, London: Free Association Books.
Binsbergen, W. M. J. van. 1981. *Religious Change in Zambia: exploratory studies*, London and Boston: Kegan Paul International.
Binsbergen, W. van and M. Schoffeleers (eds). 1985. *Theoretical Explorations in African Religion*, London and Boston: Kegan Paul International.
Blacking, J. (ed.). 1977. *The Anthropology of the Body*, ASA Monograph No. 14, London: Academic Press.
Bois, P. du. 1991. *Torture and Truth*, New York and London: Routledge.
Boone, O. 1961. *Carte ethnique du Congo, quart sud-est*, Brussels: Musée Royal de l'Afrique Central, annales 37.
Bourdieu, P. 1977. *Outline of a Theory of Practice*, Cambridge: Cambridge University Press.
Bowen, E. S. (Laura Bohannan). 1954. *Return to Laughter*, New York: Harper and Brothers.
Bradbury, M. 1976. 'The name and nature of modernism' in M. Bradbury and J. McFarlane (eds), *Modernism: 1890–1930*, Harmondsworth: Penguin.
Bradbury, M. and J. McFarlane (eds). 1976. *Modernism: 1890–1930*, Harmondsworth: Penguin.
Bullock, A. 1976. 'The double image' in M. Bradbury and J. McFarlane (eds), *Modernism: 1890–1930*, Harmondsworth: Penguin.
Burton, W. F. P. 1961. *Luba Religion and Magic in Custom and Belief*, Brussels: Musée Royal de l'Afrique Central, annales 35.
Butler, J. 1993. *Bodies that Matter: On the Discursive Limits of 'Sex'*, New York and London: Routledge.
Butler, J. 1997. *The Psychic Life of Power: theories in subjection*, Stanford CA: Stanford University Press.
Canguilhem, G. 1988. *Ideology and Rationality in the History of the Life Sciences*, Cambridge MA and London: MIT Press.
Canguilhem, G. 1991. *The Normal and the Pathological*, New York: Zone Books.
Castiglione, B. 1967. *The Book of the Courtier*, Harmondsworth: Penguin.
Certeau, M. de. 1980. 'Writing vs. time: history and anthropology in the works of Lafitau', *Yale French Studies 59, Rethinking History: Time, Myth and Writing*, 37–65.
Certeau, M. de. 1983. 'History, ethics, science and fiction' in N. Haan, R. Bellah, P. Rabinow and W. Sullivan (eds), *Social Science as Moral Enquiry*, New York: Columbia University Press.
Certeau, M. de. 1984. *The Practice of Everyday Life*, Berkeley, Los Angeles and London: University of California Press.
Certeau, M. de. 1997. *The Capture of Speech and Other Political Writings*, Minneapolis and London: University of Minnesota Press.

Chambers, R. 1984. *Story and Situation: narrative seduction and the power of fiction*, Minneapolis: University of Minnesota Press.

Chambers, R. 1991. *Room for Manoeuver: reading oppositional narrative*, Chicago and London: University of Chicago Press.

Clausewitz, C. von. 1984. *On War*, Princeton NJ: Princeton University Press.

Clifford, J. 1983. 'On ethnographic authority', *Representations* 1, 118–46, reprinted in *The Predicament of Culture*, Cambridge MA and London: Harvard University Press.

Clifford, J. 1986. 'On ethnographic allegory' in J. Clifford and G. E. Marcus (eds), *Writing Culture*, Berkeley, Los Angeles and London: University of California Press.

Clifford, J. 1988. *The Predicament of Culture: twentieth-century ethnography, literature, and art*, Cambridge MA and London: Harvard University Press.

Clifford. J. 1997. *Routes: travel and translation in the late twentieth century*, Cambridge MA and London: Harvard University Press.

Clifford, J. and G. E. Marcus (eds). 1986. *Writing Culture: the poetics and politics of ethnography*, Berkeley, Los Angeles and London: University of California Press.

Comaroff, J. 1985. *Body of Power, Spirit of Resistance: the culture and history of a South African people*, Chicago and London: University of Chicago Press.

Comaroff, J. and J. Comaroff. 1992. *Ethnography and the Historical Imagination*, Boulder, San Francisco and Oxford: Westview Press.

Comaroff, J. and J. Comaroff (eds). 1993. *Modernity and its Malcontents: ritual and power in postcolonial Africa*, Chicago and London: University of Chicago Press.

Connerton, P. 1989. *How Societies Remember*, Cambridge: Cambridge University Press.

Coombes, A. E. 1994. 'The recalcitrant object: culture contact and the question of hybridity' in F. Barker, P. Hulme and M. Iversen (eds), *Colonial Discourse/ Postcolonial Theory*, Manchester and New York: Manchester University Press.

Csordas, T. J. (ed.). 1994a. *Embodiment and Experience: the existential ground of culture and self*, Cambridge: Cambridge University Press.

Csordas, T. J. 1994b. *The Sacred Self: a cultural phenomenology of charismatic healing*, Berkeley, Los Angeles and London: University of California Press.

Cuddihy, J. M. 1987. *The Ordeal of Civility: Freud, Marx, Lévi-Strauss, and the Jewish struggle with modernity* (2nd edn), Boston: Beacon Press.

Cunnison, I. 1959. *Luapula Peoples of Northern Rhodesia*, Manchester: Manchester University Press.

Damasio, A. R. 1995. *Descarte's Error: emotion, reason and the human brain*, London: Picador.

Daniel, E. V. 1996. *Charred Lullabies: chapters in an anthropology of violence*, Princeton NJ: Princeton University Press.

Das, V. 1992. 'Our work to cry: your work to listen' in V. Das (ed.), *Mirrors of Violence: communities, riots and survivors in South Asia*, Delhi, Bombay, Calcutta, Madras: Oxford University Press.

Das, V. 1995a. 'Suffering, legitimacy and healing: the Bhopal case' and 'The anthropology of pain' both in *Critical Events: an anthropological perspective on contemporary India*, Delhi, Bombay, Calcutta, Madras: Oxford University Press.

Das, V. 1995b. *Critical Events: an anthropological perspective on contemporary India*, Delhi, Bombay, Calcutta, Madras: Oxford University Press.

Davis, C. 1995. 'Nothing to do with a corpus: only some bodies' in *The Impossible Science of Being: dialogues between anthropology and photography*, London: Photographers' Gallery.

De Boeck, F. 1994. 'Of trees and kings: politics and metaphor among the Aluund of southwestern Zaire', *American Ethnologist* 21, 451–73.

De Boeck, F. 1996. 'Postcolonialism, power and identity: local and global perspectives from Zaire' in R. Werbner and T. Ranger (eds), *Postcolonial Identities in Africa*, London: Zed Books.

De Gowan, E. and R. De Gowan. 1971. *Bedside Diagnostic Examination*, 2nd edn, London: Collier, Macmillian.

Deleuze, G. 1989. 'Coldness and cruelty' in *Masochism*, New York: Zone Books.

Deleuze, G. and F. Guattari. 1988. *A Thousand Plateaus*, London: Athlone Press.

Demos, J. 1994. *The Unredeemed Captive: a family story from early America*, New York: Alfred A. Knopf.

Dennett, D. C. 1991. *Consciousness Explained*, Boston, New York: Toronto, London: Little, Brown.

Derrida, J. 1972a. 'Structure, sign, and play in the discourse of the human sciences' in R. Macksey and E. Donato (eds), *The Structuralist Controversy*, Baltimore and London: Johns Hopkins University Press.

Derrida, J. 1972b. 'Freud and the scene of writing', *Yale French Studies* 48, *French Freud: Structural Studies in Psychoanalysis*, 74–118.

Derrida, J. 1976. *Of Grammatology*, Baltimore and London: Johns Hopkins University Press.

Derrida, J. 1978. *Writing and Difference*, Chicago: University of Chicago Press.

Desjarlais, R. R. 1992. *Body and Emotion: the aesthetics of illness and healing in the Nepal Himalayas*, Philadelphia: University of Pennsylvania Press.

Detienne, M. 1981. *The Creation of Mythology*, Chicago and London: University of Chicago Press.

Detienne, M. and J.-P. Vernant. 1974. *Les ruses d'intelligence: la metis des grecs*, Paris: Flammarion. Translated (1991) as *Cunning Intelligence in Greek Culture and Society*, Chicago: University of Chicago Press.

Devisch, R. 1993. *Weaving the Threads of Life: the* Khita *gyn-eco-logical healing cult among the Yaka*, Chicago and London: University of Chicago Press.

Devisch, R. 1996. '"Pillaging Jesus": healing churches and the villagisation of Kinshasa', *Africa* 66, 555–87.

Diprose, R. 1994. *The Bodies of Women: ethics, embodiment and sexual difference*, London and New York: Routledge.

Dorst, J. and P. Dandelot. 1969. *A Field Guide to the Larger Mammals of Africa*, Boston: Houghton Mifflin.

Douglas, M. 1975. *Implicit Meanings*, London: Routledge and Kegan Paul.

Douglas, M. and A. Wildavsky. 1982. *Risk and Culture: an essay on the selection of technological and environmental dangers*, Berkeley, Los Angeles and London: University of California Press.

Du Bois, W. E. B. 1997. *The Souls of Black Folk* (1903). Reprinted in H. L. Gates Jr and N. Y. McKay (eds), *The Norton Anthology of African American Literature*, New York and London: W. W. Norton.

Dupré, J. 1993. *The Disorder of Things: metaphysical foundations of the disunity of science*, Cambridge MA and London: Harvard University Press.

Edelman, G. 1992. *Bright Air, Brilliant Fire: on the matter of the mind*, Harmondsworth: Penguin.

Ellen, R. F. (ed.). 1984. *Ethnographic Research: a guide to general conduct*, London and New York: Academic Press.

Epstein, A. L. 1958. *Politics in an Urban African Community*, Manchester: Manchester University Press.

Epstein, A. L. 1967. *The Craft of Social Anthropology*, London: Tavistock.

Evans-Pritchard, E. E. 1937. *Witchcraft, Oracles and Magic among the Azande*, London and Oxford: Clarendon Press.

Evans-Pritchard, E. E. 1940. *The Nuer*, Oxford: Oxford University Press.

Fabian, J. 1983. *Time and the Other: how anthropology makes its object*, New York: Columbia University Press.

Fabian, J. 1990. *Power and Performance: ethnographic explorations through proverbial wisdom and theater in Shaba, Zaire*, Madison and London: University of Wisconsin Press.

Fabrega, Jr, H. 1974. *Disease and Social Behavior: an interdisciplinary perspective*, Cambridge MA and London: MIT Press.

Fabrega, Jr, H. and D. B. Silver. 1973. *Illness and Shamanistic Curing in Zinacantan: an ethnomedical analysis*, Stanford CA: Stanford University Press.

Falk, P. 1994. *The Consuming Body*, London: Thousand Oaks, New Delhi: Sage.

Fanon, F. 1967. *Black Skin, White Masks: the experiences of a black man in a white world*, New York: Grove Press.

Fardon, R. (ed.). 1990. *Localizing Strategies: regional traditions of ethnographic writing*, Edinburgh: Scottish Academic Press/Washington DC: Smithsonian Institution Press.

Fardon, R. 1995. *Counterworks: managing the diversity of knowledge*, London and New York: Routledge.

Featherstone, M., M. Hepworth and B. S. Turner (eds). 1991. *The Body: social process and cultural theory*, London, Newbury Park, New Delhi: Sage.

Feher, M. with R. Naddaff and N. Tazi (eds). 1989. *Fragments for a History of the Human Body*, 3 vols, New York: Zone Books.

Feierman, S. 1993. 'African histories and the dissolution of world history' in R. H. Bates, V. Y. Mudimbe and J. O'Barr (eds), *Africa and the Disciplines: the contributions of research in Africa to the social sciences and humanities*, Chicago and London: University of Chicago Press.

Feierman, S. and J. M. Janzen (eds). 1992. *The Social Basis of Health and Healing in Africa*, Berkeley, Los Angeles and London: University of California Press.

Feldman, A. 1991. *Formations of Violence: the narrative of the body and political terror in Northern Ireland*, Chicago and London: University of Chicago Press.

Fernandez, J. 1982. *Bwiti: an ethnography of the religious imagination in Africa*, Princeton NJ: Princeton University Press.

Fernandez, J. 1986. *Persuasions and Performances: the play of tropes in culture*, Bloomington: Indiana University Press.

Feyerabend, P. 1975. *Against Method*, London and New York: Verso.

Fischer, M. M. J. 1986. 'Ethnicity and the post-modern arts of memory' in J. Clifford and G. E. Marcus (eds), *Writing Culture*, Berkeley, Los Angeles and London: University of California Press.

Fisiy, C. and P. Geschiere. 1996. 'Witchcraft, violence and identity: different trajectories in postcolonial Cameroon' in R. Werbner and T. Ranger (eds), *Postcolonial Identities in Africa*, London: Zed Books.

Fitzsimmons, V. 1970. *A Field Guide to the Snakes of Southern Africa*, London: Collins.

Flanagan, O. 1992. *Conciousness Reconsidered*, Cambridge MA and London: MIT Press.

Foucault, M. 1970. *The Order of Things: an archaeology of the human sciences*, New York: Pantheon.

Foucault, M. 1972. *The Archaeology of Knowledge and the Discourse on Language*, New York: Pantheon.

Foucault, M. 1978. *The History of Sexuality: an introduction*, New York: Random House.

Foucault, M. 1987. *The Use of Pleasure*, Harmondsworth: Penguin.

Foucault, M. 1988. *The Care of the Self*, Harmondsworth: Penguin.

Frake, C. O. 1961. 'Diagnosis of disease among the Subanun of Mindinao', *American Anthropologist* LXIII, 113–32.

Frank, A. W. 1991. 'For a sociology of the body: an analytical review' in M. Featherstone, M. Hepworth and B. Turner (eds), *The Body: social process and cultural theory*, London, Newbury Park, New Delhi: Sage.

Frankenberg, R. 1982. *Custom and Conflict in British Society*, Manchester: Manchester University Press.

Frankl, V. E. 1985. *Man's Search for Meaning*, rev. edn, New York: Washington Square Press (First published 1946 as memoirs, then with additional analysis 1959.)

Freud, S. 1958. *The Standard Edition of the Complete Psychological Works of Sigmund Freud*, 24 vols, general ed. James Strachey, London: Hogarth Press and Institute of Psycho-Analysis.

Frye, N. 1957. *Anatomy of Criticism: four esssays*, Princeton NJ: Princeton University Press.

Gates, Jr, H. L. (ed.). 1984a. *Black Literature and Literary Theory*, New York and London: Methuen.

Gates, Jr, H. L. 1984b. 'The blackness of blackness: a critique of the sign and the signifying monkey' in H. L. Gates, Jr (ed.), *Black Literature and Literary Theory*, New York and London: Methuen.

Gates, Jr, H. L. 1988. *The Signifying Monkey: a theory of African-American literary criticism*, New York and Oxford: Oxford University Press.

Gates, Jr., H. L. and N. Y. McKay (eds). 1997. *The Norton Anthology of African American Literature*, New York and London: W. W. Norton.

Geertz, C. 1972. 'Deep play: notes on the Balinese cockfight', *Daedalus* 101, 1–37.

Geertz, C. 1973a. 'Thick description: toward an interpretive theory of culture' in *The Interpretation of Cultures*, New York: Basic Books.

Geertz, C. 1973b. *The Interpretation of Cultures*, New York: Basic Books.

Geertz, C. 1988, *Works and Lives: the anthropologist as author*, Cambridge and Oxford: Polity Press in association with Blackwell.

Genette, G. 1979. 'Valery and the poetics of language' in J. Harari (ed.), *Textual Strategies: perspectives in post-structuralist criticism*, Ithaca NY: Cornell University Press.

Geschiere, P. 1997. *The Modernity of Witchcraft: politics and the occult in postcolonial Africa*, Charlottesville and London: University Press of Virginia.

Gibson, J. W. 1986. *The Perfect War: technowar in Vietnam*, Boston and New York: Atlantic Monthly Press.

Gildea, R. 1994. *The Past in French History*, New Haven and London: Yale University Press.

Gilman, E. 1978. *The Curious Perspective: literary and pictorial wit in the seventeenth century*, New Haven and London: Yale University Press.

Gilman, S. L. 1985. *Difference and Pathology: stereotypes of sexuality, race, and madness*, Ithaca NY: Cornell University Press.

Gilman, S. L. 1993. *Freud, Race, and Gender*, Princeton NJ: Princeton University Press.

Gilroy, P. 1992. *'There Ain't No Black in the Union Jack': the cultural politics of race and nation*, London: Routledge. (First published 1987.)

Gilroy, P. 1993. *The Black Atlantic: modernity and double consciousness*, London and New York: Verso.

Ginzburg, C. 1980. *The Cheese and the Worms: the cosmos of a sixteenth-century miller*,

Baltimore and London: Johns Hopkins University Press.

Ginzburg, C. 1983. *Nightbattles: witchcraft and agrarian cults in the sixteenth and seventeenth centuries*, Baltimore and London: Johns Hopkins University Press.

Gluckman, M. 1955. *Custom and Conflict in Africa*, Oxford: Blackwell.

Gluckman, M. 1958. *Analysis of a Social Situation in Modern Zululand*, Rhodes-Livingstone Paper No. 28, Manchester: Manchester University Press.

Good, B. J. 1994. *Medicine, Rationality, and Experience: an anthropological perspective*, Cambridge: Cambridge University Press.

Good, M.-J. D., P. Brodwin, B. Good and A. Kleinman (eds). 1992. *Pain as Human Experience: an anthropological perspective*, Berkeley, Los Angeles and London: University of California Press.

Gray, C. H. 1997. *Postmodern War: the new politics of conflict*, London: Routledge.

Greenblatt, S. 1980. *Renaissance Self-Fashioning from More to Shakespeare*, Chicago and London: University of Chicago Press.

Grosz, E. 1994. *Volatile Bodies: toward a corporeal feminism*, Bloomington: Indiana University Press.

Gupta, A. and J. Ferguson (eds). 1997. *Anthropological Locations: boundaries and grounds of a field science*, Berkeley, Los Angeles and London: University of California Press.

Guyer, J. 1993. 'Wealth in people and self-realization in equatorial Africa', *Man* (n.s.) 28, 243–65.

Guyer, J. 1995. 'Wealth in people, wealth in things – introduction', *Journal of African History* 36, 83–90.

Guyer, J. and S. M. Eno Belinga. 1995. 'Wealth in people as wealth in knowledge: accumulation and composition in equatorial Africa', *Journal of African History* 36, 91–120.

Hacking, I. 1982. 'Language, truth and reason' in M. Hollis and S. Lukes (eds), *Rationality and Relativism*, Cambridge MA: MIT Press.

Hacking, I. 1983. *Representing and Intervening: introductory topics in the philosophy of natural science*, Cambridge: Cambridge University Press.

Hacking, I. 1985. 'Styles of scientific reasoning' in J. Rajchman and C. West (eds), *Post-Analytic Philosophy*, New York: Columbia University Press.

Halbwachs, M. 1992. *On Collective Memory*, Chicago and London: University of Chicago Press.

Hall, S. 1993. 'Cultural identity and diaspora' in P. Williams and L. Chrisman (eds), *Colonial Discourse and Post-Colonial Theory*, New York and London: Harvester Wheatsheaf.

Hall, S. and T. Jefferson (eds). 1993. *Resistance through Rituals: youth subcultures in post-war Britain*, London: Routledge. (First published 1976.)

Harari, J. (ed.). 1979. *Textual Strategies: perspectives in post-structuralist criticism*, Ithaca NY: Cornell University Press.

Haraway, D. J. 1991. *Simians, Cyborgs, and Women: the reinvention of nature*, New York: Routledge.

Haraway, D. J. 1992. *Primate Visions: gender, race and nature in the world of modern science*, London and New York: Verso.

Haraway, D. J. 1997. *Modest_Witness@Second_Millennium.FemaleMan©_Meets_OncoMouse™: feminism and technoscience*, New York and London: Routledge.

Harvey, D. 1990. *The Condition of Postmodernity: an enquiry into the origins of cultural change*, Oxford: Basil Blackwell.

Hayward Gallery. 1997. *Rhapsodies in Black: art of the Harlem Renaissance*, London: Hayward Gallery, International Institute of Visual Arts/Berkeley, Los Angeles and London: University of California Press.

Hebdige, D. 1994. *Subculture: the meaning of style*, London: Routledge. (First published 1979.)

Heidegger, M. 1971. 'The origin of the work of art' in *Poetry, Language, Thought*, New York: Harper & Row.

Heusch, L. de. 1971. *Pourqui l'épouser? et autres essais*, Paris: Gallimard.

Heusch, L. de. 1982. *The Drunken King, or, the Origin of the State*, Bloomington: Indiana University Press.

Heusch, L. de. 1985. *Sacrifice in Africa: a structuralist approach*, Bloomington: Indiana University Press.

Hobson, M. 1982. *The Object of Art: the theory of illusion in eighteenth-century France*, Cambridge: Cambridge University Press.

Horton, R. 1967. 'African traditional religion and western science', *Africa* 37, 50–71, 155–87. Reprinted (1970) in B. Wilson (ed.), *Rationality*, Oxford: Blackwell.

Horton, R. 1982. 'Tradition and modernity revisited' in M. Hollis and S. Lukes (eds), *Rationality and Relativism*, Cambridge MA: MIT Press.

Horton, R. and R. Finnegan. 1973. *Modes of Thought: essays on thinking in western and non-western societies*, London: Faber and Faber.

Hountondji, P. J. 1983. *African Philosophy: myth and reality*, Bloomington: Indiana University Press.

Hulme, P. 1994. 'The locked heart: the Creole family romance of *Wide Sargasso Sea*' in F. Barker, P. Hulme and M. Iversen (eds), *Colonial Discourse/Postcolonial Theory*, Manchester and New York: Manchester University Press.

Ita, J. M. 1973. 'Frobenius, Senghor and the image of Africa' in R. Horton and R. Finnegan (eds), *Modes of Thought: essays on thinking in western and non-western societies*, London: Faber and Faber.

Izard, M. and P. Smith (eds). 1979. *La fonction symbolique: essais d'anthropologie*, Paris: Gallimard.

Jackson, M. 1982. *Allegories of the Wilderness: ethics and ambiguity in Kuranko narratives*, Bloomington: Indiana University Press.

Jackson, M. 1989. *Paths Toward a Clearing: radical empiricism and ethnographic inquiry*, Bloomington and Indianapolis, Indiana University Press.

Jacobus, M., E. F. Keller and S. Shuttleworth (eds). 1990. *Body/Politics: women and the discourses of science*, New York and London: Routledge.

James, C. L. R. 1980. *The Black Jacobins: Toussaint L'Ouverture and the San Domingo revolution*, London: Allison and Busby.

Jameson, F. 1991. *Postmodernism, or, The Cultural Logic of Late Capitalism*, London and New York: Verso.

Janzen, J. 1978. *The Quest for Therapy: medical pluralism in Lower Zaire*, Berkeley, Los Angeles and London: University of California Press.

Janzen, J. 1982. *Lemba, 1650–1930: a drum of affliction in Africa and the new world*, New York and London: Garland

Janzen, J. 1992. *Ngoma: discourses of healing in Central and Southern Africa*, Berkeley, Los Angeles and Oxford: University of California Press.

Johnson, M. 1987. *The Body in the Mind: the bodily basis of meaning, imagination, and reason*, Chicago and London: University of Chicago Press.

Keller, E. F. 1995. *Refiguring Life: metaphors of twentieth-century biology*, New York: Columbia University Press.

Kesteloot, L. 1991. *Black Writers in French: a literary history of negritude*, Washington DC: Howard University Press.

Kirmayer, L. J. 1996. 'Landscapes of memory: trauma, narrative, and dissociation' in P. Antze and M. Lambek (eds), *Tense Past: cultural essays in trauma and memory*, New York and London: Routledge.

Klein, R. 1970. 'L'Éclipse de l'œuvre d'art' and 'Le thème du fou et l'ironie humaniste' both in *La forme et l'intelligible: écrits sur la renaissance et l'art moderne*, Paris: Gallimard.

Kleinman, A. 1980. *Patients and Healers in the Context of Culture: an exploration of the borderland between anthropology, medicine and psychiatry*, Berkeley, Los Angeles and London: University of California Press.

Kleinman, A. 1995. *Writing at the Margin: discourse between anthropology and medicine*, Berkeley, Los Angeles and London: University of California Press.

Kleinman, A., V. Das and M. Lock (eds). 1997. *Social Suffering*, Berkeley, Los Angeles and London: University of California Press.

Kopytoff, I. 1986. 'The cultural biography of things: commoditization as process' in A. Appadurai (ed.), *The Social Life of Things: commodities in cultural perspective*, Cambridge: Cambridge University Press.

Kuhn, T. 1962. *The Structure of Scientific Revolutions*, Chicago: University of Chicago Press. (2nd edn, enlarged, 1970.)

Lacan, J. 1972a. 'Of structure as an inmixing of an otherness prerequisite to any subject whatever' in R. Macksey and E. Donato (eds), *The Structuralist Controversy*, Baltimore and London: Johns Hopkins University Press.

Lacan, J. 1972b. 'Seminar on "The Purloined Letter"', *Yale French Studies* 48, *French Freud: Structural Studies in Psychoanalysis*, 39–73.

Lacan, J. 1977a. 'The function and field of speech and language in psychoanalysis' in *Écrits*, New York: W. W. Norton.

Lacan, J. 1977b. *Écrits*, New York: W. W. Norton.

Lacan, J. 1978. *The Four Fundamental Concepts of Psycho-Analysis*, New York: W. W. Norton.

Laclau, E. 1990. *New Reflections on the Revolution of Our Time*, London and New York: Verso.

Laderman, C. and M. Roseman. 1996. *The Performance of Healing*, New York and London: Routledge.

Lambek, M. 1993. *Knowledge and Practice in Mayotte: local discourses of Islam, sorcery, and spirit possession*, Toronto, Buffalo and London: University of Toronto Press.

Lan, D. 1985. *Guns and Rain: guerrillas and spirit mediums in Zimbabwe*, London: James Currey/Berkeley, Los Angeles and London: University of California Press.

Laplanche, J. and J.-B. Pontalis. 1973. *The Language of Psycho-Analysis*, New York: W. W. Norton.

Last, M. 1979. 'Strategies against time', *Sociology of Health and Illness* 1, 306–17.

Last, M. 1981. 'The importance of knowing about not knowing', *Social Science and Medicine* 15B, 387–92. Reprinted (1992) in S. Feierman and J. Janzen (eds), *The Social Basis of Health and Healing in Africa*, Berkeley, Los Angeles and London: University of California Press.

Lavie, S. 1990. *The Poetics of Military Occupation: Mzeina allegories of Bedouin identity under Israeli and Egyptian rule*, Berkeley, Los Angeles and London: University of California Press.

Leach, E. 1954. *Political Systems of Highland Burma*, Boston: Beacon Press.

Leder, D. 1990. *The Absent Body*, Chicago and London: University of Chicago Press.

Lévi-Strauss, C. 1963. *Structural Anthropology*, New York: Basic Books.

Lévi-Strauss, C. 1966. *The Savage Mind*, Chicago: University of Chicago Press.

Lévi-Strauss, C. 1978. *Tristes Tropiques*, New York: Atheneum.

Lindenbaum, S. and M. Lock (eds). 1993. *Knowledge, Power and Practice: the anthropology of medicine and everyday life*, Berkeley, Los Angeles and London: University of California Press.

Lingis, A. 1994. *Foreign Bodies*, New York and London: Routledge.

Lizot, J. 1985. *Tales of the Yanomami: daily life in the Venezuelan forest*, Cambridge: Cambridge University Press/Paris: Editions de la Maison des Sciences de l'Homme.

Lloyd, E. A. 1994. *The Structure and Confirmation of Evolutionary Theory*, Princeton NJ: Princeton University Press.

Lloyd, G. E. R. 1978. *Magic, Reason and Experience: studies in the origins and development of Greek science*, Cambridge: Cambridge University Press.

Lloyd, G. E. R. 1990. *Demystifying Mentalities*, Cambridge: Cambridge University Press.

Lock, M. 1993. 'Cultivating the body: anthropology and epistemologies of bodily practice and knowledge', *Annual Review of Anthropology* 22, 133–55.

Lyotard, J.-F. 1984. *The Postmodern Condition: a report on knowledge*, Minneapolis: University of Minnesota Press.

MacCannell, J. F. and L. Zakarin (eds). 1994. *Thinking Bodies*, Stanford CA: Stanford University Press.

MacGaffey, W. 1983. *Modern Kongo Prophets: religion in a plural society*, Bloomington: Indiana University Press.

MacGaffey, W. 1986. *Religion and Society in Central Africa: the BaKongo of Lower Zaire*, Chicago and London: University of Chicago Press.

MacGaffey, W. 1988. 'Complexity, astonishment and power: the visual vocabulary of Kongo Minkisi', *Journal of Southern African Studies* 14, 188–203.

MacGaffey, W. 1993. 'The eyes of understanding: Kongo Minkisi' in *Astonishment and Power*, Washington DC: National Museum of African Art.

Macksey, R. and E. Donato (eds). 1972. *The Structuralist Controversy: the languages of criticism and the sciences of man*, Baltimore and London: Johns Hopkins University Press.

Malinowski, B. 1961. *Argonauts of the Western Pacific*, New York: E. P. Dutton.

Malinowski, B. 1967. *Diary in the Strict Sense of the Word*, London: Routledge and Kegan Paul.

Mamdani, M. 1996. *Citizen and Subject: contemporary Africa and the legacy of late colonialism*, Princeton NJ: Princeton University Press/Kampala: Fountain Publishers/Cape Town: David Philip/London: James Currey.

Manuel, F. 1959. *The Eighteenth Century Confronts the Gods*, Cambridge MA: Harvard University Press.

Marcus, G. and M. Fischer. 1986. *Anthropology as Cultural Critique: an experimental moment in the human sciences*, Chicago and London: University of Chicago Press.

Markovitz, I. L. 1969. *Léopold Sédar Senghor and the Politics of Négritude*, New York: Atheneum.

Martin, E. 1987. *The Woman in the Body*, Boston: Beacon Press.

Martin, E. 1994. *Flexible Bodies: the role of immunity in American culture from the days of polio to the age of AIDS*, Boston: Beacon Press.

Masolo, D. A. 1994. *African Philosophy in Search of Identity*, Bloomington: Indiana University Press, for the International African Institute.

Matory, J. L. 1994. *Sex and the Empire That Is No More: gender and the politics of metaphor in Oyo Yoruba religion*, Minneapolis and London: University of Minnesota Press.

Mbembe, A. 1992. 'Provisional notes on the postcolony', *Africa* 62, 3–38.

McClintock, A. 1994. 'The angel of progress: pitfalls of the term "postcolonialism"' in F. Barker, P. Hulme, and M. Iversen (eds), *Colonial Discourse/Postcolonial Theory*, Manchester and New York: Manchester University Press.

McFarlane, J. 1976. 'The mind of modernism' in M. Bradbury and J. McFarlane (eds), *Modernism: 1890–1930*, Harmondsworth: Penguin.

McGee, P. 1992. *Telling the Other: the question of value in modern and postcolonial writing*, Ithaca NY: Cornell University Press.

Merleau-Ponty, M. 1962. *Phenomenology of Perception*, London and New York: Routledge.

Merleau-Ponty, M. 1968. *The Visible and the Invisible*, Evanston: Northwestern University Press.

Mudimbe, V. Y. 1985. 'African gnosis, philosophy, and the order of knowledge: an introduction', *African Studies Review* 28 (2–3), 149–231.

Mudimbe, V. Y. 1988. *The Invention of Africa: gnosis, philosophy and the order of knowledge*, Bloomington: Indiana University Press.

Mudimbe, V. Y. 1991. *Parables and Fables: exegesis, textuality, and politics in Central Africa*, Madison and London: University of Wisconsin Press.

Mudimbe, V. Y. 1992. *The Surreptitious Speech:* présence africaine *and the politics of otherness 1947–1987*, Chicago and London: University of Chicago Press.

Mudimbe, V. Y. 1994a. *Les Corps Glorieus des Mots et des Etres: esquisse d'un jardin africain à la bénédictine*, Montreal: Humanitas/Paris: Présence Africaine.

Mudimbe, V. Y. 1994b. *The Idea of Africa*, Bloomington: Indiana University Press/ London: James Currey.

Mudimbe, V. Y. 1997. *Tales of Faith: religion as political performance in Central Africa*, London and Atlantic Highlands NJ: Athlone Press.

Mudimbe, V. Y. and K. A. Appiah. 1993. 'The impact of African studies on philosophy' in R. H. Bates, V. Y. Mudimbe and J. O'Barr (eds), *Africa and the Disciplines: the contributions of research in Africa to the social sciences and humanities*, Chicago and London: University of Chicago Press.

Nandy, A. 1983. *The Intimate Enemy: loss and recovery of self under colonialism*, Delhi, Bombay, Calcutta, Madras: Oxford University Press.

Nandy, A. 1995. *The Savage Freud and Other Essays on Possible and Retrievable Selves*, Princeton NJ: Princeton University Press.

Ngubane, H. 1977. *Body and Mind in Zulu Medicine*, London, New York, San Francisco: Academic Press.

Ngugi wa Thiong'o. 1986. *Decolonizing the Mind: the politics of language in African literature*, London: James Currey/Nairobi and Portsmouth NH: Heinemann.

Ngugi wa Thiong'o. 1993. *Moving the Centre: the struggle for cultural freedoms*. London: James Currey/Nairobi: EAEP/Portsmouth NH: Heinemann.

Norval, A. 1996. *Deconstructing Apartheid Discourse*, London and New York: Verso.

Nussbaum, M. C. 1986. *The Fragility of Goodness: luck and ethics in Greek tragedy and philosophy*, Cambridge: Cambridge University Press.

Owusu, M. 1978. 'The ethnography of Africa: the usefulness of the useless', *American Anthropologist* 80, 310–34.

Palmié, S. 1995. 'Against syncretism: "Africanizing" and "Cubanizing" discourses in North American òrìsà worship' in R. Fardon (ed.), *Counterworks: managing the diversity of knowledge*, London and New York: Routledge.

Parkin, D. 1995. 'Latticed knowledge: eradication and dispersal of the unpalatable in Islam, medicine and anthropological theory' in R. Fardon (ed.), *Counterworks: managing the diversity of knowledge*, London and New York: Routledge.

Pinney, C., C. Wright and R. Poignant. 1995. 'The impossible science' in *The Impossible Science of Being: dialogues between anthropology and photography*, London: The Photographers' Gallery.

Pool, R. 1994. *Dialogue and the Interpretation of Illness: conversations in a Cameroon village*, Oxford and Providence: Berg.

Rabinow, P. 1977. *Reflections on Fieldwork in Morocco*, Berkeley, Los Angeles and London: University of California Press.

Rabinow, P. 1986. 'Representations are social facts: modernity and post-modernity in anthropology' in J. Clifford and G. E. Marcus (eds), *Writing Culture*, Berkeley, Los Angeles and London: University of California Press.

Radley, A. 1993. *Worlds of Illness: biographical and cultural perspectives on health and disease*, London and New York: Routledge.

Rajchman, J. and C. West (eds). 1985. *Post-Analytic Philosophy*, New York: Columbia University Press.

Rebhorn, W. A. 1978. *Courtly Performances: masking and festivity in Castiglione's Book of the Courtier*, Detroit: Wayne State University Press.

Reisman, P. 1977. *Freedom in Fulani Social Life: an introspective ethnography*, Chicago and London: University of Chicago Press.

Reynolds, P. 1996. *Traditional Healers and Childhood in Zimbabwe*, Athens OH: Ohio University Press.

Reznek, L. 1987. *The Nature of Disease*, London and New York: Routledge and Kegan Paul.

Richards, A. I. 1935. 'A modern movement of witch-finders', *Africa* VIII (4), 448–61.

Richards, A. I. 1956. *Chisungu: a girl's initiation ceremony among the Bemba of Northern Rhodesia*, London: Faber and Faber.

Richards, A. I. 1969. *Land, Labour and Diet in Northern Rhodesia*, London: Oxford University Press, for the International African Institute [reprinted 1995].

Ricoeur P. 1970. *Freud and Philosophy: an essay on interpretation*, New Haven and London: Yale University Press.

Ricoeur P. 1974. *The Conflict of Interpretations*, Evanston: Northwestern University Press.

Ricoeur P. 1981. *Hermeneutics and the Human Sciences*, Cambridge: Cambridge University Press/Paris, Éditions de la Maison des Sciences de L'Homme.

Roberts, A. F. 1980. 'Heroic Beasts, Beastly Heroes', unpublished doctoral dissertation, Department of Anthropology, University of Chicago.

Roberts, C. D. 1985. 'Consciousness in extremity: discourse on madness among the Tabwa of Zaire', *International Journal of Psychology* 20, 569–81.

Rorty, R. 1982. 'Philosophy as a kind of writing: an essay on Derrida' in *Consequences of Pragmatism (Essays: 1972–1980)*, Minneapolis: University of Minnesota Press.

Rorty, R. 1989. *Contingency, Irony, and Solidarity*, Cambridge: Cambridge University Press.

Ross, A. 1989. *No Respect: intellectuals and popular culture*, New York and London: Routledge.

Ryan, M. and A. Gordon. 1994. *Body Politics: diseae, desire, and the family*, Boulder, San Francisco and Oxford: Westview Press.

Said, E. W. 1975. *Beginnings: intention and method*, Baltimore and London: Johns Hopkins University Press.

Sapir, J. D. 1977. 'The anatomy of metaphor' in J. David Sapir and Christopher Crocker (eds), *The Social Use of Metaphor*, Philadelphia: University of Pennsylvania Press.

Sartre, J.-P. 1965. *Anti-Semite and Jew*, New York: Schocken Books.

Scarry, E. 1985. *The Body in Pain: the making and unmaking of the world*, Oxford: Oxford University Press.

Scheper-Hughes, N. 1992. *Death Without Weeping: the violence of everyday life in Brazil*, Berkeley, Los Angeles and London: University of California Press.

Scheper-Hughes, N. and M. Lock. 1986. 'Speaking "truth" to illness: metaphors, reification, and a pedagogy for patients', *Medical Anthropology Quarterly* 17, 137–140.

Scheper-Hughes, N. and M. Lock. 1987. 'The mindful body', *Medical Anthropology Quarterly* 1, 6–41.

Schiebinger, L. 1993. *Nature's Body: sexual politics and the making of modern science*, Boston: Beacon Press.

Serequeberhan, T. 1991. *African Philosophy: the essential readings*, New York: Paragon House.

Showalter, E. 1997. *Hystories: hysterical epidemics and modern culture*, London: Picador.

Simmel, G. 1971. *On Individuality and Social Forms*, Chicago and London: University of Chicago Press.

Sontag, S. 1966. 'The anthropologist as hero' in *Against Interpretation*, New York: Delta Books.

Sorabji, R. 1980. *Necessity, Cause and Blame: perspectives on Aristotle's theory*, Ithaca NY: Cornell University Press.

Spivak, G. C. 1985. 'Three women's texts and a critique of imperialism', *Critical Inquiry* 12, guest ed., H. L. Gates, Jr, *'Race,' Writing, and Difference*, 243–62.

Stafford, B. M. 1991. *Body Criticism: imaging the unseen in enlightenment art and medicine*, Cambridge MA and London: MIT Press.

Stewart, S. 1993. *On Longing: narratives of the miniature, the gigantic, the souvenir, the collection*, Durham and London: Duke University Press.

Steyn, D. G. 1931. *The Toxicology of Plants in Southern Africa*, Central News Agency.

Stocking, Jr., G. W. (ed.) 1991. *Colonial Situations: essays on the contextualisation of ethnographic knowledge*, History of Anthropology, Vol. 7, Madison: University of Wisconsin Press.

Stocking, Jr, G. W. 1992. *The Ethnographer's Magic and Other Essays in the History of Anthropology*, Madison and London: University of Wisconsin Press.

Stoller, P. and C. Olkes. 1987. *In Sorcery's Shadow: a memoir of apprenticeship among the Songhay of Niger*, Chicago and London: University of Chicago Press.

Strathern, M. 1985. 'Dislodging a world view: challenge and counter-challenge in the relationship between feminism and anthropology', *Australian Feminist Studies Journal* 1, 1–25.

Strathern, M. 1987. 'An awkward relationship: the case of feminism and anthropology', *Signs: Journal of Women in Culture and Society*, 12(2), 276–92.

Tambiah, S. J. 1973. 'Form and meaning of magical acts: a point of view' in R. Horton and R. Finnegan (eds), *Modes of Thought: essays on thinking in western and non-western societies*, London: Faber and Faber.

Tambiah, S. J. 1985. *Culture, Thought, and Social Action: an anthropological perspective*, Cambridge MA and London: Harvard University Press.

Tambiah, S. J. 1990. *Magic, Science, Religion, and the Scope of Rationality*, Cambridge: Cambridge University Press.

Taussig, M. 1980. 'Reification and the consciousness of the patient', *Social Science and Medicine* 14B, 3–13.

Taussig, M. 1987. *Shamanism, Colonialism, and the Wild Man: a study in terror and healing*, Chicago and London: University of Chicago Press.

Taussig, M. 1993. *Mimesis and Alterity: a particular history of the senses*, New York and London: Routledge.

Thomas, K. 1971. *Religion and the Decline of Magic*, New York: Charles Scribner's Sons.

Tsing, A. L. 1993. *In the Realm of the Diamond Queen*, Princeton NJ: Princeton University Press.

Turner, B. S. 1991. 'Recent developments in the theory of the body' in M. Featherstone, M. Hepworth, and B. Turner (eds), *The Body: social process and cultural theory*, London, Newbury Park, New Delhi: Sage.

Turner, B. S. 1992. *Regulating Bodies: essays in medical sociology*, London and New York: Routledge.

Turner, B. S. 1996. *The Body and Society*, 2nd edn, London, Thousand Oaks, New Delhi: Sage.

Turner, G. 1996. *British Cultural Studies: an introduction*, 2nd edn, London and New York: Routledge.

Turner, V. 1957. *Schism and Continuity in an African Society: a study in Ndembu village life*, Manchester: Manchester University Press.

Turner, V. 1967a. *The Forest of Symbols*, Ithaca NY: Cornell University Press.

Turner, V. 1967b. 'Mukanda: rite of circumcision' in *Forest of Symbols*, Ithaca NY: Cornell University Press.

Turner, V. 1967c. 'A Ndembu doctor in practice' in *Forest of Symbols*, Ithaca NY: Cornell University Press.

Turner, V. 1968. *The Drums of Affliction: a study of religious processes among the Ndembu of Zambia*, Oxford: Oxford University Press and the International African Institute.

Turner, V. 1975. *Revelation and divination in Ndembu Ritual*, Ithaca NY: Cornell University Press.

Valéry, P. 1972. 'Leonardo' (comprising 'Introduction to the method of Leonardo da Vinci', 'Note and digression' and 'Leonardo and the philosophers') in *Leonardo, Poe and Mallarmé*, Vol. 8 of the collected works of Paul Valéry, Bollingen Series XLV, Princeton NJ: Princeton University Press.

Vansina, J. 1990. *Paths in the Rainforests: toward a history of political tradition in equatorial Africa*, London: James Currey.

Vaughan, M. 1991. *Curing their ills: colonial power and African illness*, Cambridge: Polity Press.

Verdecourt, B. and E. C. Trump. 1969. *Common poisonous plants of East Africa*. London: Collins.

Vernant, J. P., L. Vandermeersh, J. Gernet, J. Bottéro, R. Crahay, L. Brisson, J. Carlier, D. Grodzynski and A. Retel-Laurentin. 1974. *Divination et Rationalité*, Paris: Éditions du Seuil.

Vickers, B. (ed.). 1984. *Occult and Scientific Mentalities in the Renaissance*, Cambridge: Cambridge University Press.

Volosinov, V. N. 1987. 'Discourse in life, discourse in art' in *Freudianism: a critical sketch*, Bloomington: Indiana University Press.

Wallman, S. 1997. 'Appropriate anthropology and the risky inspiration of "Capability Brown"' in A. James, J. Hockey and A. Dawson (eds), *After Writing Culture*, ASA Monograph 34, London and New York: Routledge.

Watt, I. 1979. *Conrad in the Nineteenth Century*, Berkeley and Los Angeles: University of California Press.

Watt, J. M. and M. G. Breyer-Brandwijk. 1962. *Medicinal and Poisonous Plants of Southern and Eastern Africa*, Edinburgh: E. & S. Livingstone.

Werbner, R. 1990. 'South–Central Africa: the Manchester School and after' in R. Fardon (ed.), *Localizing Strategies*, Edinburgh: Scottish Academic Press.

Werbner, R. 1991. *Tears of the Dead: the social biography of an African Family*, Edinburgh: Edinburgh University Press, for the International African Institute.

Werner, D. 1971. 'Some developments in Bemba religious history', *Religion in Africa* IV(1), 1–24.

West, C. 1985. 'The politics of American neo-pragmatism' in J. Rajchman and C. West (eds), *Post-Analytic Philosophy*, New York: Columbia University Press.

Williams, P. and L. Chrisman (eds). 1993. *Colonial Discourse and Post-Colonial Theory*, New York and London: Harvester Wheatsheaf.

Wilson, B. (ed.). 1970. *Rationality*, Oxford: Blackwell.

Winkler, J. J. 1990. *The Constraints of Desire: The anthropology of sex and gender in ancient Greece*, New York and London: Routledge.

Yates, F. 1966. *The Art of Memory*, London and New York: Routledge and Kegan Paul.

Young, A. 1982. 'The anthropologies of illness and sickness', *Annual Review of Anthropology* 11: 257–85.

Young, A. 1993. 'A description of how ideology shapes knowledge of a mental disorder (posttraumatic stress disorder)' in S. Lindenbaum and M. Lock (eds), *Knowledge, Power and Practice: the anthropology of medicine and everyday life*, Berkeley, Los Angeles and London: University of California Press.

Young, A. 1995. *The Harmony of Illusions: inventing post-traumatic stress disorder*, Princeton NJ: Princeton University Press.

Young, R. 1990. *White Mythologies: writing history and the west*, London and New York: Routledge.

Zamora, M. 1988. *Language, Authority and Indigenous History in the* Comentarios Reales de los Incas, Cambridge: Cambridge University Press.

INDEX

aardvark, 281, 294
adulterous, 52–4, 56, 58, 60, 75, 144, 176, 178, 260
adulterous sex, as uncontrolled transformation, 56
adultery, 4, 52, 53, 55, 57, 58, 60, 66, 75, 96, 100, 114, 115, 118, 119, 122, 135, 144, 177, 178, 181, 182, 184, 185, 289
  and cause of illness, 175, 176
  as cause of death, 181
  as cause of illness, 52
aetiology
  and narrative, 93
  and problematic illness, 94
  types of, 95
alienation, 9, 106, 107, 109, 117, 168, 173
ambiguity, and uncertainty, 158
amulets, and intention, 292, 293
an 'other', 10
  and writing practice, 14
anaemia, 228, 229
anatomy, 39, 40, 44, 45, 65, 234
anger, 61, 105–7, 171, 172, 255, 281, 289, 297
antagonism, and ethnographic knowledge, 17
Antidesma sp., 271
antidote, 186, 236
ants, 270
Arbus precatorius L. ssp. africanus Verdc., 278
archive, 13, 14
arrogance, 6, 66, 114
arrogance (*kiburi*), and fear of death, 66
ash heap, 61–4, 67, 241
asira, 61, 105, 106, 297
asyndeton, 25
authentication
  divination and, 126
  of ethnographic knowledge, 10, 11
avenging ghost, 135
  and throwing the person in the bush, 260

  as cause of illness, 125, 150
avenging ghosts (*vibanda*), and problematic illness, 95

baendo, 193, 195, 243, 277, 299
BaMbwela, 32
banda, 262, 264, 271
baridi, 44, 48, 64
bat, 270
Bathybates vittatus, 32
bazuzi, 104
bela, 43
Bemba, 12, 27, 28, 30, 266, 274, 278
Bembe, 27
bilumbu, 28, 277, 278, 280, 283, 285–7, 297, 299
biomedicine, 33, 43, 70, 77, 80, 83, 93, 247
birth, 48–50, 54, 77, 116, 118, 134–6, 139, 144, 168, 170, 171, 173, 174, 178–80, 183–5, 193, 194, 235, 250, 252, 254–6, 301
Bitis arientans arientans, 269
Bitis gabonica gabonica, 269
bitterness, 96, 105, 184, 192, 201, 203
black mamba, 269
blind, 21, 40, 45, 71, 259, 270
blindness
  causes of, 40
  ignorance as, 259
blood, 40–4, 47, 48, 50, 52–4, 62, 64, 65, 75, 85, 86, 94, 108, 143, 145, 198, 203, 220, 222, 224, 227, 237, 238, 252, 259, 266–8, 272, 275, 295
bodily events, 247, 258
bodily therapy, 245
body, 5, 7, 12, 20, 21, 35, 39–45, 47, 48, 50–2, 55–62, 64–6, 68, 72, 77–80, 83, 93, 94, 103, 106–11, 136, 139, 140, 142–4, 156, 163, 170, 172, 174–6, 178, 188, 198, 207, 223, 224, 227, 228, 231, 234–8, 244–6, 248, 251–4, 258, 264, 266, 269, 275, 283, 287–9, 293–5, 300
  as communicative subject, 78